THE COMPLEXITY
OF ADOLESCENT OBESITY

Causes, Correlates, and Consequences

THE COMPLEXITY
OF ADOLESCENT OBESITY

Causes, Correlates, and Consequences

Edited by
Peter D. Vash, MD, MPH

Apple Academic Press

TORONTO   NEW JERSEY

Apple Academic Press Inc. | Apple Academic Press Inc.
3333 Mistwell Crescent | 9 Spinnaker Way
Oakville, ON L6L 0A2 | Waretown, NJ 08758
Canada | USA

© 2015 by Apple Academic Press, Inc.

First issued in paperback 2021

Exclusive worldwide distribution by CRC Press, a member of Taylor & Francis Group

No claim to original U.S. Government works

ISBN 13: 978-1-77463-373-1 (pbk)
ISBN 13: 978-1-77188-097-8 (hbk)

Library of Congress Control Number: 2014950949

Library and Archives Canada Cataloguing in Publication

The complexity of adolescent obesity : causes, correlates, and consequences/edited by Peter D. Vash, M.D., M.P.H.

Includes bibliographical references and index.
ISBN 978-1-77188-097-8 (bound)
1. Obesity in adolescence. 2. Obesity in adolescence--Etiology.
I. Vash, Peter D., editor

RJ399.C6C64 2015   618.92'398   C2014-906460-8

Apple Academic Press also publishes its books in a variety of electronic formats. Some content that appears in print may not be available in electronic format. For information about Apple Academic Press products, visit our website at **www.appleacademicpress.com** and the CRC Press website at **www.crcpress.com**

ABOUT THE EDITOR

PETER D. VASH, MD, MPH

Peter D. Vash, MD, MPH, FACE, Assistant Clinical Professor of Medicine at U.C.L.A. Medical Center and Fellow of the American Association of Clinical Endocrinologists, is a board-certified internist specializing in endocrinology and metabolism and a Diplomat in Obesity Medicine. He is the past president of the American Society of Bariatric Physicians and served on the Board of the North American Society for the Study of Obesity (NASSO). Dr. Vash works in private practice with patients suffering from obesity and eating disorders and has lectured extensively nationally and internationally on the medical management and treatment of obesity. He has been an invited expert witness to speak before a Senate subcommittee and the FTC (US Federal Trade Commission) concerning medical weight-loss issues and the safety and impact of commercial weight-loss programs. He has written four books—*The Fat to Muscle Diet, The Dieter's Dictionary, A Matter of Fat: A Physician's Program,* and *Lose It and Keep It Off.* He has served on the board of *Shape Magazine,* writing numerous articles regarding health, fitness and weight problems. Dr. Vash has worked closely in consultation with the media (TV, radio, print), aiding them with information and explanations of issues regarding obesity and eating disorders. He is currently the Executive Medical Director of the Lindora Medical Clinics, the largest and oldest medical weight-loss clinic in Southern California..

CONTENTS

ACKNOWLEDGMENT AND HOW TO CITE

The editor and publisher thank each of the authors who contributed to this book, whether by granting their permission individually or by releasing their research as open source articles or under a license that permits free use, provided that attribution is made. The chapters in this book were previously published in various places in various formats. To cite the work contained in this book and to view the individual permissions, please refer to the citation at the beginning of each chapter. Each chapter was read individually and carefully selected by the editor; the result is a book that provides a nuanced study of adolescent obesity. The chapters included examine the following topics:

- Understanding the prevalence of the problem is the vital first step to seeking solutions. The obesity epidemic is common knowledge in our world today, but Chapter 1 is a good overview of the problem specific to the adolescent population, a demographic that is less often researched and discussed in isolation from childhood obesity.
- The role of the television is tremendous in adolescent obesity, yet poorly understood. Chapter 2 also focuses on how cultural and ethnic variations play a role.
- Adolescents are chronically late to bed, a fact that is often accepted as a given. However, this lifestyle habit has direct implications on obesity and overweight, as described in Chapter 3. As the rest of the world lies sleeping, there are few activities available to the wakeful adolescent aside from staring at a screen and snacking—two activities we already know correlate with a higher incidence of obesity.
- It is a good idea to sometimes look past Western scholarship in order to garner information from other areas of the world. In Chapter 4, we have the opportunity to apply research from Malaysian adolescents: breakfast is the meal most often skipped. Individuals who were awake and eating at midnight, are likely to be rushed and unhungry in the morning before school, and thus breakfast is easily dispensed with. The question placed before clinicians is this: how can we help our adolescent patients and their parents restructure their lives to support healthier lifestyles with daily habits less likely to contribute to obesity and overweight?

- All obesity is not equivalent. The research in Chapter 5 promotes a deeper understanding of particular dietary factors' correlation with body-fat distribution.
- Chapter 6 is another important look at a non-Western perspective. China's overall obesity rates is less than 5 percent in rural areas but greater than 20 percent in many cities, where people—and especially adolescents—are adopting the West's food and exercise culture. The great size of China's population means that more than one-fifth of the billion obese people in the world come from China, underscoring the importance of obesity research conducted in this nation.
- Chapter 7 provides interesting information on the way physical characteristics can correlate with obesity. However, the focus drawn from this research should be directed toward intervention strategies.
- In Chapter 8, we again must keep in mind that correlations like this are only useful in so far that they offer greater insight into aggressive action against adolescent obesity. It is, however, important to understand the factors that contribute to this problem, in order to sort out the possible solutions that offer the most practical hope.
- Although Chapter 9 is confined to one city, it's findings offer useful information regarding the precise connections between weight and behavior.
- In a world that puts great stress on academic performance, Chapter 10 provides an important reminder of the practical connections between an adolescent's mind and body.
- Obesity and eating disorders may seem to inhabit separate and contradictory worlds, but that is not the case. Chapter 11 is a good primary foundation for understanding some of the connections and overlap between the two dangerous conditions.
- When obesity's health risks are discussed, joint pain is often considered a long-term consequence, usually suffered by older people. The reality, as described in Chapter 12, is that many adolescents experience this as a result of the extra weight they carry. It should be considered a very real consideration for clinicians working with adolescent patients.
- The role that genetics plays in obesity, a role in part described in Chapter 13, cannot be denied and needs to be understood. However, like other "nature" versus "nurture" considerations, it is important to remember that we have less control over the nature side of the equation, and thus research there should engender strategies that can be applied on the equation's nurture side.
- As we face this serious health condition as regional, national, and worldwide societies, we are not helpless. There are very real and practical steps we can take against adolescent obesity. The research offered in Chapter 14 provides a vital and realistic intervention at the regional level.

- Obesity has reached epidemic proportions in India, as well as in several other developing countries, due to the fact that high-sugar foods and beverages have become much more accessible with the nations' integration into the global food market. This, combined with rising middle class incomes, is increasing the average caloric intake per individual among the middle classes. The research in Chapter 15 offers a practical action plan at the national level to begin to combat this trend.
- At the conclusion of this book, it is vital to look at our topic from the widest perspective. Understanding and combating adolescent obesity is not so simple as educating and encouraging teens to have healthier diets and exercise more. The research in Chapter 16 encourages us to take a look at the realities that rule the global food market. The article's conclusions provide a foundation for policymakers and governments to make changes that will contribute to the health of our adolescents.

LIST OF CONTRIBUTORS

Michal Abrahamowicz
McGill University, Montreal, Canada

S. Abreu
Research Centre in Physical Activity, Health and Leisure, Faculty of Sport, University of Porto, Porto, Portugal

Kristi B. Adamo
Healthy Active Living and Obesity Research Group, Children's Hospital of Eastern Ontario Research Institute, Ontario, Canada

Sutapa Agrawal
South Asia Network for Chronic Disease, Public Health Foundation of India, New Delhi, India

Lene F. Andersen
Department of Nutrition, Faculty of Medicine, University of Oslo, Oslo, Norway

Sigmund A. Anderssen
Department of Sports Medicine, Norwegian School of Sport Sciences, Oslo, Norway

Eric Artiges
Institut National de la Santé et de la Recherche Médicale, INSERM CEA Unit 1000 'Imaging & Psychiatry', University of Paris-Sud, Paris, France and AP-HP Department of Adolescent Psychopathology and Medicine, Maison de Solenn, University Paris Descartes, Paris, France

R. Autran
Research Centre in Physical Activity, Health and Leisure, Faculty of Sport, University of Porto, Porto, Portugal

Tobias Banaschewski
Central Institute of Mental Health, Mannheim, Germany

Gareth J. Barker
Institute of Psychiatry, London, UK

Daheia J. Barr-Anderson
Department of Epidemiology and Biostatistics, University of South Carolina, Columbia, South Carolina, USA

Sanjay Basu
Prevention Research Center; Centers for Health Policy, Primary Care and Outcomes Research; Center on Poverty and Inequality; and Cardiovascular Institute, Stanford University, Stanford, California, United States of America and Department of Public Health and Policy, London School of Hygiene & Tropical Medicine, London, United Kingdom

Katherine W. Bauer
Temple University, Philadelphia, Pennsylvania

L. A. Baur
The Children's Hospital at Westmead Clinical School, University of Sydney, Sydney, Australia

Kevin Belanger
Healthy Active Living and Obesity Research Group, Children's Hospital of Eastern Ontario Research Institute, Ontario, Canada

Ingunn H. Bergh
Department of Coaching and Psychology, Norwegian School of Sport Sciences, Oslo, Norway

Manon Bernard
The Hospital for Sick Children, University of Toronto, Toronto, Canada

Mona Bjelland
Department of Nutrition, Faculty of Medicine, University of Oslo, Oslo, Norway

Sharon Bout-Tabaku
Department of Pediatrics, Division of Rheumatology, Nationwide Children's Hospital, 700 Children's Drive, Columbus, OH, USA, The Ohio State University College of Medicine, Columbus, USA, and Center for Clinical Epidemiology and Biostatistics, University of Pennsylvania School of Medicine, Philadelphia, USA

Rüdiger Brühl
Physikalisch-Technische Bundesanstalt, Berlin, Germany

Christian Büchel
Universitaetsklinikum Hamburg Eppendorf, Hamburg, Germany

M. E. Calle
Department of Preventive Medicine and Public Health and History of Science, Faculty of Medicine, Complutense University of Madrid, Madrid, Spain

R. Castillo
Department of Basic Psychology, School of Psychology, University of Malaga, Spain

M. Mallar Chakravarty
Rotman Research Institute, Toronto, Canada and Kimel Family Translational Imaging-Genetics Laboratory, Research Imaging Centre, Centre for Addiction and Mental Health, Toronto, Canada

Jean-Philippe Chaput
Healthy Active Living and Obesity Research Group, Children's Hospital of Eastern Ontario Research Institute, Ontario, Canada

Peijie Chen
Key Laboratory of Exercise and Health Sciences of Ministry of Education at the Shanghai University of Sport, #650 Qingyuanhuan Road, Shanghai 200438, China

Patricia Conrod
Institute of Psychiatry, London, UK and Department of Psychiatry, CHU Ste Justine Hospital, Universite de Montreal,Montreal, Canada

C. T. Cowell
The Children's Hospital at Westmead Clinical School, University of Sydney, Sydney, Australia, Kids Research Institute, The Children's Hospital at Westmead, Westmead, Australia, and Institute of Endocrinology and Diabetes, The Children's Hospital at Westmead, Westmead, Australia

Patrick Dawes
Department of Surgical Sciences, University of Otago, Dunedin, New Zealand

Maria del Mar Bibiloni
Research Group on Community Nutrition and Oxidative Stress, University of Balearic Islands, 07122 Palma de Mallorca, Spain and CIBERobn (Fisiopatología de la Obesidad y la Nutrición CB12/03/30038), Instituto de Salud Carlos III, 15706 Santiago de Compostela, Spain

Shah Ebrahim
South Asia Network for Chronic Disease, Public Health Foundation of India, New Delhi, India and Department of Non-Communicable Disease Epidemiology, London School of Hygiene & Tropical Medicine, London, United Kingdom

Herta Flor
Central Institute of Mental Health, Mannheim, Germany and University of Heidelberg, Heidelberg, Germany

Leng Huat Foo
Program of Nutrition, School of Health Sciences, Universiti Sains Malaysia, Health Campus, Kubang Kerian, Kelantan, Malaysia

Vincent Frouin
Neurospin, Commissariat à l'Energie Atomique, Paris, France

Barbara Galland
Department of Women's and Children's Health, University of Otago, Dunedin, New Zealand

Jürgen Gallinat
Department of Psychiatry and Psychotherapy, Campus Charité Mitte, Charité—Universitätsmedizin Berlin, Berlin, Germany

Binghong Gao
Key Laboratory of Exercise and Health Sciences of Ministry of Education at the Shanghai University of Sport, #650 Qingyuanhuan Road, Shanghai 200438, China

Hugh Garavan
Institute of Neuroscience, Trinity College Dublin, Dublin, Ireland

S. P. Garnett
The Children's Hospital at Westmead Clinical School, University of Sydney, Sydney, Australia, Kids Research Institute, The Children's Hospital at Westmead, Westmead, Australia, and Institute of Endocrinology and Diabetes, The Children's Hospital at Westmead, Westmead, Australia

Daniel Gaudet
Community Genomic Centre, Chicoutimi Hospital, Université de Montréal, Montreal, Canada

Jesse Gillis
Centre for High-Throughput Biology and Department of Psychiatry, University of British Columbia, Vancouver, Canada

S. Gómez-Martínez
Immunonutrition Research Group, Department of Metabolism and Nutrition, Institute of Food Science and Technology and Nutrition, Spanish National Research Council (CSIC), Madrid, Spain

M. González-Gross
ImFINE Research Group, Department of Health and Human Performance, Faculty of Physical Activity and Sport Sciences (INEF), Universidad Politécnica de Madrid, Spain

L. Graves
Sydney Medical School, University of Sydney, Sydney, Australia and The Children's Hospital at Westmead Clinical School, University of Sydney, Sydney, Australia

May Grydeland
Department of Nutrition, Faculty of Medicine, University of Oslo, Oslo, Norway and Department of Sports Medicine, Norwegian School of Sport Sciences, Oslo, Norway

Kajuandra A. Harris
Private nutrition and health consultant, Auburn, AL, USA

Dione Healey
Department of Psychology, University of Otago, Dunedin, New Zealand

Andreas Heinz
Department of Psychiatry and Psychotherapy, Campus Charité Mitte, Charité—Universitätsmedizin Berlin, Berlin, Germany

Inge Huybrechts
Dietary Exposure Assessment Group, International Agency for Research on Cancer (IARC), Lyon, France and Department of Public Health, Ghent University, Ghent, Belgium

Knut-Inge Klepp
Department of Nutrition, Faculty of Medicine, University of Oslo, Oslo, Norway

Sarah B. Klieger
Department of Pediatrics, Division of Infection Diseases, The Children's Hospital of Philadelphia, Philadelphia, USA

Mark Lathrop
Centre National de Génotypage, Paris, France

Eva Lattka
Research Unit of Molecular Epidemiology, Helmholtz Zentrum München, Munich, Germany

D. A. Lawlor
MRC Centre for Causal Analyses in Translational Epidemiology, School of Social and Community Medicine, University of Bristol, Bristol, UK

Clare M. Lenhart
East Stroudsburg University, East Stroudsburg, Pennsylvania. At the time of the study, Dr Lenhart was affiliated with Lehigh Valley Health Network, Allentown, Pennsylvania.

Gabriel T. Leonard
Montreal Neurological Institute, McGill University, Montreal, Canada

Nanna Lien
Department of Nutrition, Faculty of Medicine, University of Oslo, Oslo, Norway

Dongmei Liu
Key Laboratory of Exercise and Health Sciences of Ministry of Education at the Shanghai University of Sport, #650 Qingyuanhuan Road, Shanghai 200438, China

Eva Loth
Institute of Psychiatry, London, UK and MRC Social, Genetic and Developmental Psychiatry (SGDP) Centre, London, UK

Anbarasu Lourdusamy
Institute of Psychiatry, London, UK

Karl Mann
Central Institute of Mental Health, Mannheim, Germany

A. Marcos
Immunonutrition Research Group, Department of Metabolism and Nutrition, Institute of Food Science and Technology and Nutrition, Spanish National Research Council (CSIC), Madrid, Spain

Adilson Marques
Interdisciplinary Center for the Study of Human Performance, Faculty of Human Kinetics, University of Lisbon, Estrada da Costa, 1499-002 Cruz-Quebrada, Portugal

Sandra Martins
Faculty of Physical Education and Sport, Lusophone University of Humanities and Technologies, Lisbon, Portugal

D. Martínez-Gómez
Immunonutrition Research Group, Department of Metabolism and Nutrition, Institute of Food Science and Technology and Nutrition, Spanish National Research Council (CSIC), Madrid, Spain and Department of Physical Education, Sport and Human Movement, Faculty of Education and Teaching Training, Autónoma University of Madrid, Madrid, Spain

William J. McCarthy
Division of Cancer Prevention and Control Research and Psychology Department, University of California, Los Angeles, USA

Melkaye G. Melka
The Hospital for Sick Children, University of Toronto, Toronto, Canada

Cláudia Minderico
Interdisciplinary Center for the Study of Human Performance, Faculty of Human Kinetics, University of Lisbon, Estrada da Costa, 1499-002 Cruz-Quebrada, Portugal

C. Moreira
Research Centre in Physical Activity, Health and Leisure, Faculty of Sport, University of Porto, Porto, Portugal

P. Moreira
Research Centre in Physical Activity, Health and Leisure, Faculty of Sport, University of Porto, Porto, Portugal, Faculty of Nutrition and Food Science, University of Porto, Porto, Portugal, and Institute of Public Health, University of Porto, Porto, Portugal

J. Mota
Research Centre in Physical Activity, Health and Leisure, Faculty of Sport, University of Porto, Porto, Portugal

A. Ness
School of Oral and Dental Sciences, University of Bristol, Bristol, UK

Marion Nestle
Department of Nutrition, Food Studies, and Public Health, New York University, New York, New York, United States of America andDepartment of Nutritional Sciences, Cornell University, Ithaca, New York, United States of America

Abdullah Nurul-Fadhila
Program of Nutrition, School of Health Sciences, Universiti Sains Malaysia, Health Campus, Kubang Kerian, Kelantan, Malaysia

Yngvar Ommundsen
Department of Coaching and Psychology, Norwegian School of Sport Sciences, Oslo, Norway

F. B. Ortega
Department of Physical Education and Sport, School and Sports Sciences, University of Granada, Granada, Spain and Department of Medical Physiology, School of Medicine, University of Granada, Spain

António Palmeira
Interdisciplinary Center for the Study of Human Performance, Faculty of Human Kinetics, University of Lisbon, Estrada da Costa, 1499-002 Cruz-Quebrada, Portugal and Faculty of Physical Education and Sport, Lusophone University of Humanities and Technologies, Lisbon, Portugal

Freda Patterson
Department of Public Health, Temple University College of Health Professions and Social Work, 1301 Cecil B. Moore Ave, 963 Ritter Annex, Philadelphia, PA 19122

Tomáš Paus
Rotman Research Institute, Toronto, Canada and Montreal Neurological Institute, McGill University, Montreal, Canada

Zdenka Pausova
The Hospital for Sick Children, University of Toronto, Toronto, Canada

Paul Pavlidis
Centre for High-Throughput Biology and Department of Psychiatry, University of British Columbia, Vancouver, Canada

Michel Perron
Université du Québec à Chicoutimi, Chicoutimi, Canada

Antoni Pons
Research Group on Community Nutrition and Oxidative Stress, University of Balearic Islands, 07122 Palma de Mallorca, Spain and CIBERobn (Fisiopatología de la Obesidad y la Nutrición CB12/03/30038), Instituto de Salud Carlos III, 15706 Santiago de Compostela, Spain

Barry Popkin
School of Public Health, University of North Carolina at Chapel Hill and the Carolina Population Center, Chapel Hill, North Carolina, United States of America

Louis Richer
Université du Québec à Chicoutimi, Chicoutimi, Canada

Marcella Rietschel
Central Institute of Mental Health, Mannheim, Germany

P. C. Santos
Research Centre in Physical Activity, Health and Leisure, Faculty of Sport, University of Porto, Porto, Portugal and Department of Physical Therapy, School of Health Technology of Porto, Polytechnic Institute of Porto, Vila Nova de Gaia, Portugal

R. Santos
Research Centre in Physical Activity, Health and Leisure, Faculty of Sport, University of Porto, Porto, Portugal and Maia Institute of Higher Education, Maia, Portugal

Luís B. Sardinha
Interdisciplinary Center for the Study of Human Performance, Faculty of Human Kinetics, University of Lisbon, Estrada da Costa, 1499-002 Cruz-Quebrada, Portugal

N. Sattar
Metabolic Medicine, University of Glasgow, Glasgow, UK

Elizabeth Schaughency
Department of Psychology, University of Otago, Dunedin, New Zealand

Gunter Schumann
Institute of Psychiatry, London, UK and MRC Social, Genetic and Developmental Psychiatry (SGDP) Centre, London, UK

Yannick Schwartz
Neurospin, Commissariat à l'Energie Atomique, Paris, France

David D. Sherry
Department of Pediatrics, Division of Rheumatology, The Children's Hospital of Philadelphia, Philadelphia, USA and University of Pennsylvania School of Medicine, Philadelphia, USA

Michael N. Smolka
Department of Psychiatry and Psychotherapy and Neuroimaging Center, Department of Psychology, Technische Universität Dresden,Dresden, Germany

L. Soares-Miranda
Research Centre in Physical Activity, Health and Leisure, Faculty of Sport, University of Porto, Porto, Portugal

Nicolas Stettler
The Lewin Group, Falls Church, USA

Andreas Ströhle
Department of Psychiatry and Psychotherapy, Campus Charité Mitte, Charité—Universitätsmedizin Berlin, Berlin, Germany

Maren Struve
Central Institute of Mental Health, Mannheim, Germany and University of Heidelberg, Heidelberg, Germany

David Stuckler
Department of Sociology, University of Cambridge, Cambridge, United Kingdom and Department of Public Health & Policy, London School of Hygiene & Tropical Medicine, London, United Kingdom

Evan Tan
Department of Women's and Children's Health, University of Otago, Dunedin, New Zealand

Pey Sze Teo
Program of Nutrition, School of Health Sciences, Universiti Sains Malaysia, Health Campus, Kubang Kerian, Kelantan, Malaysia

Josep A. Tur
Research Group on Community Nutrition and Oxidative Stress, University of Balearic Islands, 07122 Palma de Mallorca, Spain and CIBERobn (Fisiopatología de la Obesidad y la Nutrición CB12/03/30038), Instituto de Salud Carlos III, 15706 Santiago de Compostela, Spain

S. Vale
Research Centre in Physical Activity, Health and Leisure, Faculty of Sport, University of Porto, Porto, Portugal

O. L. Veiga
Department of Physical Education, Sport and Human Movement, Faculty of Education and Teaching Training, Autónoma University of Madrid, Madrid, Spain

Sukumar Vellakkal
South Asia Network for Chronic Disease, Public Health Foundation of India, New Delhi, India

Suzanne Veillette
Université du Québec à Chicoutimi, Chicoutimi, Canada

A. M. Veses
Immunonutrition Research Group, Department of Metabolism and Nutrition, Institute of Food Science and Technology and Nutrition, Spanish National Research Council (CSIC), Madrid, Spain

G. Vicente-Rodriguez
Growth, Exercise, Nutrition and Development (GENUD) Research Group, Universidad de Zaragoza, Zaragoza, Spain

Melanie Waldenberger
Research Unit of Molecular Epidemiology, Helmholtz Zentrum München, Munich, Germany

Ru Wang
Key Laboratory of Exercise and Health Sciences of Ministry of Education at the Shanghai University of Sport, #650 Qingyuanhuan Road, Shanghai 200438, China

Xueqiang Wang
Key Laboratory of Exercise and Health Sciences of Ministry of Education at the Shanghai University of Sport, #650 Qingyuanhuan Road, Shanghai 200438, China

Shanna Wilson
Healthy Active Living and Obesity Research Group, Children's Hospital of Eastern Ontario Research Institute, Ontario, Canada

Brian H. Wrotniak
Department of Physical Therapy, D'Youville College, Buffalo, USA and Center for Clinical Epidemiology and Biostatistics, University of Pennsylvania School of Medicine, Philadelphia, USA

Nana Wu
Key Laboratory of Exercise and Health Sciences of Ministry of Education at the Shanghai University of Sport, #650 Qingyuanhuan Road, Shanghai 200438, China

Weihua Xiao
Key Laboratory of Exercise and Health Sciences of Ministry of Education at the Shanghai University of Sport, #650 Qingyuanhuan Road, Shanghai 200438, China

Antronette (Toni) K. Yancey
Department of Health Services, University of California, Los Angeles, USA

Michelle Yore
Private statistical consultant, Orlando, FL, USA

Babette S. Zemel
Department of Pediatrics, Division of Gastroenterology and Nutrition, The Children's Hospital of Philadelphia, Philadelphia, USA and University of Pennsylvania School of Medicine, Philadelphia, USA

INTRODUCTION

Obesity has become an epidemic, a fact frequently discussed in the media, with many references to both childhood obesity and adult. These discussions overlook an important demographic: the adolescent who is obese or overweight. The road from childhood obesity into adolescent obesity and from there into adult obesity is now a well-travelled path for individuals around the world. To omit adolescent obesity from our discussions is to miss many of the vital factors that contribute to the obesity epidemic.

The road that leads through adolescent obesity is littered with the signposts of causation: increased consumption of high carbohydrate snacks; eating too much, too fast, and too frequently; eating high-fat, cheap, convenient, and readily assessable foods; increased sedentary activities, such as TV watching and video games, accompanied by decreased physical activity; parents' and schools' lack of nutrition vigilance; and the commercial incentives to sell calorie-dense foods aggressively and relentlessly. Understanding these "obesogenic" signposts is the first step toward helping health-care professionals redirect overweight and obese adolescent youth down a different road toward a goal of a stable weight.

The research contained in this compendium offers a much-needed perspective on one of the most dangerous health crises our world faces today. The authors' investigations offer critical insights into the forces and factors that result in the numerous metabolic and psychological consequences of adolescent obesity.

Peter Vash, MD, MPH

The objective of Chapter 1, by Biblioni and colleagues, was to review the extant literature on the prevalence of overweight and obesity in adolescents (10–19 years old) of both sexes. The search was carried out using

Medline and Scopus considering articles published from the establishment of the databanks until June 7, 2012. Data on the prevalence of children being overweight and obese from the International Obesity Task Force (IOTF) website was also reviewed. Only original articles and one National Health Report were considered. Forty studies met the inclusion criteria. Results. Twenty-five of these studies were nationally representative, and ten countries were represented only by regional data. The study concluded that the prevalence of overweight and obesity among adolescents world-wide is high, and obesity is higher among boys. The IOTF criterion is the most frequently used method to classify adolescents as overweighed or obese in public health research.

Chapter 2, by Barr-Anderson and colleagues, aimed to examine the cross-sectional and longitudinal relationships between television viewing and preferred food choices in a sample of ethnic minority, low income adolescents. A sample of predominantly minority students (n=133) completed surveys at two time points, six months apart. Linear regression models examined television viewing and eating associations. Participants watched >3.5 hours/day of television, which is similar to the national average. Positive cross-sectional relationships existed between television viewing with fast food and sweetened beverage intakes at Time 1 and with snack food intake at both time points (p<0.01). The longitudinal association between change in snack food intake and change in average television hours/day approached significance after adjusting for baseline measure (β=0.305, p=0.017), as did the relationship with family meals (β=-0.20, p=0.02). No other longitudinal relationships were significant. If interventions reduced adolescents' television viewing time, such interventions could positively impact eating habits and thereby reduce adolescent's risk for obesity.

In Chapter 3, Adamo and colleagues examined if sleep timing (combination of bedtime and wake up time) is associated with energy intake and physical activity/sedentary behaviour in obese adolescents. Participants included in this cross-sectional examination were 26 (13 females) obese volunteers (BMI ≥ 95th percentile) with a mean age of 13.6 ± 0.5 years and valid data on self-reported sleep, food intake (dietary record), physical activity and sedentary time (accelerometer), screen time (self-reported), and anthropometry (BMI). The authors categorized participants as "late sleepers" (midpoint of sleep >3:30 a.m., n=13) and participants as "normal sleepers" (midpoint of sleep ≤ 2:30 a.m., n=13). As expected, wake-up time and bedtime were different between sleep timing groups (p<0.01); however, total sleep duration was the same (9.23 ± 1.14 vs. 9.16 ± 1.28 hours for normal and late sleepers, respectively, p=0.88). There was no significant BMI difference between late sleepers and normal sleepers. Total daily caloric intake was 27% higher in late sleepers (425 kcal) compared to normal sleepers (p=0.04). Using a linear regression model in the whole sample we observed that later sleep timing was associated with greater total caloric intake, independent of age, sex, BMI, moderate-to-vigorous physical activity (MVPA) and sleep duration (β=368.6, p=0.01). No association was found between sleep timing and MVPA or sedentary time. However, later sleep timing was related to greater screen time, independent of age, sex, BMI and sleep duration (β=105.7, p<0.01). The present study is the first to report that later bedtime is associated with greater caloric intake and screen time in obese adolescents independent of total sleep duration.

Unhealthy dietary pattern increases the risk of obesity and metabolic disorders in growing children and adolescents. However, the way the habitual pattern of breakfast consumption influences body composition and risk of obesity in adolescents is not well defined. Thus, the aim of Chapter 4, by Nurul-Fadhilah and colleagues was to assess any associations between breakfast consumption practices and body composition profiles in 236 apparently healthy adolescents aged 12 to 19 years. A self-administered questionnaire on dietary behaviour and lifestyle practices and a dietary food frequency questionnaire were used. Body composition and adiposity indices were determined using standard anthropometric measurement protocols and dual energy χ-ray absorptiometry (DXA). Mean age of the participants was 15.3±1.9 years. The majority of participants (71.2%) fell in the normal body mass index (BMI) ranges. Breakfast consumption patterns showed that only half of the participants (50%) were consuming breakfast daily. Gender-specific multivariate analyses (ANCOVA) showed that in both boys and girls, those eating breakfast at least 5 times a week had significantly lower body weight, body mass index (BMI), BMI z-scores, waist circumference, body fat mass and percent body fat (%BF) compared to infrequent breakfast eaters, after adjustment for age, household income, pubertal status, eating-out and snacking practices, daily energy intakes, and daily physical activity levels. The present findings indicate that infrequent breakfast consumption is associated with higher body adiposity and abdominal obesity. Therefore, daily breakfast consumption with healthy food choices should be encouraged in growing children and adolescents to prevent adiposity during these critical years of growth.

Diet and physical activity (PA) are recognized as important factors to prevent abdominal obesity (AO), which is strongly associated with chronic diseases. Some studies have reported an inverse association between milk consumption and AO. Chapter 5, by Abreu and colleagues, examined the association between milk intake, PA and AO in adolescents. A cross-sectional study was conducted with 1209 adolescents, aged 15–18 from the Azorean Archipelago, Portugal in 2008. AO was defined by a waist circumference at or above the 90th percentile. Adolescent food intake was measured using a semi-quantitative food frequency questionnaire, and milk intake was categorized as 'low milk intake' (<2 servings per day) or 'high milk intake' (≥2 servings per day). PA was assessed via a self-report questionnaire, and participants were divided into active (>10 points) and low-active groups (≤10 points) on the basis of their reported PA. They were then divided into four smaller groups, according to milk intake and PA: (i) low milk intake/low active; (ii) low milk intake/active; (iii) high milk intake/low active and (iv) high milk intake/active. The association between milk intake, PA and AO was evaluated using logistic regression analysis, and the results were adjusted for demographic, body mass index, pubertal stage and dietary confounders. In this study, the majority of adolescents consumed semi-skimmed or skimmed milk (92.3%). The group of adolescents with high level of milk intake and active had a lower proportion of AO than did other groups (low milk intake/low active: 34.2%; low milk intake/active: 26.9%; high milk intake/low active: 25.7%; high milk intake/active: 21.9%, P=0.008). After adjusting for confounders, low-active and active adolescents with high levels of milk intake were less likely to have AO, compared with low-active adolescents with low milk intake (high milk intake/low active, odds ratio [OR]=0.412, 95% confidence intervals [CI]: 0.201–0.845; high milk intake/active adolescents, OR=0.445, 95% CI: 0.235–0.845). High milk intake seems to have a protective effect on AO, regardless of PA level.

Exercise and diet are the cornerstones for the treatment of obesity in obese children and adolescents. However, compensatory changes in appetite and energy expenditure elicited by exercise and dieting make it hard to maintain a reduced weight over the longterm. The anorexic effect of hypoxia can be potentially utilized to counteract this compensatory increase, thereby enhancing the success of weight loss. Wang and colleagues' purpose in Chapter 6 is to assess the effectiveness of four week intermittent hypoxia exposure added to a traditional exercise and diet intervention on inducing short- and longterm weight loss in obese adolescents. In this randomized parallel group controlled clinical trial, 40 obese adolescents (20 boys and 20 girls, 11 to 15-years-old), will be recruited from a summer weight loss camp at the Shanghai University of Sport, China. Participants will be stratified by gender and randomly assigned to either the control group or the hypoxia group. During the four-week intervention period, both groups will exercise and eat a balanced diet. Additionally, the control group will sleep in normal conditions, while the hypoxia group will sleep in a normobaric hypoxia chamber (sleep high and train low). The primary outcome will be body composition and the main secondary outcomes will be the circulating levels of appetite regulatory gastrointestinal hormones. All the outcome measures will be assessed at baseline, after the four-week intervention, and at two months follow-up. This study will be the first to evaluate the effectiveness of 'sleep high and train low' on short- and long-term weight loss among obese adolescents. A potential mechanism for the appetite regulatory effect of hypoxia will also be explored. The results of the study will provide an evidence-based recommendation for the use of hypoxia in a weight loss intervention among obese children and adolescents. Furthermore, the clarification of mechanisms leading to weight loss in 'sleep high and train low' might provide information for the development of new strategies in combating obesity.

Chapter 7, by Graves and colleagues aimed to examine the associations between body mass index (BMI) and waist-to-height ratio (WHtR) measured in childhood and adolescence and cardiometabolic risk factors in adolescence.Secondary data analysis of the Avon Longitudinal Study of Parents and Children, a population based cohort. Data from 2858 adolescents aged 15.5 (standard deviation 0.4) years and 2710 of these participants as children aged 7–9 years were used in this analysis. Outcome measures were cardiometabolic risk factors, including triglycerides, low density lipoprotein cholesterol, high density lipoprotein cholesterol, insulin, glucose and blood pressure at 15 years of age. Both BMI and WHtR measured at ages 7–9 years and at age 15 years were associated with cardiometabolic risk factors in adolescents. A WHtR ≥0.5 at 7–9 years increased the odds by 4.6 [95% confidence interval 2.6 to 8.1] for males and 1.6 [0.7 to 3.9] for females of having three or more cardiometabolic risk factors in adolescence. Cross-sectional analysis indicated that adolescents who had a WHtR ≥0.5, the odds ratio of having three or more cardiometabolic risk factors was 6.8 [4.4 to 10.6] for males and 3.8 [2.3 to 6.3] for females. The WHtR cut-point was highly specific in identifying cardiometabolic risk co-occurrence in male children and adolescents as well as female children (90 to 95%), but had poor sensitivity (17 to 53%). Similar associations were observed when BMI was used to define excess adiposity. The study concludes that WHtR is a simple alternative to age and sex adjusted BMI for assessing cardiometabolic risk in adolescents.

The relationship between obstructive sleep apnoea (OSA) and poorer neurobehavioural outcomes in school-age children is well established, but the relationship in obese children and adolescents, in whom OSA is more common, is not so well established. In Chapter 8, Tane and colleagues aimed to investigate this relationship in 10–18-year-olds. Thirty-one participants with a mean body mass index (BMI) of 32.3 ± 4.9 enrolled. BMI-for-age cut-offs were used to define obesity. Participants underwent polysomnography and were classified into OSA (apnoea-hypopnoea index (AHI) > 2 per hour) and non-OSA (AHI ≤ 2) groups. Intelligence, memory and learning, academic achievement, behaviour and executive functioning were assessed using the Wechsler Abbreviated Scale of Intelligence, Wide Range Assessment of Memory and Learning 2, Wechsler Individual Achievement Test II (WIAT-II), Behavioural Assessment System for Children 2 and Behaviour Rating Inventory of Executive Function, respectively. Forty-eight per cent (15/31) were classified as having OSA, and 52% (16/31) as non-OSA. The obese cohort performed below the average of normative data on several neurobehavioural measures. WIAT-II maths scores were significantly lower (P = 0.034) in the OSA group than in the non-OSA group (means 84.5 vs. 94.6, respectively), losing significance after adjustment for IQ, age and gender. Self-reported school problems were significantly worse in the OSA group before and after multivariate adjustment (P = 0.010, Cohen's d = 1.02). No other significant differences were found. Results suggest that OSA may increase risk for some poorer educational and behavioural outcomes. The findings are reasonably consistent with and add to the evidence base of the few studies that have explored this relationship.

The prevalence of obesity among youth may be stabilizing and even declining in some areas of the United States. Lenhard and colleagues' objective in Chapter 9 was to examine whether the stabilization in obesity prevalence among Philadelphia high school students was accompanied by changes in weight-management behaviors. The authors evaluated changes in self-reported weight status and weight-management behaviors by using data collected by the Youth Risk Behavior Survey in 2007, 2009, and 2011. The study used multivariable regression models controlling for race/ethnicity and age to estimate prevalence. Although the proportion of overweight and obese students did not change significantly during the study period, the authors found that approximately half of female students and 30% of male students reported trying to lose weight. Among female students, they observed significant increases in the proportion engaging in 5 or more days of physical activity per week (26.0% in 2007 to 31.9% in 2011; P = .003) and significant decreases in the proportion consuming at least 1 soda per day (31.1% in 2007 to 22.5% in 2011, P = .001). The proportion of female students who fasted for weight loss also increased significantly during the study period (12.2% in 2007 to 17.0% in 2011,P = .02). The study found no significant changes in behavior among male students. Although the prevalence of obesity and overweight may have reached a plateau among Philadelphia high school students, most students still failed to meet recommendations for healthful weight-management behaviors. Continued public health initiatives are necessary to promote participation in healthful weight-management behaviors.

In addition to the benefits on physical and mental health, cardiorespiratory fitness has shown to have positive effects on cognition. Chapter 10, by Sardinha and colleagues, aimed to investigate the relationship between cardiorespiratory fitness and body weight status on academic performance among seventh-grade students.Participants included 1531 grade 7 students (787 male, 744 female), ranging in age from 12 to 14 years

(Mage=12.3±0.60), from 3 different cohorts. Academic performance was measured using the marks students had, at the end of their academic year, in mathematics, language (Portuguese), foreign language (English), and sciences. To assess cardiorespiratory fitness the Progressive Aerobic Cardiovascular Endurance Run, from Fitnessgram, was used as the test battery. The relationship between academic achievement and the independent and combined association of cardiorespiratory fitness/weight status was analysed, using multinomial logistic regression. Cardiorespiratory fitness and weight status were independently related with academic achievement. Fit students, compared with unfit students had significantly higher odds for having high academic achievement (OR=2.29, 95% CI: 1.48-3.55, p<0.001). Likewise, having a normal weight status was also related with high academic achievement (OR=3.65, 95% CI: 1.82-7.34, p<0.001). Cardiorespiratory fitness and weight status were independently and combined related to academic achievement in seventh-grade students independent of the different cohorts, providing further support that aerobically fit and normal weight students are more likely to have better performance at school regardless of the year that they were born.

Eating disorders together with the overweight and obesity are important health concerns in adolescents. Chapter 11, by Veses and colleagues, aimed to analyse the individual and combined influence of overweight and physical fitness on the risk of developing eating disorders in Spanish adolescents. The sample consisted of 3571 adolescents (1864 females), aged 13 to 18.5 years, from Spain who participated in the AVENA and AFINOS studies. The risk of eating disorders was evaluated using the SCOFF questionnaire. Body mass index was calculated and the adolescents were classified into two groups: overweight (including obesity) and non-overweight according to Cole's cut-off points. Cardiorespiratory fitness in the AVENA Study was assessed by the 20-m shuttle-run test and the overall physical fitness level was self-reported in the AFINOS Study. Overweight adolescents had a higher risk of developing eating disorders than non-overweight adolescents (odds ratio [OR]=4.91, 95% confidence interval [CI]: 3.63–6.61 in the AVENA Study and OR=2.45, 95% CI: 1.83–3.22 in the AFINOS Study). Also, adolescents with medium and low levels of physical fitness had a higher risk of developing eating disorders (OR=1.51, 95% CI: 1.05–2.16, and OR=2.25, 95% CI: 1.60–3.19, respectively, in the AVENA Study, and OR=1.73, 95% CI: 1.37–2.17, and OR=4.11 95% CI: 2.98–5.65, respectively, in the AFINOS Study) than adolescents with high levels of physical fitness. In both studies, the combined influence of overweight and physical fitness showed that adolescents with lower levels of physical fitness had an increased risk of developing eating disorders in both non-overweight and overweight groups. The authors concluded that physical fitness might attenuate the influence of overweight on the development of eating disorders in adolescents.

Obesity associated with joint pain of the lower extremities is likely due to excessive mechanical load on weight bearing joints. Additional mechanical factors may explain the association between obesity and joint pain. In Chapter 12, Bout-Tabaku and colleagues characterized the association between obesity and non-traumatic lower extremity (LE) joint pain in adolescents and examined the modifying effect of hypermobility on this association. The authors performed a cross-sectional analysis of data from subjects enrolled in a clinical trial examining the impact of weight loss on bone health in adolescents. Anthropometric data were collected and body mass index (BMI=kg/m^2) was calculated. Subjects were categorized as obese or healthy weight controls based on CDC 2000 growth curves for age and gender. We assessed any musculoskeletal pain and LE pain by the PEDS™ Pediatric Pain Questionnaire™. Hypermobility was assessed with the modified Beighton scoring system. Multivariate logistic regression models adjusted for covariates were performed to examine the association between weight status and joint pain. Out of 142 subjects, 91 were obese and 51 were healthy weight. Obesity was not associated with any musculoskeletal pain (OR 0.86, CI 0.49-1.50), LE pain (OR 1.02, CI 0.49-2.15) or hypermobility (OR 1.23, CI 0.72-2.14, p=0.3). There was no effect modification on the association between obesity and any musculoskeletal pain (OR 0.80, CI 0.45 -1.42) or LE pain (OR 0.98, CI 0.46 - 2.08) by hypermobility status. The authors found no association between LE pain and obesity, and hypermobility did not modify this association.

Genetic variations in fat mass- and obesity (FTO)-associated gene, a well-replicated gene locus of obesity, appear to be associated also with reduced regional brain volumes in elderly. In Chapter 13, Melka and colleagues examined whether FTO is associated with total brain volume in adolescence, thus exploring possible developmental effects of FTO. The authors studied a population-based sample of 598 adolescents recruited from the French Canadian founder population in whom we measured brain volume by magnetic resonance imaging. Total fat mass was assessed with bioimpedance and body mass index was determined with anthropometry. Genotype–phenotype associations were tested with Merlin under an additive model. We found that the G allele of FTO (rs9930333) was associated with higher total body fat [TBF ($P = 0.002$) and lower brain volume ($P = 0.005$)]. The same allele was also associated with higher lean body mass ($P = 0.03$) and no difference in height ($P = 0.99$). Principal component analysis identified a shared inverse variance between the brain volume and TBF, which was associated with FTO at $P = 5.5 \times 10^{-6}$. These results were replicated in two independent samples of 413 and 718 adolescents, and in a meta-analysis of all three samples (n = 1729 adolescents), FTO was associated with this shared inverse variance at $P = 1.3 \times 10^{-9}$. Co-expression networks analysis supported the possibility that the underlying FTO effects may occur during embryogenesis. In conclusion, FTO is associated with shared inverse variance between body adiposity and brain volume, suggesting that this gene may exert inverse effects on adipose and brain tissues. Given the completion of the overall brain growth in early childhood, these effects may have their origins during early development.

Inconsistent effects of school-based obesity prevention interventions may be related to how different subgroups receive them. The aim of Chapter 14, by Bjelland and colleagues, was to evaluate the effect of an intervention program, including fact sheets to parents and classroom components, on intake of sugar-sweetened beverages (SSB) and screen time. Further, to explore whether potential effects and parental involvement varied by adolescents' gender, weight status (WS) and parental educational level. In total, 1465 11-year-olds participated at the pre-test and the 8 month mid-way assessment of the HEIA study. Parents (n = 349) contributed with process evaluation data. Self-reported intake of SSB was collected from the 11-year-olds assessing frequency and amount, while time used on watching TV/DVD and computer/game-use (weekday and weekend day) were assed by frequency measures. Data on awareness of the intervention and dose received were collected from parents. Covariance analyses (ANCOVA) were conducted testing for effects by gender and for moderation by WS and parental education. Time spent on TV/

DVD (week p = 0.001, weekend p = 0.03) and computer/game-use (week p = 0.004, weekend p <.001), and the intake of SSB during weekend days (p = 0.04), were significantly lower among girls in the intervention group compared to the control group girls after 8 months. Girls' WS did not moderate these findings. However, no significant effects of the intervention were found for boys, but moderation effects were found for WS (week days: TV/DVD, p = 0.03 and computer/games, p = 0.02). There were no moderating effects of parental education for neither boys nor girls with respect to intake of SSB, time used for watching TV/DVD and computer/game-use. Parental awareness of the intervention was significantly higher among the parents of girls, while the parents of boys were more satisfied with the fact sheets. The preventive initiatives appeared to change behaviour in girls only. This study suggests that exploration of potential beneficial or negative effects of intervention in subgroups is important. In formative evaluation of obesity prevention studies it seems warranted to include issues related to gender, WS and parental involvement in order to enhance the effectiveness of preventive initiatives.

Taxing sugar-sweetened beverages (SSBs) has been proposed in high-income countries to reduce obesity and type 2 diabetes. In Chapter 15, Basu and colleagues sought to estimate the potential health effects of such a fiscal strategy in the middle-income country of India, where there is heterogeneity in SSB consumption, patterns of substitution between SSBs and other beverages after tax increases, and vast differences in chronic disease risk within the population. Using consumption and price variations data from a nationally representative survey of 100,855 Indian households, the authors first calculated how changes in SSB price alter per capita consumption of SSBs and substitution with other beverages. They then incorporated SSB sales trends, body mass index (BMI), and diabetes incidence data stratified by age, sex, income, and urban/rural residence into a validated microsimulation of caloric consumption, glycemic load, overweight/obesity prevalence, and type 2 diabetes incidence among Indian subpopulations facing a 20% SSB excise tax. The 20% SSB tax was anticipated to reduce overweight and obesity prevalence by 3.0% (95% CI 1.6%–5.9%) and type 2 diabetes incidence by 1.6% (95% CI 1.2%–1.9%) among various Indian subpopulations over the period 2014–2023, if SSB consumption continued to increase linearly in accordance with secular trends. However, acceleration in SSB consumption trends consistent with industry marketing models would be expected to increase the impact efficacy of taxation, averting 4.2% of prevalent overweight/obesity (95% CI 2.5–10.0%) and 2.5% (95% CI 1.0–2.8%) of incident type 2 diabetes from 2014–2023. Given current consumption and BMI distributions, our results suggest the largest relative effect would be expected among young rural men, refuting our a priori hypothesis that urban populations would be isolated beneficiaries of SSB taxation. Key limitations of this estimation approach include the assumption that consumer expenditure behavior from prior years, captured in price elasticities, will reflect future behavior among consumers, and potential underreporting of consumption in dietary recall data used to inform the calculations. The authors concluded that sustained SSB taxation at a high tax rate could mitigate rising obesity and type 2 diabetes in India among both urban and rural subpopulations.

Chapter 16, by Stuckler and Nestle, is taken from the PLoS Medicine series on Big Food. The essay argues that global food systems are not keeping up with dietary needs, and argues that a different approach to engaging with food industries is necessary.

PART I

THE PREVALENCE
OF ADOLESCENT OBESITY

CHAPTER 1

PREVALENCE OF OVERWEIGHT AND OBESITY IN ADOLESCENTS: A SYSTEMATIC REVIEW

MARIA DEL MAR BIBILONI, ANTONI PONS, AND JOSEP A. TUR

1.1 INTRODUCTION

The prevalence of overweight and obesity among children and adolescents has widely increased worldwide [1, 2], making it one of the most common chronic disorders in this age group and in adulthood.

The use of body mass index (BMI) for age to define being overweight and obese in children and adolescents is well established for both clinical and public health applications, because of their feasibility under clinical settings and in epidemiological studies [3, 4]. In children and adolescents, the natural increases in BMI that occur with age necessitate the use of age-sex-specific thresholds. The most widely used growth charts

Prevalence of Overweight and Obesity in Adolescents: A Systematic Review. © del Mar Bibiloni M, Antoni Pons A, and Tur JA. ISRN Obesity, 2013 (2013). http://dx.doi.org/10.1155/2013/392747. Licensed under Creative Commons Attribution 3.0 Unported License, http://creativecommons.org/licenses/by/3.0/.

are the Centers for Disease Control and Prevention (CDC-2000) [5], the International Task Force (IOTF) [6], and the 2007 growth references for 5 to 19 year olds produced by the World Health Organization (WHO-2007) [7].

The CDC-2000 growth charts were developed to evaluate the nutritional status of US children and were originated from five cross-sectional representative surveys carried out in the US between 1963 and 1994. These growth charts are routinely applied to identify children and adolescents with a BMI greater than the 85th or 95th percentiles following the advice of the US Expert Committee on Childhood Obesity [8]. However, the appropriateness of an American dataset for defining overweight in young people from other countries is questionable [9].

The IOTF reference also uses age-sex-specific BMI percentiles, and overweight and obesity definition corresponds to an adult BMI of 25 and $30 \, kg/m^2$, respectively, and reflects values in children tracking to overweight and obesity in adults [6]. This reference is based on six large international cross-sectional representative datasets, identifying the BMI values that extrapolate to childhood.

The WHO-2007 growth references were created to replace the National Center for Health Statistics (NCHS) references [10, 11]. This reference was constructed using data from the 1977 NCHS/WHO growth reference (1 to 24 years old) merged with data from the 2006 WHO Child Growth Standards for preschool children (under 5 years of age) using state-of-the-art statistical methods [7].

Although valuable information has been appearing in the literature or online, such as works from the Health Behaviour of School-aged Children study which is mainly related to social determinants of health and well-being among young people [12], no systematic review has been conducted to understand the worldwide magnitude of the overweight and obesity problem among the adolescent population. Thus, the objective of this study was to systematically review the literature regarding the prevalence of overweight and obesity in adolescents (10–19 years old) of both sexes published in the past 12 academic years (1999–2011).

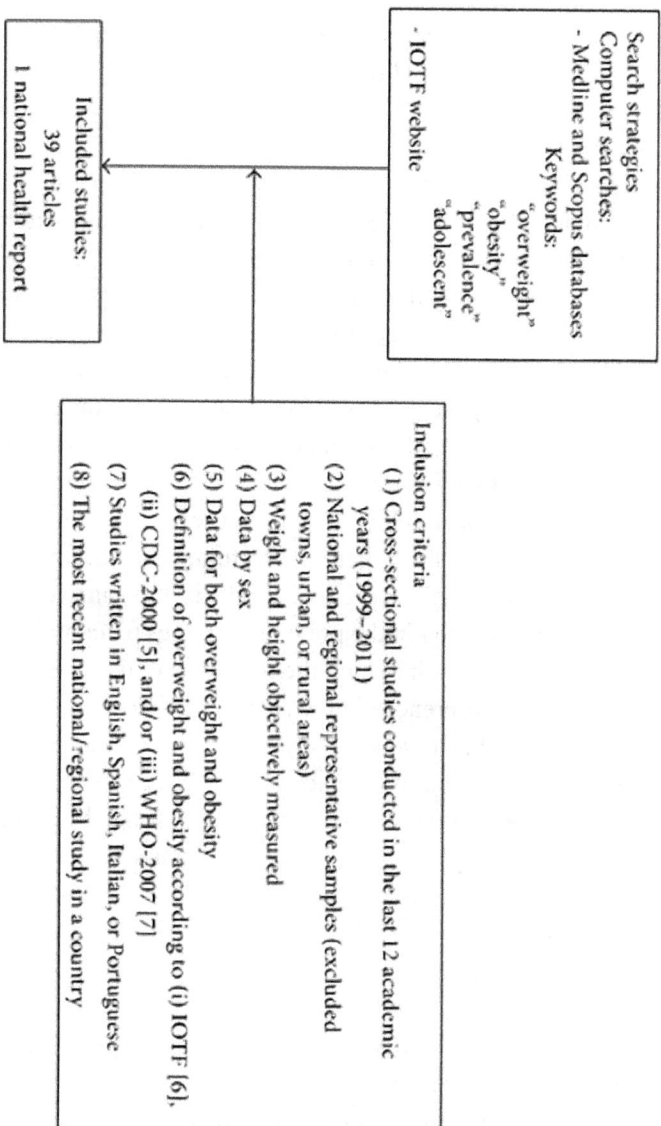

FIGURE 1: Flow diagram of study selection.

Search strategies
Computer searches:
- Medline and Scopus databases
  Keywords:
    "overweight"
    "obesity"
    "prevalence"
    "adolescent"

- IOTF website

Inclusion criteria

(1) Cross-sectional studies conducted in the last 12 academic
    years (1999–2011)

(2) National and regional representative samples (excluded
    towns, urban, or rural areas)

(3) Weight and height objectively measured

(4) Data by sex

(5) Data for both overweight and obesity

(6) Definition of overweight and obesity according to (i) IOTF [6],
    (ii) CDC-2000 [5], and/or (iii) WHO-2007 [7]

(7) Studies written in English, Spanish, Italian, or Portuguese

(8) The most recent national/regional study in a country

Included studies:
39 articles
1 national health report

1.2 METHODS

A systematic literature search was performed which ended on June 7, 2012 (see Figure 1). The literature search was conducted in Medline and Scopus using the following MeSH terms: "overweight"; "obesity"; "prevalence"; "adolescent". In total, 2537 articles were selected. We also reviewed the data on the prevalence of childhood overweight and obesity on the International Obesity Task Force Website at http://www.iaso.org/iotf/. To find the articles included in this review, the following inclusion criteria were used: (1) cross-sectional studies conducted in the last 12 years (1999–2011)— when the original study did not report the survey year, it was not included; (2) national and regional representative samples, but articles published on the prevalence of overweight in towns, urban, or rural areas in a country were excluded; (3) weight and height objectively measured; (4) results presented by sex; (5) and for both overweight and obesity prevalence; (6) the definition of overweight and obesity using the (i) CDC-2000 [5], (ii) IOTF [6], and (iii) WHO-2007 [7] growth references; and (7) studies written in English, Spanish, Italian, or Portuguese. Moreover, if there were more than one national or regional study in the same country, the most recent one was included in the prevalence tables (except for USA [13] and Canada [14], countries in which the most recent data was not included in the tables due to differences in the representativeness of the samples [13] and the impossibility to calculate a single prevalence of overweight and obesity for adolescents' boys and girls [14]; however, no differences in prevalence were observed between studies as it has been indicated in the discussion). The final number of articles included in this review was 39 articles related to overweight and obesity and also a study on the latest statistics on the prevalence of overweight and obesity in South Africa [15].

Potentially relevant papers were selected by (1) screening the titles; (2) screening the abstracts, and (3) if abstracts were not available or did not provide sufficient data, the entire article was retrieved and screened to determine whether it met the inclusion criteria. Full-text articles were assessed by 2 authors (M. M. Bibiloni and J. A. Tur). Any matter of doubt was discussed by at least two of the reviewers (M. M. Bibiloni, A. Pons, and J. A. Tur).

TABLE 1: Descriptive analysis of the studies reviewed.

Area	Continent	Country, region	Date of survey study[1]	Total n of study[1]	Total n of adolescents[1]	Age (years)/ school grade	Proportion of girls	Number of definition	Definition	Reference
National	Africa	Seychelles	2004	4,854	2,177	7th, 10th	51.5%	1	IOTF	Bovet et al., 2006 [16]
		South Africa	2008	9,862	9,862	13–15	50.9%	1	IOTF	Reddy et al., 2010 [15]
		Tunisia	2004	2,872	2,872	15–19	54.9%	1	IOTF	Aounallah-Skhiri et al., 2008 [17]
	America	Canada	2004	8,661	4,099	12–17	—	3	IOTF, CDC, WHO	Shields and Tremblay, 2010 [18]
		Mexico	2006	48,304	13,219	12–18	50.7%	1	IOTF	Bonvecchio et al., 2009 [19]
		USA	2007	44,101	44,101	10–17	—	1	CDC	Singh et al., 2010 [20]
	Asia	Bahrain	2000	506	506	12–17	50.8%	1	IOTF	Al-Sendi et al., 2003 [21]
		China	2002	44,880	12,475	13–17	47.7%	1	IOTF	Li et al., 2008 [22]
		Iran	2003-04	21,111	16,035	10–18	51.3%	2	IOTF, CDC	Kelishadi et al., 2008 [23]
		Israel	2003-04	5,588	5,588	11–19	55.1%	1	CDC	Nitzan Kaluski et al., 2009 [24]

TABLE 1: *Cont.*

Area	Continent	Country, region	Date of survey	Total n of study[1]	Total n of adolescents[1]	Age (years)/ school grade	Proportion of girls	Number of definition	Definition	Reference
		Jordan	2009	5,640	637	13–18	55.7%	1	IOTF	Khader et al., 2011 [25]
		Qatar	2003–04	3,923	3,923	12–17	49.8%	1	IOTF	Bener, 2006 [26]
		Saudi Arabia	2005	19,317	7,251	13–18	49.2%	2	CDC, WHO	El Mouzan et al., 2010 [27]
		Taiwan	2003	72,789	58,424	10–18	49.0%	1	IOTF	Liou et al., 2009 [28]
		United Arab Emirates	2009–10	1,007	276	11–18	—	1	IOTF	Ng et al., 2011 [29]
	Europe	Cyprus	1999–2000	2,467	1,694	10–17	50.7%	1	IOTF	Savva et al., 2002 [30]
		Czech Republic	2005	1,417	957	11–17	49.4%	1	IOTF	Kunesova et al., 2007 [31]
		Germany	2008	40,622	5,623	12–16	46.7%	1	IOTF	Blüher et al., 2011 [32]
		Greece	2003	14,456	14,456	13–19	53.8%	1	IOTF	Tzotzas et al., 2008 [33]
		Italy	2002	4,386	4,386	11, 13, 15	51.6%	1	IOTF	Vieno et al., 2005 [34]
		Republic of Ireland	2003	17,499	7,294	11–16	50.6%	1	IOTF	Whelton et al., 2007 [35]

TABLE 1: *Cont.*

Area	Continent	Country, region	Date of survey	Total n of study[1]	Total n of adolescents[1]	Age (years)/ school grade	Proportion of girls	Number of definition	Definition	Reference
		Northern Ireland	2003	2,039	964	11–15	51.5%	1	IOTF	Whelton et al., 2007 [35]
		Portugal	2008	22,048	22,048	10–18	51.5%	2	IOTF, WHO	Sardinha et al., 2011 [36]
		Sweden	2001	1,732	1,732	10, 13, 16	48.3%	1	IOTF	Ekblom et al., 2004 [37]
	Oceania	Australia	2004	5,407	1,771	8th, 10th	45.6%	1	IOTF	Booth et al., 2007 [38]
		New Zealand	2007	8,796	8,796	13–17	45.4%	2	IOTF, WHO	Utter et al., 2010 [39]
Regional	Africa	South Africa, Eastern Cape	2008	926	926	13–19	52.1%	1	IOTF	Reddy et al., 2010 [15]
		South Africa, Free State	2008	1,236	1,236	13–19	49.1%	1	IOTF	Reddy et al., 2010 [15]
		South Africa, Gauteng	2008	931	931	13–19	52.1%	1	IOTF	Reddy et al., 2010 [15]
		South Africa, KwaZulu-Natal	2008	910	910	13–19	52.1%	1	IOTF	Reddy et al., 2010 [15]
		South Africa, Limpopo	2008	1,140	1,140	13–19	50.5%	1	IOTF	Reddy et al., 2010 [15]
		South Africa, Mpumalanga	2008	1,238	1,238	13–19	49.8%	1	IOTF	Reddy et al., 2010 [15]

TABLE 1: *Cont.*

Area	Continent	Country, region	Date of survey	Total n of study[1]	Total n of adolescents[1]	Age (years)/ school grade	Proportion of girls	Number of definition	Definition	Reference
		South Africa, Northern Cape	2008	1,088	1,088	13–19	48.6%	1	IOTF	Reddy et al., 2010 [15]
		South Africa, North West	2008	1,234	1,234	13–19	48.6%	1	IOTF	Reddy et al., 2010 [15]
		South Africa, Western Cape	2008	1,159	1,159	13–19	56.4%	1	IOTF	Reddy et al., 2010 [15]
	America	USA, 52 States[2]	2007	—	—	10–17	—	1	CDC	Singh et al., 2010 [20]
		Brazil, Pernambuco State	2006	4,210	4,210	14–19	59.8%	1	IOTF	Tassitano et al., 2009 [40]
	Asia	China, Hong Kong	2003-04	2,098	2,098	11–18	53.2%	2	IOTF, CDC	Ko et al., 2008 [41]
		India, Manipur	2005-06	3,356	3,356	12–19	56.2%	1	IOTF	Bishwalata et al., 2010 [42]
		Jordan, Irbid Governorate	2007	1,355	1,355	13–16	55.6%	1	CDC	Abu Baker and Daradkeh, 2010 [43]
	Europe	Denmark, Greater Copenhagen area and 3 municipalities outside the Capital Region	2007-09	7,541	7,541	14–16	50.1%	1	IOTF	Søren and Jo, 2010 [44]

TABLE 1: *Cont.*

Area	Continent	Country, region	Date of survey	Total n of study[1]	Total n of adolescents[1] school grade	Age (years)/	Proportion of girls	Number of definition	Definition	Reference
		France, Aquitaine Region	2004-05	2,385	2,385	11–18	49.1%	1	IOTF	Thibault et al., 2010 [45]
		Greece, Crete	2005-06	481	481	10–12	54.0%	1	IOTF	Manios et al., 2011 [46]
		Hungary, Szeged and Szolnok regions	2005-2006	14,290	14,290	11–16	48.1%	1	IOTF	Baráth et al., 2010 [47]
		Italy, 5 residence regions[3]	2002	4,386	4,386	11–15	51.6%	1	IOTF	Vieno et al., 2005 [34]
		Italy, Sardinia	1999-2001	3,946	3,946	11–15	49.0%	1	IOTF	Velluzzi et al., 2007 [48]
		Italy, Sicily	1999-2001	48,897	48,897	11–15	50.7%	1	CDC	Baratta et al., 2006 [49]
		Poland, Kujawsko-Pomorskie	2005	—	—	13–15	—	1	IOTF	Jodkowska et al., 2010 [50]
		Poland, Lubuskie	2005	—	—	13–15	—	1	IOTF	Jodkowska et al., 2010 [50]
		Poland, Malopolskie	2005	—	—	13–15	—	1	IOTF	Jodkowska et al., 2010 [50]
		Poland, Podlaskie	2005	—	—	13–15	—	1	IOTF	Jodkowska et al., 2010 [50]
		Poland, Pomorskie	2005	—	—	13–15	—	1	IOTF	Jodkowska et al., 2010 [50]

Area	Continent	Country, region	Date of survey	Total n of study[1]	Total n of adolescents[1]	Age (years)/ school grade	Proportion of girls	Number of definition	Definition	Reference
		Spain, Balearic Islands	2007-08	1,231	1,231	12–17	53.4%	1	WHO	Bibiloni et al., 2010 [51]
		Spain, Grand Canary	2004-05	1,002	1,002	12–14	50.0%	1	IOTF	Henríquez Sánchez et al., 2008 [52]
		Switzerland, Canton of Vaud	2005-06	5,207	5,207	10–14	49.7%	2	IOTF, CDC	Lasserre et al., 2007 [53]
		Turkey, Edirne Province	2001	989	989	12–17	48.1%	1	IOTF	Öner et al., 2004 [54]

[1]Only subjects with anthropometric measurements were included in each country.
[2]There are 52 states in the USA, but no information about total number of subjects was included in each state.
[3]Vieno et al. [34] assessed the overall overweight and obesity prevalence among Italian adolescents, and also according to the geographic region: North-West, North-East, Center, South, and Islands, but no information about total number of subjects was included in each region.
IOTF: International Obesity Task Force; CDC: Center for Disease Control and Prevention; WHO: World Health Organization.

1.3 RESULTS

1.3.1 LITERATURE SEARCH

A total of thirty-nine articles and a National Health Report were eligible according to the inclusion criteria established for this review. Table 1 presents a description of the forty studies selected for this review including the continent and the country where it was performed (and region for not national studies), year of publishing, total number of participants in the study, number of adolescents, age range, proportion of girls, and number and definition for overweight and obesity classification used. All the articles were published after the year of 2002. Nationally representative data were obtained in twenty-five countries (including Northern Ireland) [15–39], and ten countries were represented only by regional data [40, 42, 44, 45, 47, 50–54].

1.3.2 PREVALENCE AND CRITERIA FOR CLASSIFICATION

Table 2 shows overweight and obesity prevalence from the twenty-five national studies (one of them including data from Northern Ireland) that were included in this review according to the continent and the country where it was performed, year of survey, study population, age range, criteria used for classifying overweight and obesity used, and along with total data by sex. There were thirty-two different prevalence levels described in the included articles, because five countries presented data using at least two different criteria for overweight and obesity classification [18, 23, 27, 36, 39]. The IOTF cut-off was used to classify overweight and obesity in twenty-three of the twenty-five national studies considered in the present review.

There was a broad range of overweight and obesity prevalence noted. In general, the prevalence of overweight plus obesity was higher in America [18–20], Oceania [38, 39] and Europe [30–37] and lower in Africa [15–17] and certain parts of Asia [21–29] (in China [22] and Iran [23] the total prevalence was less than 10% by the IOTF cut-offs). Overall, about 30% of American adolescents and 22%–25% of European adolescents (excepting the Czech Republic and Italian adolescents' which showed a prevalence of 13.7% and 17.9%, resp.) were overweight or obese. Among Oceanian adolescents the prevalence ranged from 23.2% in Australia in 2004 to 34.2% in New Zealand in 2007. In Africa, the overall prevalence of overweight and obesity was lower than 20%. Among Asian adolescents there was a broad range of overweight plus obesity. Using IOTF cut-off, the prevalence of being overweight or obese for Asian boys and girls ranged from 5.2% in China in 2002 to 36.4% in Bahrain in 2000.

Table 3 shows regional data prevalence of overweight and obesity from fifteen countries. Specific prevalence from all the geographic regions was included in this review from three countries: South Africa (nine provinces) [15], USA (fifty two states) [20], and Italy (five regions) [34]. In Europe, data from islands of Greece (Crete) [46] and Italy (Sicily and Sardinia) [48, 49] and Spain (Balearic Islands' archipelago [51]; and the Grand Canary Island [52]) were also included. On the other hand, regional but not national data was found for eleven countries (Italy [34], Brazil [40], India [42], Jordan [43], Denmark [44], France [45], Hungary [47], Poland [48], Spain [51, 52], Switzerland [53], and Turkey [54]). The IOTF cut-off was used to classify overweight and obesity in fourteen of the eighteen selected studies that included regional data. In one study [51], data was presented using only the WHO-2007 growth charts and in two studies using only the CDC-2000 growth reference [20, 43].

In South Africa and USA, substantial geographic variations in adolescent overweight and obesity existed. In 2008, overweight and obesity prevalence varied in South Africa from 13.5% in Limpopo to 25.5% in KwaZulu-Natal. In 2007, overweight and obesity varied in USA from 23.1% in Utah and Minnesota to 44.5% in Mississippi. In 2002, the prevalence of overweight and obesity in Southern Italy and Italian islands was higher among boys. In Southern Italy, the overweight prevalence among girls also was higher than in the other geographic regions.

Comparison between the islands from Greece (Crete), Italy (Sicily and Sardinia), and Spain (Balearic Islands and Grand Canary Island) which were included in this review showed that Crete had the highest prevalence of overweight and obesity—despite data were presented using different definition. In Spain, using the IOTF cut-off (data not shown for Balearic Islands but given by authors), the prevalence of overweight plus obesity was higher in the Grand Canary Island (29.1%) than in the Balearic Islands (24.7%).

TABLE 2: Description of overweight and obesity prevalence (%) along with total data by sex from each national study that was included in the review according to year of survey, study population, age range, and classification criteria used.

Continent	Country	Date of survey	Study population	Age (years)/school grade	Criteria	Overweight (%)			Obesity (%)			Reference
						All	Boys	Girls	All	Boys	Girls	
Africa	Seychelles	2004	School-based survey	7th, 10th	IOTF[1]	12.0	9.5	14.3	5.1	4.2	6.0	Bovet et al., 2006 [16]
	South Africa	2008	2008 SA YRBS	13–19	IOTF[1]	14.4	7.9	20.6	5.3	3.3	7.2	Reddy et al., 2010 [15]
	Tunisia	2004	Household-based survey	15–19	IOTF[1]	12.4	11.0	14.1	2.6	1.9	3.2	Aounallah-Skhiri et al., 2008 [17]
America	Canada	2004	2004 CCHS	12–17	IOTF[1]	19.8	21.2	18.4	9.4	11.1	7.4	Shields and Tremblay, 2010 [18]
					CDC-2000[2]	15.9	17.0	14.7	12.1	14.3	9.6	
					WHO-2007[3]	20.8	21.9	19.6	12.4	15.1	9.4	
	Mexico	2006	Household-based survey	12–18	IOTF[1]	21.2	20.1	22.3	8.9	9.2	8.6	Bonvecchio et al., 2009 [19]
	USA	2007	2007 NSCH	10–17	CDC-2000[2]	15.2	15.3	15.2	16.4	19.2	13.5	Singh et al., 2010 [20]
Asia	Bahrain	2000	School-based survey	12–17	IOTF[1]	20.0	15.3	24.5	16.4	14.9	17.9	Al-Sendi et al., 2003 [21]
	China	2002	2002 CNNHS survey	13–17	IOTF[1]	4.6	4.6	4.6	0.6	0.7	0.5	Li et al., 2008 [22]
	Iran	2003–04	CASPIAN Study	10–18	IOTF[1]	5.9	5.7	6.0	1.3	1.5	1.1	Kelishadi et al., 2008 [23]

TABLE 2: *Cont.*

Continent	Country	Date of survey	Study population	Age (years)/ school grade	Criteria	Overweight (%)			Obesity (%)			Reference
						All	Boys	Girls	All	Boys	Girls	
					CDC-2000²	4.5	4.3	4.7	1.9	2.3	1.6	
	Israel	2003-04	MABAT Youth Survey	11–19	CDC-2000²	12.9	12.7	13.0	5.6	7.4	4.1	Nitzan Kaluski et al., 2009 [24]
	Jordan	2009	Household-based survey	13–18	IOTF¹	13.7	11.3	15.5	10.0	12.4	8.2	Khader et al., 2011 [25]
	Qatar	2003-04	School-based survey	12–17	IOTF¹	23.8	28.6	18.9	6.3	7.9	4.7	Bener, 2006 [26]
	Saudi Arabia	2005	Household-based survey	13–18	CDC-2000²	17.9	16.5	19.6	7.0	8.2	5.5	El Mouzan et al., 2010 [27]
					WHO-2007³	16.0	13.6	18.4	10.6	11.2	10.0	
	Taiwan	2003	School-based survey	10–18	IOTF¹	16.3	18.4	14.2	6.2	8.1	4.2	Liou et al., 2009 [28]
	United Arab Emirates	2009-10	Household-based survey	11–18	IOTF¹	—	16.2	20.5	—	11.7	19.7	Ng et al., 2011 [29]
Europe	Cyprus	1999-00	School-based survey	10–17	IOTF¹	18.9	21.3	16.5	5.8	7.1	4.5	Savva et al., 2002 [30]
	Czech Republic	2005	Lifestyle and Obesity Study	6–17	IOTF¹	12.3	16.6	8.0	1.4	1.7	1.0	Kunesova et al., 2007 [31]
	Germany	2008	CrescNet database	12–16	IOTF¹	18.2	19.3	17.0	6.2	7.6	4.6	Blüher et al., 2011 [32]

TABLE 2: *Cont.*

Continent	Country	Date of survey	Study population	Age (years)/ school grade	Criteria	Overweight (%)			Obesity (%)			Reference
						All	Boys	Girls	All	Boys	Girls	
	Greece	2003	School-based survey	13–19	IOTF¹	18.3	23.3	14.0	4.3	6.1	2.7	Tzotzas et al., 2008 [33]
	Italy	2002	HBSC Study	11, 13, 15	IOTF¹	15.6	20.9	10.6	2.3	3.5	1.2	Vieno et al., 2005 [34]
	Republic of Ireland	2003	School-based survey	11–16	IOTF¹	18.5	17.8	19.2	5.8	5.6	6.1	Whelton et al., 2007 [35]
	Northern Ireland	2003	School-based survey	11–15	IOTF¹	18.2	18.5	17.8	5.9	6.0	5.7	Whelton et al., 2007 [35]
	Portugal	2008	School-based survey	10–18	IOTF¹	17.4	17.7	17.0	5.2	5.8	4.6	Sardinha et al., 2011 [36]
					WHO-2007	21.8	20.4	23.1	9.9	10.3	9.6	
	Sweden	2001	School-based survey	10, 13, 16	IOTF¹	15.8	14.6	16.9	4.4	5.0	3.6	Ekblom et al., 2004 [37]
Oceania	Australia	2004	2004 SPANS	8th, 10th	IOTF¹	17.9	19.4	16.2	5.3	6.7	3.6	Booth et al., 2007 [38]
	New Zealand	2007	Youth'07 Survey	13–17	IOTF¹	24.0	23.3	24.7	10.2	10.8	9.5	Utter et al., 2010 [39]
					WHO-2007	25.9	25.9	26.0	13.5	14.6	12.1	

TABLE 2: *Cont.*

Overweight and obesity, all adolescents with BMI-for-age ≥25 kg/m2 and <30 kg/m2 and ≥30 kg/m², respectively, according to the IOTF [6].
Overweight and obesity, all adolescents with BMI-for-age ≥P85th and <P95th and ≥P95th, respectively, according to the CDC [5].
Overweight and obesity, all adolescents with BMI-for-age >+1SD and <+2SD and >+2SD, respectively, according to the WHO [7].
IOTF: International Obesity Task Force; CDC: Center for Disease Control and Prevention; WHO: World Health Organization; 2008 SA YRBS: 2008 South African National Youth Risk Behaviour; 2004 CCHS: 2004 Canadian Community Health Survey; 2007 NSCH: National Survey of Children's Health; 2002 CNNHS: 2002 China National Nutrition and Health Survey; CASPIAN Study: Childhood and Adolescence Surveillance and Prevention of Adult Non-communicable disease; HBSC: Health Behaviour in School-aged Children; 2004 SPANS: 2004 NSW Schools Physical Activity and Nutrition Survey.

1.3.3 GENDER DIFFERENCES

According to national data, the prevalence of overweight among boys was ≥10% higher than girls in nine countries (Canada [18], Qatar [26], Taiwan [28], Cyprus [30], Czech Republic [31], Germany [32], Greece [33], Italy [34], Australia [38], Denmark [44], and Hungary [47]) and among girls ≥10% higher than boys in seven of the twenty-five countries (South Africa [15], Seychelles [16], Tunisia [17], Mexico [19], Bahrain [21], Saudi Arabia [27], and Sweden [37]). The obesity prevalence was ≥10% higher among boys in seventeen countries (Canada [18], USA [20], China [22], Iran [23], Israel [24], Qatar [26], Saudi Arabia [27], Taiwan [28], Cyprus [30], Czech Republic [31], Germany [32], Greece [33], Italy [34], Portugal [36], Sweden [37], Australia [38], New Zealand [39], Denmark [44], and Hungary [47]) and ≥10% higher among girls in four of the twenty-five countries (South Africa [14], Seychelles [16], Tunisia [17], and Bahrain [21]).

1.4 DISCUSSION

The aim of this study was to review systematically the literature on overweight and obesity prevalence among adolescents worldwide. Thirty-nine articles and one National Health Report that met the inclusion criteria were considered. The overweight and obesity prevalence in the included studies ranged widely. In sixteen of the twenty-three countries with national representative data using the IOTF cut-off, overweight and obesity prevalence higher than 20% were found, five countries showed prevalence above 30%, and just in two countries prevalence was lower than 10%.

Regarding national data, when prevalence was analysed according to sex, it was observed that boys showed a higher prevalence of overweight in almost half of the countries and a higher prevalence of obesity in almost all countries. These results are consistent with previous studies that pointed out a high prevalence of abdominal obesity among boys [55]. Differences of prevalence of overweight and obesity between genders have been related to geopolitical and cultural conditions [55].

Eight articles compared data between 1980s and/or 1990s with 2000s [16, 19, 20, 22, 28, 32, 37, 50] and pointed out an increased prevalence of overweight and obesity in both sexes over this period. However, among Australian adolescents [38] the overweight and obesity prevalence increased significantly among boys but not among girls over the period 1997–2004. In the Australian National Children's Nutrition and Physical Activity Survey 2007 (NCNPAS07) [14], 25% of boys and 30% of girls aged 9- to 13-year-olds and 25% of boys and 23% of girls aged 14- to 16-year-olds were overweight or obese using the IOTF criteria. A comparison of the 1985, 1995, and 2007 Australian national surveys of 7- to 15-year-olds indicated that Australian children are changing body shape to a more central fat distribution [14]. In USA, overweight and obesity prevalence among adolescents increased 4% in 2003 and 10% in 2007. Overweight and obesity prevalence increased by 3% and 18% among USA girls over this period. However, a cross-sectional analyses of a representative sample of the USA child and adolescent population (birth through 19 years of age) with data from the National Health and Nutrition Examination Survey 2009-10 (NHANES) indicated a prevalence of overweight and obesity among adolescents aged 12 through 19 years of 15.2% and 18.4%, respectively. Analyses of trends in obesity prevalence for the last two NHANES surveys (2007-08 and 2009-10) indicated that the prevalence of obesity in children and adolescents has not changed in 2009-10 compared with 2007-08 [13]. On the other hand, since 2004 the overweight and obesity trends were stabilized or decreased among German adolescents [32].

In USA, substantial geographic disparities in adolescent overweight and obesity were found, with an apparent shift toward higher prevalence in 2007 for several states [20]. Generally, overweight and obesity prevalence was also higher in southern USA in 2007. Lobstein et al. [56] reported that children in Northern Europe countries generally tended to have lower overweight and obesity prevalence (10–20%) than in Southern Europe (20–35%). Also within the same country, the prevalence and trends of overweight and obesity may not be homogeneous according to different geographic regions [57]. In Italy, a north-south gradient in overweight and obesity prevalence among boys but also in overweight prevalence among girls was also reported [34]. A higher prevalence of overweight and obesity has been reported in Southern Spain in both children [58] and adults [59].

It is important to note that the choice of a reference and a cut-off point will determine the absolute prevalence of overweight and obesity and its trends, and hence different information will be obtained from the papers [60]. The IOTF classification for adolescent overweight and obesity [6] is the most frequently used. Cole et al. [6] argued that the reference they published, supported by the IOTF, is less arbitrary and more international than others and recommended its use in international comparisons. Lately, Monasta et al. [61] suggested that the IOTF reference and cut-offs could be preferable to identify overweight and obesity both at individual and population levels because they are at least based on a crude association with ill and health later in life, namely, the definition of overweight and obesity at age 18 years. However, the IOTF cut-offs have been not recommended for clinical use when assessing an individual child's growth [9, 62–64]. Furthermore, recent findings suggested that a universal BMI classification system for childhood and adolescent overweight and obesity may not correspond to a comparable level of body fatness in all populations [9]. The prevalence estimates may not accurately characterize the population groups most at risk of health disadvantages because the correlation of BMI with adiposity is highly variable and dependent on ethnic group [9, 60, 65, 66].

1.5 LIMITATIONS OF THE STUDY

The comparisons of overweight and obesity prevalence need interpretation with caution due to the difference in survey sampling methods, sample sizes, age range of subjects, quality of data in terms of height and weight measurement, and whether national programmes or strategies to tackle overweight and obesity are in place [57]. Even within the same country, the prevalence and trends of overweight and obesity may not be homogenous in view of different ethnicities, geographic regions, and socioeconomic status [57]. Only articles in English, Spanish, Italian, and Portuguese were included in this review.

1.6 CONCLUSIONS

The results of this review allow the following conclusions: (1) overweight and obesity prevalence is high; (2) obesity is higher among boys, although it is not clear which sex has a higher proportion of adolescents with overweight; (3) despite that there is no consensus about criteria to be used to classify adolescents as overweighed or obese, the most frequently used was the IOTF reference [6]. However, the international reference charts for monitoring the secular trends in childhood obesity need to be continually refined and evaluated [56]. The results of this study would contribute to guiding health planners and administrators to develop proper tools for adolescent obesity management.

REFERENCES

1. C. B. Ebbeling, D. B. Pawlak, and D. S. Ludwig, "Childhood obesity: public-health crisis, common sense cure," The Lancet, vol. 360, no. 9331, pp. 473–482, 2002.
2. I. Lissau, M. D. Overpeck, W. J. Ruan, P. Due, B. E. Holstein, and M. L. Hediger, "Body mass index and overweight in adolescents in 13 European Countries, Israel, and the United States," Archives of Pediatrics and Adolescent Medicine, vol. 158, no. 1, pp. 27–33, 2004.

3. A. Must and S. E. Anderson, "Body mass index in children and adolescents: considerations for population-based applications," International Journal of Obesity, vol. 30, no. 4, pp. 590–594, 2006.

4. J. J. Reilly, "Diagnostic accuracy of the BMI for age in paediatrics," International Journal of Obesity, vol. 30, no. 4, pp. 595–597, 2006.

5. R. J. Kuczmarski, C. L. Ogden, S. S. Guo et al., "2000 CDC Growth Charts for the United States: methods and development," Vital and Health Statistics, no. 246, pp. 1–190, 2002.

6. T. J. Cole, M. C. Bellizzi, K. M. Flegal, and W. H. Dietz, "Establishing a standard definition for child overweight and obesity worldwide: international survey," British Medical Journal, vol. 320, no. 7244, pp. 1240–1243, 2000.

7. M. De Onis, A. W. Onyango, E. Borghi, A. Siyam, C. Nishida, and J. Siekmann, "Development of a WHO growth reference for school-aged children and adolescents," Bulletin of the World Health Organization, vol. 85, no. 9, pp. 660–667, 2007.

8. S. E. Barlow and W. H. Dietz, "Obesity evaluation and treatment: expert Committee recommendations. The Maternal and Child Health Bureau, Health Resources and Services Administration and the Department of Health and Human Services," Pediatrics, vol. 102, no. 3, article E29, 1998.

9. J. S. Duncan, E. K. Duncan, and G. Schofield, "Accuracy of body mass index (BMI) thresholds for predicting excess body fat in girls from five ethnicities," Asia Pacific Journal of Clinical Nutrition, vol. 18, no. 3, pp. 404–411, 2009.

10. A. Must, G. E. Dallal, and W. H. Dietz, "Reference data for obesity: 85th and 95th percentiles of body mass index (wt/ht2) and triceps skinfold thickness," American Journal of Clinical Nutrition, vol. 53, no. 4, pp. 839–846, 1991.

11. A. Must, G. E. Dallal, and W. H. Dietz, "Reference data for obesity: 85th and 95th percentiles of body mass index (wt/ht2)—a correction," American Journal of Clinical Nutrition, vol. 54, no. 5, article 773, 1991.

12. "Health Behaviour of School-aged Children study," http://www.hbsc.org/.

13. C. L. Ogden, M. D. Carroll, B. K. Kit, and K. M. Flegal, "Prevalence of obesity and trends in body mass index among US children and adolescents, 1999–2010," Journal of the American Medical Association, vol. 307, no. 5, pp. 483–490, 2012.

14. "Commonwealth Scientific Industrial Research Organisation (CSIRO), University of South Australia: user Guide: 2007 Australian National Children's Nutrition and Physical Activity Survey," http://www.health.gov.au/internet/main/publishing.nsf/Content/phd-nutrition-childrens-survey-userguide.

15. S. P. Reddy, S. James, R. Sewpaul, et al., "Umthente Uhlaba Usamila—The South African Youth Risk Behaviour. South African Medical Research Council," 2010, http://www.mrc.ac.za/healthpromotion/yrbs_2008_final_report.pdf.

16. P. Bovet, A. Chiolero, G. Madeleine, A. Gabriel, and N. Stettler, "Marked increase in the prevalence of obesity in children of the Seychelles, a rapidly developing country, between 1998 and 2004," International Journal of Pediatric Obesity, vol. 1, no. 2, pp. 120–128, 2006.

17. H. Aounallah-Skhiri, H. B. Romdhane, P. Traissac et al., "Nutritional status of Tunisian adolescents: associated gender, environmental and socio-economic factors," Public Health Nutrition, vol. 11, no. 12, pp. 1306–1317, 2008.

18. M. Shields and M. S. Tremblay, "Canadian childhood obesity estimates based on WHO, IOTF and CDC cut-points," International Journal of Pediatric Obesity, vol. 5, no. 3, pp. 265–273, 2010.

19. A. Bonvecchio, M. Safdie, E. A. Monterrubio, T. Gust, S. Villalpando, and J. A. Rivera, "Overweight and obesity trends in Mexican children 2 to 18 years of age from 1988 to 2006," Salud Pública de México, vol. 51, supplement 4, pp. S586–S594, 2009.

20. G. K. Singh, M. D. Kogan, and P. C. Van Dyck, "Changes in state-specific childhood obesity and overweight prevalence in the United States from 2003 to 2007," Archives of Pediatrics and Adolescent Medicine, vol. 164, no. 7, pp. 598–607, 2010.

21. A. M. Al-Sendi, P. Shetty, and A. O. Musaiger, "Prevalence of overweight and obesity among Bahraini adolescents: a comparison between three different sets of criteria," European Journal of Clinical Nutrition, vol. 57, no. 3, pp. 471–474, 2003.

22. Y. Li, E. G. Schouten, X. Hu, Z. Cui, D. Luan, and G. Ma, "Obesity prevalence and time trend among youngsters in China, 1982–2002," Asia Pacific Journal of Clinical Nutrition, vol. 17, no. 1, pp. 131–137, 2008.

23. R. Kelishadi, G. Ardalan, R. Gheiratmand et al., "Thinness, overweight and obesity in a national sample of Iranian children and adolescents: CASPIAN Study," Child, vol. 34, no. 1, pp. 44–54, 2008.

24. D. Nitzan Kaluski, G. Demem Mazengia, T. Shimony, R. Goldsmith, and E. M. Berry, "Prevalence and determinants of physical activity and lifestyle in relation to obesity among schoolchildren in Israel," Public Health Nutrition, vol. 12, no. 6, pp. 774–782, 2009.

25. Y. S. Khader, A. Batieha, H. Jaddou, Z. Batieha, M. El-Khateeb, and K. Ajlouni, "Metabolic abnormalities associated with obesity in children and adolescents in Jordan," International Journal of Pediatric Obesity, vol. 6, no. 3-4, pp. 215–222, 2011.

26. A. Bener, "Prevalence of obesity, overweight, and underweight in Qatari adolescents," Food and Nutrition Bulletin, vol. 27, no. 1, pp. 39–45, 2006.

27. M. I. El Mouzan, P. J. Foster, A. S. Al Herbish et al., "Prevalence of overweight and obesity in Saudi children and adolescents," Annals of Saudi Medicine, vol. 30, no. 6, pp. 203–208, 2010, Erratum in: Annals of Saudi Medicine, vol. 30, 500–502, 2010.

28. T.-H. Liou, Y.-C. Huang, and P. Chou, "Prevalence and secular trends in overweight and obese Taiwanese children and adolescents in 1991–2003," Annals of Human Biology, vol. 36, no. 2, pp. 176–185, 2009.

29. S. W. Ng, S. Zaghloul, H. Ali et al., "Nutrition transition in the United Arab Emirates," European Journal of Clinical Nutrition, vol. 65, no. 12, pp. 1328–1337, 2011.

30. S. C. Savva, Y. Kourides, M. Tornaritis, M. Epiphaniou-Savva, C. Chadjigeorgiou, and A. Kafatos, "Obesity in children and adolescents in Cyprus. Prevalence and predisposing factors," International Journal of Obesity, vol. 26, no. 8, pp. 1036–1045, 2002.

31. M. Kunesova, J. Vignerova, A. Steflová et al., "Obesity of Czech children and adolescents: relation to parental obesity and socioeconomic factors," Journal of Public Health, vol. 15, no. 3, pp. 163–170, 2007.

32. S. Blüher, C. Meigen, R. Gausche et al., "Age-specific stabilization in obesity prevalence in German children: a cross-sectional study from 1999 to 2008," International Journal of Pediatric Obesity, vol. 6, no. 2, pp. e199–e206, 2011.

33. T. Tzotzas, E. Kapantais, K. Tziomalos et al., "Epidemiological survey for the prevalence of overweight and abdominal obesity in Greek adolescents," Obesity, vol. 16, no. 7, pp. 1718–1722, 2008.

34. A. Vieno, M. Santinello, and M. C. Martini, "Epidemiology of overweight and obesity among Italian early adolescents: relation with physical activity and sedentary behaviour," Epidemiologia e Psichiatria Sociale, vol. 14, no. 2, pp. 100–107, 2005.

35. H. Whelton, J. Harrington, E. Crowley, V. Kelleher, M. Cronin, and I. J. Perry, "Prevalence of overweight and obesity on the island of Ireland: results from the North South Survey of Children's Height, Weight and Body Mass Index, 2002," BMC Public Health, vol. 7, article 187, 2007.

36. L. B. Sardinha, R. Santos, S. Vale et al., "Prevalence of overweight and obesity among Portuguese youth: a study in a representative sample of 1018-year-old children and adolescents," International Journal of Pediatric Obesity, vol. 6, no. 2, pp. e124–e128, 2011.

37. Ö. B. Ekblom, K. Oddsson, and B. T. Ekblom, "Prevalence and regional differences in overweight in 2001 and trends in BMI distribution in Swedish children from 1987 to 2001," Scandinavian Journal of Public Health, vol. 32, no. 4, pp. 257–263, 2004.

38. M. L. Booth, T. Dobbins, A. D. Okely, E. Denney-Wilson, and L. L. Hardy, "Trends in the prevalence of overweight and obesity among young Australians, 1985, 1997, and 2004," Obesity, vol. 15, no. 5, pp. 1089–1095, 2007.

39. J. Utter, S. Denny, S. Crengle et al., "Overweight among New Zealand adolescents: associations with ethnicity and deprivation," International Journal of Pediatric Obesity, vol. 5, no. 6, pp. 461–466, 2010.

40. R. M. Tassitano, M. V. G. D. Barros, M. C. M. Tenório, J. Bezerra, and P. C. Hallal, "Prevalence of overweight and obesity and associated factors among public high school students in Pernambuco State, Brazil," Cadernos de Saúde Pública, vol. 25, no. 12, pp. 2639–2652, 2009.

41. G. T. C. Ko, R. Ozaki, G. W. K. Wong et al., "The problem of obesity among adolescents in Hong Kong: a comparison using various diagnostic criteria," BMC Pediatrics, vol. 8, article 10, 2008.

42. R. Bishwalata, A. B. Singh, A. J. Singh, L. U. Devi, and R. K. Bikramjit Singh, "Overweight and obesity among schoolchildren in Manipur, India," National Medical Journal of India, vol. 23, no. 5, pp. 263–266, 2010.

43. N. N. Abu Baker and S. M. Daradkeh, "Prevalence of overweight and obesity among adolescents in irbid governorate, Jordan," Eastern Mediterranean Health Journal, vol. 16, no. 6, pp. 657–662, 2010.

44. K. Søren and C. Jo, "The prevalence of overweight and obesity among Danish school children," Obesity Reviews, vol. 11, no. 7, pp. 489–491, 2010.

45. H. Thibault, B. Contrand, E. Saubusse, M. Baine, and S. Maurice-Tison, "Risk factors for overweight and obesity in French adolescents: physical activity, sedentary behavior and parental characteristics," Nutrition, vol. 26, no. 2, pp. 192–200, 2010.

46. Y. Manios, P. D. Angelopoulos, G. Kourlaba et al., "Prevalence of obesity and body mass index correlates in a representative sample of Cretan school children," International Journal of Pediatric Obesity, vol. 6, no. 2, pp. 135–141, 2011.

47. Á. Baráth, K. Boda, M. Tichy, É. Károly, and S. Túri, "International comparison of blood pressure and BMI values in schoolchildren aged 11–16 years," Acta Paediatrica, International Journal of Paediatrics, vol. 99, no. 2, pp. 251–255, 2010.

48. F. Velluzzi, A. Lai, G. Secci et al., "Prevalence of overweight and obesity in Sardinian adolescents," Eating and Weight Disorders, vol. 12, no. 2, pp. e44–e50, 2007.

49. R. Baratta, C. Degano, D. Leonardi, R. Vigneri, and L. Frittitta, "High prevalence of overweight and obesity in 11–15-year-old children from Sicily," Nutrition, Metabolism and Cardiovascular Diseases, vol. 16, no. 4, pp. 249–255, 2006.

50. M. Jodkowska, A. Oblacinska, and I. Tabak, "Overweight and obesity among adolescents in Poland: gender and regional differences," Public Health Nutrition, vol. 13, no. 10, pp. 1688–1692, 2010.

51. M. M. Bibiloni, E. Martinez, R. Llull, M. D. Juarez, A. Pons, and J. A. Tur, "Prevalence and risk factors for obesity in Balearic Islands adolescents," British Journal of Nutrition, vol. 103, no. 1,z pp. 99–106, 2010.

52. P. Henríquez Sánchez, J. Doreste Alonso, P. Laínez Sevillano et al., "Prevalence of obesity and overweight in adolescents from Canary Islands, Spain. Relationship with breakfast and physical activity," Medicina Clínica, vol. 130, pp. 606–610, 2008.

53. A. M. Lasserre, A. Chiolero, F. Cachat, F. Paccaud, and P. Bovet, "Overweight in Swiss children and associations with children's and parents' characteristics," Obesity, vol. 15, no. 12, pp. 2912–2919, 2007.

54. N. Öner, Ü. Vatansever, A. Sari et al., "Prevalence of underweight, overweight and obesity in Turkish adolescents," Swiss Medical Weekly, vol. 134, no. 35-36, pp. 529–533, 2004.

55. A. C. F. De Moraes, R. P. Fadoni, L. M. Ricardi et al., "Prevalence of abdominal obesity in adolescents: a systematic review," Obesity Reviews, vol. 12, no. 2, pp. 69–77, 2011.

56. T. Lobstein, L. Baur, and R. Uauy, "Obesity in children and young people: a crisis in public health," Obesity Reviews, vol. 5, supplement 1, pp. 4–85, 2004.

57. S. Low, M. C. Chin, and M. Deurenberg-Yap, "Review on epidemic of obesity," Annals of the Academy of Medicine Singapore, vol. 38, no. 1, pp. 57–59, 2009.

58. L. Serra Majem, L. Ribas Barba, J. Aranceta Bartrina, C. Pérez Rodrigo, P. Saavedra Santana, and L. Peña Quintana, "Childhood and adolescent obesity in Spain. Results of the enKid study (1998–2000)," Medicina Clinica, vol. 121, no. 19, pp. 725–732, 2003.

59. J. Aranceta, C. Pérez Rodrigo, L. Serra Majem, et al., "Prevalencia de la obesidad en España: resultados del estudio SEEDO, 2000," Medicina Clínica, vol. 120, pp. 608–612, 2003.

60. J. Kain, R. Uauy, F. Vio, and C. Albala, "Trends in overweight and obesity prevalence in Chilean children: comparison of three definitions," European Journal of Clinical Nutrition, vol. 56, no. 3, pp. 200–204, 2002.

61. L. Monasta, T. Lobstein, T. J. Cole, J. Vignerová, and A. Cattaneo, "Defining overweight and obesity in pre-school children: IOTF reference or WHO standard?" Obesity Reviews, vol. 12, no. 4, pp. 295–300, 2011.

62. L. A. Moreno, M. G. Blay, G. Rodríguez et al., "Screening performances of the International Obesity Task Force body mass index cut-off values in adolescents," Journal of the American College of Nutrition, vol. 25, no. 5, pp. 403–408, 2006.

63. M. De Onis and T. Lobstein, "Defining obesity risk status in the general childhood population: which cut-offs should we use?" International Journal of Pediatric Obesity, vol. 5, no. 6, pp. 458–460, 2010.

64. J. J. Reilly, J. Kelly, and D. C. Wilson, "Accuracy of simple clinical and epidemiological definitions of childhood obesity: systematic review and evidence appraisal," Obesity Reviews, vol. 11, no. 9, pp. 645–655, 2010.

65. D. S. Freedman, J. Wang, J. C. Thornton et al., "Racial/ethnic differences in body fatness among children and adolescents," Obesity, vol. 16, no. 5, pp. 1105–1111, 2008.

66. J. J. Reilly, "Obesity in childhood and adolescence: evidence based clinical and public health perspectives," Postgraduate Medical Journal, vol. 82, no. 969, pp. 429–437, 2006.

Table 3 is not available in this version of the article. To view this additional information, please use the citation on the first page of this chapter.

PART I

CAUSES AND CORRELATIONS

CHAPTER 2

TELEVISION VIEWING AND FOOD CHOICE PATTERNS IN A SAMPLE OF PREDOMINANTLY ETHNIC MINORITY YOUTH

DAHEIA J. BARR-ANDERSON, WILLIAM J. MCCARTHY,
MICHELLE YORE, KAJUANDRA A. HARRIS,
AND ANTRONETTE (TONI) K. YANCEY

2.1 INTRODUCTION

Eleven to fourteen year olds watch 3+ hours of television daily [1] and are exposed to ~25,000 television advertisements annually [2]. It has been suggested that television viewing influences obesity risk because advertising disproportionately promotes high-calorie, low-nutrient food that lead to increased energy intake [3].

The higher rates of overweight in minority children [4] may be partially explained by their greater volume of television viewing as compared to white youth [1]. This increased exposure is potentially compounded in that more nutrient-poor food advertisements (i.e., fast food/candy/soda) appear during programs that target ethnic minorities than programs for the

Television Viewing and Food Choice Patterns in a Sample of Predominantly Ethnic Minority Youth. © *Barr-Anderson DJ, McCarthy WJ, Yore M, Harris KA, and Yancey AK.* Child and Adolescent Behavior, *1,2 (2013). http://dx.doi.org/10.4172/jcalb.1000106. Licensed under Creative Commons Attribution License, http://creativecommons.org/licenses/by/3.0/.*

general public [5]. However, the longitudinal associations between screen time and snacking have not been fully examined in minority children.

This study examined cross-sectional and longitudinal relationships between television viewing and food choices/behaviors in a sample of minority, low-income adolescents. We hypothesize that minority youth who watch more hours of television will report poor eating habits. To our knowledge, no other published research has examined the prospective relationship between television viewing and food choices/behaviors in minority youth.

2.2 METHODS

2.2.1 PARTICIPANTS

Data from predominantly Latino and African American 6th grade students who participated in the Community Steps to Minority Youth Fitness project [6] were used for the current study. This intervention substituted activity-focused physical education (PE) classes for usual, "stand-and-watch" PE, and provided brief nutrition lessons with healthy snacks. Intervention behavior change targets did not include efforts to change television viewing behavior, which is the focus of the current study. Students' PE instructors and parents provided consent and students provided assent. UCLA's Human Subjects Protection Committee provided IRB approval for study protocol. Students who completed follow-up surveys at 12 months (Time 1) and 18 months (Time 2) were included (n=198; mean age=11.5 years). Anyone (n=65) who had missing data at either time point for television viewing were excluded.

2.2.2 MEASURES

Television viewing, eating, and physical activity behaviors were assessed using a self-administered survey with questions patterned from the Youth Risk Behavior Survey [7]. Participants were asked about the number of hours spent watching television on a typical school day from 3 pm to 11 pm and on a typical weekend day. Food choice/behavior patterns were assessed from questions that inquired about how often over the past month did the participant eat/drink a variety of items, and ate breakfast and meals with family. Physical activity was defined by participation in at least 20 minutes of vigorous and at least 30 minutes of moderate intensity exercises.

TABLE 1: Descriptive statistics for television viewing, food and beverage choice behaviors, and family meals.[1]

	Time 1		Time 2		
	mean	SD	mean	SD	p-value[2]
Daily TV viewing (hours)					
Weekday	3.6	2.1	3.9	2.3	0.06
Weekend (Saturday)	4.3	2.4	4.1	2.4	0.37
Average/day	3.8	2.0	3.9	2.1	0.06
Dietary intake (daily servings)					
Fruit	1.70	1.7	1.49	1.5	0.12
Green salad 0.94	1.3	0.79	1.2	0.15	
Potato[3]	0.76	1.1	0.61	1.0	0.16
Carrots	0.98	1.4	0.62	1.0	0.004
Other vegetables	1 05	1.4	1.18	1.5	0.35
Total fruits & vegetables[4]	4.70	4.3	4.09	4.0	0.05
Milk	1.44	1.7	1.09	1.4	0.02
Fast food	0.63	1.2	0.52	1.0	0.35
Snack food	1.31	1.4	1.33	1.5	0.87
Juice	1.91	1.8	1.50	1.6	0.03
Sweetened beverage	1.41	1.5	0.66	1.0	<0.0001
Number of family meals per week	1.65	1.7	1.69	1.7	0.82
Number of breakfast per week	4.62	2.7	4.59	2.7	0.92

[1]*Estimates are unadjusted*
[2]*P-values generated from paired t-tests*
[3]*Potato servings exclude French fries, fried potatoes, and potato chips*
[4]*Total fruits & vegetable servings exclude potato servings*

TABLE 2: Association between television viewing (hours/day) and food choice intake (servings/day) at Time 1, Time 2, and longitudinally (Time 2 - Time 1).[1]

Dietary intake (daily servings)	Cross-sectional at Time 1			Cross-sectional at Time 2			Longitudinal		
	β	t	P	β	t	P	β	t	P
Fruit	-0.05	-0.68	0.50	0.0	1.72	0.09	-0.01	-0.12	0.90
Green salad	0.01	0.12	0.91	0.021	0.43	0.67	-0.11	-2.03	0.04
Potato[2]	0.01	0.14	0.89	0.04	1.13	0.26	-0.03	-0.45	0.66
Carrots	0.07	1.08	0.28	0.02	0.38	0.70	-0.08	-1.21	0.23
Other vegetables	0.01	0.13	0.89	-0.16	-0.26	0.80	0.08	1.14	0.26
Total vegetables[3]	0.03	0.17	0.87	0.12	0.76	0.45	-0.12	-0.75	0.46
Milk	0.03	0.35	0.73	-0.09	-0.86	0.39	-0.06	-0.87	0.39
Fast food	0.13	2.56	0.01	0.03	0.86	0.39	-0.10	-1.75	0.08
Snack food[4]	0.20	3.35	<0.01	0.26	4.35	<0.01	0.30	2.14	0.02
Juice	0.04	0.46	0.65	0.04	0.58	0.56	-0.12	-1.35	0.18
Sweetened beverage	0.20	2.93	<0.01	0.04	0.94	0.35	-0.39	-0.53	0.60
Family meals[5]	0.10	1.36	0.18	0.08	1.18	0.24	-0.20	-2.36	0.02
Breakfast[6]	0.23	1.91	0.06	0.07	0.61	0.54	-0.22	-1.50	0.14

[1]*t-test and p-value from linear regression models (note: only p<0.01 was considered statistically significant to correct for the multiplicity of tests)*
[2]*Potato servings exclude French fries, fried potatoes, and potato chips*
[3]*Total fruits and vegetable servings exclude potato servings*
[4]*In cross-time analysis, baseline snacking was included as a covariate*
[5]*Data represent number of reported family meals per week*
[6]*Data represent reported number of times respondents eat breakfast per week*

Height and weight were measured by trained research staff. Body Mass Index (BMI) was calculated and BMI percentiles categories (average weight/overweight/obese) were defined using CDC age and sex-adjusted growth chart [8,9]. Students self-reported sex, race/ ethnicity, and school grades.

2.2.3 DATA ANALYSIS

Descriptive statistics (frequencies, means) were calculated. The association between television viewing and food choice behaviors was examined using linear regression and evaluated at Time 1, Time 2, and the change between Time 1 and Time 2 (Time 2 minus Time 1 controlling for Time 1). Models were adjusted for sex, race/ethnicity, BMI, school grades, and physical activity. To control for multiple comparisons, a more conservative alpha level ($p<0.01$) was used.

List wise deletion of cases with missing values was employed in regressing outcomes of interest on television viewing, resulting in an analytical sample of n=114 for the cross-time analyses. Those cases that were dropped because of missing values on 1+ variables included in the regression models were not significantly different on any outcome measures except for baseline snack food intake, where subjects retained in the analysis reported less frequent snacking than subjects dropped from the analysis ($t(147)=2.04$, $p=0.044$). Cross-time regression of follow-up snacking on television viewing included baseline snacking as a covariate, partly to control for this difference. There were also proportionately more girls retained in the regression analyses than boys, consistent with the literature, so findings may be more pertinent to girls than boys ($t(225)=-2.48$, $p=0.014$).

2.3 RESULTS AND DISCUSSION

The sample was majority female (61%) and primarily minority (56% Latino, 32% African American). At both time points, ~40% was overweight/obese and participated in ~4 days/week of moderate-to-vigorous physical activity. Few differences between Time 1 and Time 2 in television viewing and eating behaviors existed (Table 1). Fewer carrot and sweetened beverage servings were consumed at Time 2 than Time 1 ($p=0.004$ and $p<0.0001$, respectively).

There was a positive cross-sectional relationship between snack food intake and television viewing at both Time 1 and Time 2 ($p<0.01$; Table 2). The longitudinal association between change in snack food intake and change in average television hours/day approached significance (β=0.305, p=0.017). Fast food intake and sweetened beverage consumption were associated with television viewing at Time 1 (p=0.01 and p<0.01, respectively) and change in family meals with change in television viewing was approaching significance (p=0.02). No other relationships between television viewing and eating behavior were significant.

Significant cross-sectional associations between snack food intake and television viewing were found in this sample of predominantly Latino and African American middle school students. These associations were expected and similar results have been found in less ethnically diverse student populations [10]. Fast food intake and sweetened beverage consumption were associated with television viewing at Time 1, but other expected cross-sectional associations between eating behaviors and television viewing were not statistically significant in this sample. Numerous other studies [11-16] found an inverse relationship between healthful eating behaviors and television viewing in adolescents in different grade levels (i.e., elementary through college).

None of the longitudinal associations were significant, although the cross-time relationships between increased television viewing with increased snack food intake and decreased family meals did approach significance. Few studies have examined the relationship between diet and television viewing over time in adolescents [10,17], and both studies found a positive association between hours of television viewing and poorer food choices. Among middle schoolers, each hour increase in television viewing was associated with increased consumption of baked sweet snacks, candy, fast food, fried potatoes, salty snack foods, and sweetened beverages [10]. High school students who watched 5+ hours of television while in middle school reported lower fruit intake and higher sweetened beverage consumption than those who watched less television [17]. Family meals are associated both crosssectionally and longitudinally with better food choice intake and that watching television during dinner may have a negative influence on the quality of food choices [18]. Among middle and high school students who reported having at least three family meals/ week, those students who reported often watching television during dinner had a higher intake of sweetened beverages and lower intakes of vegetables and grains than students who had regular family meals but did not watch television during mealtime [19]. The current study confirmed a positive, cross-sectional relationship between television viewing and poor food choices at each measurement point. However, longitudinal associations only approached significance, likely due to sample size and multiple comparisons. Due to social desirability, students may have underreported food intake of foods of minimum nutritional value, which may have hampered the relationship with television viewing.

Latino and African American youth have among the highest rates of obesity and report higher television viewing than white adolescents. Television viewing has been linked consistently with an increased risk for obesity. Future research should include intervention methods to decrease television viewing in this population and more longitudinal research examining mechanisms that could explain the relationship between adolescent obesity risk and television viewing.

REFERENCES

1. Rideout VJ, Foehr UG, Roberts DF (2010) Generation M2: Media in the Lives of 8- to 18-Year Olds. A Kaiser Family Foundation Study, Menlo Park.
2. Lacey JV Jr, Chia VM, Rush BB, Carreon DJ, Richesson DA, et al. (2012) Incidence rates of endometrial hyperplasia, endometrial cancer and hysterectomy from 1980 to 2003 within a large prepaid health plan. Int J Cancer 131: 1921-1929.
3. Zimmerman FJ, Bell JF (2010) Associations of television content type and obesity in children. Am J Public Health 100: 334-340.
4. Ogden CL, Carroll MD, Kit BK, Flegal KM (2012) Prevalence of obesity and trends in body mass index among US children and adolescents, 1999-2010. JAMA 307: 483-490.
5. Henderson VR, Kelly B (2005) Food advertising in the age of obesity: content analysis of food advertising on general market and african american television. J Nutr Educ Behav 37: 191-196.
6. McCarthy WJ, Yancey AK, Siegel JM, Wong WK, Ward A, et al. (2008) Correlation of obesity with elevated blood pressure among racial/ethnic minority children in two Los Angeles middle schools. Prev Chronic Dis 5: A46.
7. Kolbe LJ, Kann L, Collins JL (1993) Overview of the Youth Risk Behavior Surveillance System. Public Health Rep 108: 2-10.
8. Barlow SE (2007) Expert committee recommendations regarding the prevention, assessment, and treatment of child and adolescent overweight and obesity: summary report. Pediatrics 120: 164-192.
9. Kuczmarski RJ, Ogden CL, Grummer-Strawn LM, Flegal KM, Guo SS, et al. (2000) CDC growth charts: United States. Adv Data 314: 1-27.

10. Wiecha JL, Peterson KE, Ludwig DS, Kim J, Sobol A, et al. (2006) When children eat what they watch: impact of television viewing on dietary intake in youth. Arch Pediatr Adolesc Med. 160: 436-442.

11. Boynton-Jarrett R, Thomas TN, Peterson KE, Wiecha J, Sobol AM, et al. (2003) Impact of television viewing patterns on fruit and vegetable consumption among adolescents. Pediatrics 112: 1321-1326.

12. Coon KA, Goldberg J, Rogers BL, Tucker KL (2001) Relationships between use of television during meals and children's food consumption patterns. Pediatrics 107: E7.

13. Kremers SP, van der Horst K, Brug J (2007) Adolescent screen-viewing behaviour is associated with consumption of sugar-sweetened beverages: the role of habit strength and perceived parental norms. Appetite 48: 345-350.

14. Lowry R, Wechsler H, Galuska DA, Fulton JE, Kann L (2007) Television viewing and its associations with overweight, sedentary lifestyle, and insufficient consumption of fruits and vegetables among US high school students: differences by race, ethnicity, and gender. J Sch Health 72: 413-421.

15. Matheson DM, Killen JD, Wang Y, Varady A, Robinson TN (2004) Children's food consumption during television viewing. Am J Clin Nutr 79: 1088-1094.

16. Utter J, Scragg R, Schaaf D (2006) Associations between television viewing and consumption of commonly advertised foods among New Zealand children and young adolescents. Public Health Nutr 9: 606-612.

17. Barr-Anderson DJ, Larson NI, Nelson MC, Neumark-Sztainer D, Story M (2009) Does television viewing predict dietary intake five years later in high school students and young adults? Int J Behav Nutr Phys Act 6: 7.

18. Neumark-Sztainer D, Larson NI, Fulkerson JA, Eisenberg ME, Story M (2010) Family meals and adolescents: what have we learned from Project EAT (Eating Among Teens)? Public Health Nutr 13: 1113-1121.

19. Feldman S, Eisenberg ME, Neumark-Sztainer D, Story M (2007) Associations between watching tv during family meals and dietary intake among adolescents. J Nutr Educ Behav 39: 257-263.

CHAPTER 3

LATER BEDTIME IS ASSOCIATED WITH GREATER DAILY ENERGY INTAKE AND SCREEN TIME IN OBESE ADOLESCENTS INDEPENDENT OF SLEEP DURATION

KRISTI B. ADAMO, SHANNA WILSON, KEVIN BELANGER, AND JEAN-PHILIPPE CHAPUT

3.1 INTRODUCTION

Childhood obesity has been widely identified as a complex condition, with a plethora of factors that are associated with its development. Accumulating evidence suggests that short sleep duration may be an additional determinant of obesity [1,2]. The mechanisms by which short sleep duration influence body weight are under investigation and might involve both sides of the energy balance equation. Experimental sleep restriction has been reported to increase appetite via an up-regulation of appetite-stimulating hormones [3]. Lack of sleep could also lead to weight gain and obesity by increasing the time available for eating and by making the maintenance of a healthy, physically active lifestyle more difficult [4]. In an environment where energy-dense foods are highly palatable and readily available, caloric intake may be directly proportional to the time spent awake, especially if most of wakefulness is spent in screen-based sedentary activities where snacking is common [5]. Furthermore, the increased fatigue and tiredness associated with not having enough sleep may impact overall physical activity participation [6].

In addition to the duration of sleep, sleep timing may also play an important role in energy metabolism and recent studies have set out to investigate the effects of misaligned sleep timing on health [7,8]. For example, an animal model experiment has shown that feeding mice at the "wrong time", i.e. when they are supposed to sleep, can lead to weight gain [9]. Interestingly, a 2011 observational study involving 52 adults has shown that "late sleepers" (midpoint of sleep $\geq$ 5:30 a.m.) consumed on average 248 more calories per day than "normal sleepers" (midpoint of sleep <5:30 a.m.), with the majority of the excess calories occurring at dinner and after 8:00 p.m. [10]. This finding suggests that greater caloric consumption in the evening may be a behaviour that links later sleep timing to obesity risk. Likewise, two recent cross-sectional studies by Australian researchers have shown that late bedtimes and late wake up times are associated with a higher risk of obesity and poorer diet quality in children and adolescents, independent of sleep duration, physical activity level and sociodemographic characteristics [11,12]. More specifically, children with a later bedtime/later wake time engaged in less Moderate-to-Vigorous Physical Activity (MVPA) and in more screen time compared to a group of early bedtime/early wake time children, despite having similar sleep duration [12]. Similarly, the same authors found that children with a later bedtime/later wake time had a higher Body Mass Index (BMI) Z-score and consumed more nutrient poor foods than the early bedtime/early wake time group [11]. Although the literature is still sparse, these novel findings suggest that sleep timing, particularly time to sleep, is an important factor to consider for health outcomes and behaviours that is distinct and separate from total sleep duration.

A better understanding of children's sleep timing behaviours is thus needed to determine whether children with late-to-bed behaviours engage in more sedentary time and/or consume excess energy, two behaviours that may impact body weight. To our knowledge, the present study is the first to investigate sleep timing and its relationship with caloric consumption and activity patterns in a population of obese children and adolescents. The primary objective of this study was to determine whether sleep timing is associated with energy intake and physical activity/sedentary behaviour of obese children and adolescents. We hypothesized that obese children and adolescents with later sleep timing would have greater daily energy intake, lower MVPA and greater sedentary time than those going to bed earlier, independent of total sleep duration and other potential confounding factors.

3.2 SUBJECTS AND METHODS

3.2.1 PARTICIPANTS

A sample of 62 obese children and adolescents aged between 8 and 18 years with a BMI greater than the 95th percentile [13] were recruited from the Children's Hospital of Eastern Ontario (Ottawa, Canada) endocrinology clinic to participate in the Physiological and Psychological Predictors and Determinants of Metabolic Complications of Pediatric Obesity (POC) study between 2008-2010. All new patients visiting the pediatric endocrinology clinic for an obesity assessment were eligible to participate in the POC study and 26 of the original 62 met the eligibility criteria for the current cross-sectional analysis. These included having 5 or more days of self-reported sleep data (time to bed and time to wake), 3 days of complete dietary recording and at least 4 days of valid accelerometer data for assessment of their sleeping, eating and physical activity behaviours, respectively. Further details of the study subjects are displayed in Table 1. The POC protocol was approved by the Children's Hospital of Eastern Ontario's Research Ethics Board and written informed consent (>16 years) or parental consent and child assent ($\leq$ 16 years) were obtained before study initiation as required by the institutional ethics board.

3.2.2 ANTHROPOMETRIC ASSESSMENT

Weight was measured to the nearest 0.1 kg using a medical grade SECA 634 calibrated digital scale. Standing height was measured to the nearest

0.5 cm using a wall-mounted SECA 222 stadiometer. Body mass index (BMI) was calculated as weight in kilograms divided by height in meters squared and BMI Z- scores were computed. These measurements were performed by trained research assistants according to standardized methods [14].

TABLE 1: Descriptive characteristics of participants (n = 26).

	Normal sleepers (n=13)	Late sleepers (n=13)	p value
Age (years)	13.3 ± 3.1	13.9 ± 2.0	0.53
Sex			
Boys	5 (38)	8 (62)	0.24
Girls	8 (62)	5 (38)	
Height (cm)	157.4 ± 12.0	164.4 ± 11.7	0.15
Body weight (kg)	91.6 ± 27.8	96.4 ± 19.6	0.61
Body mass index (kg/m2)	36.4 ± 8.1	35.6 ± 6.4	0.77
Wake-up time (hour:min)	7:08 ± 0:41	8:06 ± 0:47	<0.01
Bedtime (hour:min)	21:54 ± 0:34	23:01 ± 0:55	<0.01
Sleep duration (hour)	9.23 ± 1.14	9.16 ± 1.28	0.88
Daily energy intake (kcal/day)	1590 ± 468	2015 ± 543	0.04
% Protein	19.3 ± 5.9	19.2 ± 4.3	0.94
% Carbohydrate	49.6 ± 8.0	48.1 ± 7.1	0.61
% Fat	31.1 ± 7.4	32.7 ± 7.5	0.57
MVPA (min/day)	28.2 ± 10.0	42.9 ± 4.9	0.03
Sedentary time (min/day)	575.6 ± 17.1	560.3 ± 26.4	0.64
Screen time (min/day)	137.5 ± 17.2	225.3 ± 52.4	0.13

Normal sleepers are participants with a midpoint of sleep ≤ 2:30 a.m. and late sleepers are those with a midpoint of sleep > 3:30 a.m. Statistical significance was assessed by using an independent t-test with continuous variables and by a chi-squared test with categorical variables.

3.2.3 SLEEP ASSESSMENT

Participants were asked to self-report their respective time to sleep and time to wake for a 7-day period, and the average over 7 days was computed (bedtime, wake time, and sleep duration). Previous studies have found good agreement between self-reported sleep timing and objective measures such as actigraphy [11,15].

3.2.4 CLASSIFICATION OF SLEEP TIMING GROUPS

Midpoint of sleep for each participant was calculated by subtracting half of the total sleep duration from time to wake (e.g., 8:00 a.m. wake time- ½ 10 h slept = 3:00 a.m. midpoint). Participants were categorized a priori into two age-specific groups; children (≤ 12 years) and adolescents (≥ 13 years). The rationale for this stratification is based on the different sleep needs in these two groups [16]. In both age groups, "late sleepers" were defined as having a midpoint of sleep greater than the median and participants with a midpoint of sleep less than or equal to the median were classified as "normal sleepers" for subsequent analyses. The two normal sleep groups, initially stratified by age, were amalgamated into one group (normal sleepers, midpoint of sleep ≤ 2:30 a.m., n=13), and the same procedure was replicated for the late sleepers (midpoint of sleep >3:30 a.m., n=13).

3.2.5 FOOD INTAKE ASSESSMENT

All participants were instructed to complete a 3-day dietary record, including 2 week days and 1 weekend day. Participants were shown how to complete the record by the research coordinator who provided instructions about measuring the quantities of ingested foods. Subjects were instructed to log when they ate and what they ate at each meal and snack, during the 3-day period. If time for snack and meals were reported simultaneously, the two meals were merged for consistency. Mean energy and macronutrient intake was calculated using the ESHA food processor SQL dietary analysis software (ESHA Research, USA), with the 2007 Canadian Nutrient File. This method of dietary assessment has been shown to provide a relatively reliable measure of diet in this population [17]. Of note, the 3 days of dietary record data were matched to sleep data for each participant.

3.2.6 PHYSICAL ACTIVITY AND SEDENTARY BEHAVIOUR ASSESSMENT

Participants were asked to wear an Actical accelerometer over the right side of their hip on an elasticized belt during waking hours for 7 consecutive days. The Actical device measures and records timestamped movement in all directions and provides an assessment of physical activity level. A valid day was defined as at least 10 hours of wear time; respondents with 4 or more valid days were retained for analyses [18]. For each minute, the level of movement intensity (sedentary, light, and moderate-to-vigorous physical activity—MVPA) was based on published cut-points: sedentary equating to wear-time zeros plus observations less than 100 counts per minute (cpm) [19]; MVPA equating to 1,500 cpm or more [20]. For each child, minutes at each intensity level were summed for each day and averaged for all valid days. Further details on how the MVPA and sedentary time were derived from the accelerometers can be found elsewhere [18,21].

While accelerometers can accurately classify participant's behaviours as sedentary, they do not provide information about the type of sedentary behaviour or context. For this reason, daily screen time values were derived as a mean score of reported time spent watching TV/movies, playing seated videogames and spending time on computers outside of school or homework over a 7 day period. Although self-report measures provide reliable estimates of screen time, their validity remains untested [22].

3.2.7 STATISTICAL ANALYSIS

Since there was no statistically significant gender interaction between sleep timing and the outcome variables, data for both sexes were combined to improve clarity and maximize power. Independent t-tests were used to test for differences between groups (late sleepers vs. normal sleepers). A chi-squared test was also used to assess statistical significance with categorical variables. Furthermore, we conducted a linear regression analysis to examine the association between sleep timing and daily energy intake, MVPA and sedentary behaviour. In the adjusted analysis, age, sex, BMI, MVPA (when not the outcome) and sleep duration were entered into the model to determine whether the association is independent of these covariates. All statistical analyses were performed using the Statistical Package for Social Science for Windows software (SPSS 20, IBM, USA). A two-tailed p value of less than 0.05 was considered to indicate statistical significance.

3.3 RESULTS

Baseline characteristics of participants by sleep timing category are shown in Table 1. The midpoint of sleep for the children ($\leq$ 12 years) was 2:48 a.m., whereas the midpoint of sleep for the adolescents ($\geq$ 13 years) was 3:08 a.m. We observed no significant difference in the anthropometric measurements between sleep timing groups. As expected, time to wake and time to bed were significantly different between child and adolescent groups; however, total sleep duration was not different.

Total daily caloric intake was 27% higher in late sleepers (425 kcal) compared to normal sleepers, p=0.04, with no difference in macronutrient distribution. Figure 1 provides a visual representation of cumulative calorie intake across the day for a sub-sample, n=16, of participants for whom we had complete data on meal timing. Albeit not statistically significant due to the small sample size, this illustrates a tendency for greater food intake later in the evening (after dinner). MVPA was nevertheless significantly higher in late sleepers; however, late sleepers engaged in 88 min more daily screen time on average, p=0.13, than their counterparts categorized as normal sleepers.

The relationship between sleep timing in the whole sample and daily energy intake is shown in Table 2. We observed that later sleep timing behaviour was associated with greater total caloric intake in this cohort of obese adolescents, independent of sleep duration and other covariates. In the adjusted model (model b), 25% of the variance in daily caloric intake was explained by sleep timing and a 1-hour change in sleep timing was associated with a 369 kcal/day change in energy intake. However, when screen time was entered into the model the association became non- significant. We did not find any association between sleep timing and BMI Z-score (data not shown).

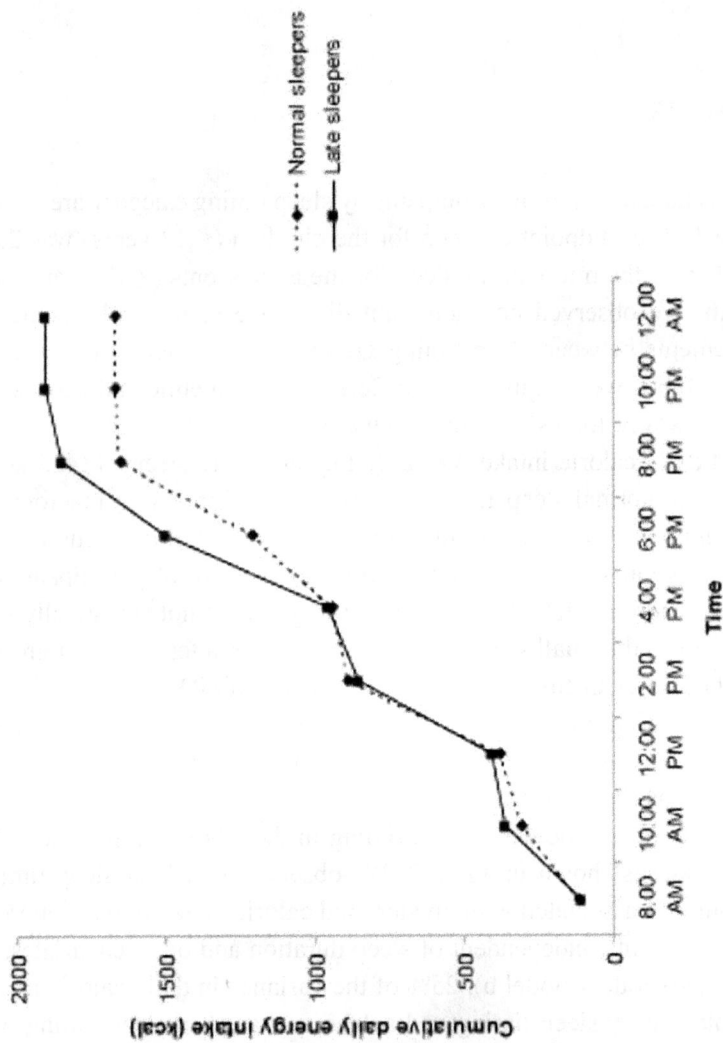

FIGURE 1: Cumulative daily caloric intake according to sleep timing (n=16 with complete data on meal timing).

As shown in Table 3, the linear regression analysis did not identify a significant association between sleep timing and daily MVPA or sedentary time in this cohort. Later sleep timing was however related to greater screen time, independent of sleep duration and other covariates, p<0.01. In the adjusted model, 31% of the variance in screen time was explained by sleep timing and a 1-hour change in sleep timing was associated with a 106 min/day change in screen time.

3.4 DISCUSSION

Collectively, this study showed that daily caloric intake was 425 kcal higher in late sleepers (midpoint of sleep >3:30 a.m.) compared to normal sleepers (midpoint of sleep ≤ 2:30 a.m.). Furthermore, later sleep timing was associated with greater daily energy intake, independent of sleep duration, BMI, and MVPA; however, the association became non significant after further adjustment for screen time, suggesting that screen time may be a possible mediator of the relationship between sleep timing and increased food consumption. Although sleep timing was not associated with MVPA, we observed that later sleep timing was associated with more screen time regardless of total sleep duration. These findings imply that sleep timing is an important aspect to consider with regards to eating and screen time behaviours in obese children and adolescents and that a narrow focus on sleep duration alone may not be enough.

Our results are concordant with those recently published by other researchers [10-12] showing that later sleep timing is associated with increased food intake and greater screen time engagement. Studies have also repeatedly reported that screen time promotes overconsumption of food [5], suggesting that it may not be surprising to observe a higher food intake later in the day if a large proportion of this time is spent in screen-time sedentary behaviour. However, previous studies in the field have mainly reported that short sleep duration (or experimental sleep restriction) is associated with increased food intake, possibly due to an up-regulation of appetite-stimulating hormones and a longer period of time spent awake [1-3]. The finding that later bedtimes and later wake up times are associated with greater food intake independent of total sleep duration is a novel

The Complexity of Adolescent Obesity

observation and suggests that sleep timing is also an important additional aspect to consider in the control of energy balance. For instance, a later bedtime likely allows for more unprotected time (i.e. time not spent in school or engaged in a specific activity) for a child or adolescent to access and subsequently consume food or drink.

TABLE 2: Association between sleep timing and daily energy intake in obese adolescents.

	Beta	95% CI	r	p
Unadjusted model	359.8	59.7; 660.0	0.45	0.02
Adjusted model[a]	368.6	101.2; 636.0	0.50	0.01
Adjusted model[b]	141.9	-143.1; 426.8	0.21	0.31

[a]*Model adjusted for age, sex, body mass index, moderate-to-vigorous physical activity and sleep duration.*
[b]*Model adjusted for screen time in addition to age, sex, body mass index, moderateto-vigorous physical activity and sleep duration.*
The beta coefficients represent the change in daily energy intake (kcal) for a 1-hour change in sleep timing. CI, confidence interval. N=26.

TABLE 3: Association of sleep timing with moderate-to-vigorous physical activity and sedentary behaviour in obese adolescents.

	Beta	95% CI	r	p
MVPA (min/day) Unadjusted model	7.43	-1.88; 16.74	0.40	0.10
	6.36	-1.71; 14.4	0.39	0.11
Sedentary time (min/day) Unadjusted model	11.1	-34.5; 56.8	0.13	0.61
Adjusted model[a]	4.7	-20.9; 30.4	0.10	0.70
Screen time (min/day) Unadjusted model	125.7	42.1; 209.2	0.55	<0.01
Adjusted modela	105.7	36.4; 175.1	0.56	<0.01

[a]*Model adjusted for age, sex, body mass index, and sleep duration. The beta coefficients represent the change in moderate-to-vigorous physical activity or sedentary behaviour (min) for a 1-hour change in sleep timing.*
MVPA, moderate-to-vigorous physical activity. N=26.

In contrast to recent findings published by Olds and coworkers [12], we did not find an association of sleep timing with adiposity indices and MVPA in the present study. The most plausible explanation for the lack of association between sleep timing and anthropometric measurements is the fact that the present study was conducted only in an obese sample of children and adolescents, thereby significantly reducing the inter-individual variability in body size. Additionally, the fact that short sleep duration was the same for both sleep timing groups suggests that sleep duration may be more important in predicting adiposity, as previously reported [1], but that sleep timing may still negatively influence eating and screen time behaviours without necessarily impacting body weight. This observation is reinforced by the fact that late sleepers engaged in more MVPA than normal sleepers, thus suggesting that certain unhealthy behaviours (i.e. greater food intake and screen time) can be compensated for by a greater participation in physical activity so that the net impact on body weight is not different between both sleep timing groups.

Although counterintuitive, the observation showing that late sleepers engaged in more MVPA than normal sleepers is in line with recent studies showing large inter-individual variations in physical activity levels across different sleep patterns [23]. It is possible that physical activity participation is more related to individual motivation than to sleep timing per se. For example, restricted sleep has been shown to increase [24,25], decrease [6,26], or have no effect [27,28] on physical activity level in previous studies. Thus, the higher MVPA in late sleepers compared to normal sleepers can be seen as a balancing force for them; however, adjusting for MVPA did not reduce the association between sleep timing and daily energy intake (i.e. no change in the beta coefficient), suggesting that MVPA is not a major explanatory variable. In contrast, further adjusting for screen time substantially reduced the beta coefficient, suggesting that an important portion of the extra 425 kcal ingested by late sleepers may be attributed to snacking while engaging in screen time. In addition, a projected weekly accumulation of 2,975 extra kilocalories for late sleepers would not be fully compensated for by their approximately 98 extra minutes of weekly MVPA approximating less than 1,000 kcal. The residual positive caloric balance is not inconsequential.

The present study has limitations that warrant discussion. First, the cross-sectional nature of this investigation limits causal inferences. Second, the small sample size and preliminary nature of this study preclude any definitive conclusion and generalization of our findings. This is the first study to explore sleep timing and its relationship with caloric consumption and activity patterns in a population of wellphenotyped obese children and adolescents and the fact that many of our associations were significant despite the small sample suggests that the reported relationships are meaningful and relevant. Third, there are the commonly acknowledged limitations associated with self-reported measures (e.g. recall and social desirability bias). Finally, residual confounding is always a limitation in observational studies and the possibility that some unmeasured variables could influence the reported associations (e.g. maturation, socio-economic status, and family characteristics) is always a possibility.

In summary, the present study shows that later bedtime is associated with greater caloric intake and screen time in obese children and adolescents independent of total sleep duration. These substantial differences suggest that that bedtime is an important factor to consider that is separate and distinct from total sleep duration. Given that the higher energy intake associated with later bedtime appears to be partly explained by screen time, future studies should examine whether reducing screen time can positively influence feeding behaviour of late sleepers.

REFERENCES

1. Chaput JP, Tremblay A (2012) Insufficient sleep as a contributor to weight gain: an update. Curr Obes Rep 1: 245-256.
2. Nielsen LS, Danielsen KV, Sørensen TI (2011) Short sleep duration as a possible cause of obesity: critical analysis of the epidemiological evidence. Obes Rev 12: 78-92.
3. Leproult R, Van Cauter E (2010) Role of sleep and sleep loss in hormonal release and metabolism. Endocr Dev 17: 11-21.
4. Chaput JP, Klingenberg L, Sjödin A (2010) Do all sedentary activities lead to weight gain: sleep does not. Curr Opin Clin Nutr Metab Care 13: 601-607.
5. Chaput JP, Klingenberg L, Astrup A, Sjödin AM (2011) Modern sedentary activities promote overconsumption of food in our current obesogenic environment. Obes Rev 12: e12-20.

6. Schmid SM, Hallschmid M, Jauch-Chara K, Wilms B, Benedict C, et al. (2009) Short-term sleep loss decreases physical activity under free-living conditions but does not increase food intake under time-deprived laboratory conditions in healthy men. Am J Clin Nutr 90: 1476-1482.

7. Johnston JD, Frost G, Otway DT (2009) Adipose tissue, adipocytes and the circadian timing system. Obes Rev 10 Suppl 2: 52-60.

8. Rüger M, Scheer FA (2009) Effects of circadian disruption on the cardiometabolic system. Rev Endocr Metab Disord 10: 245-260.

9. Arble DM, Bass J, Laposky AD, Vitaterna MH, Turek FW (2009) Circadian timing of food intake contributes to weight gain. Obesity (Silver Spring) 17: 2100-2102.

10. Baron KG, Reid KJ, Kern AS, Zee PC (2011) Role of sleep timing in caloric intake and BMI. Obesity (Silver Spring) 19: 1374-1381.

11. Golley RK, Maher CA, Matricciani L, Olds TS (2013) Sleep duration or bedtime? Exploring the association between sleep timing behaviour, diet and BMI in children and adolescents. Int J Obes (Lond) 37: 546-551.

12. Olds TS, Maher CA, Matricciani L (2011) Sleep duration or bedtime? Exploring the relationship between sleep habits and weight status and activity patterns. Sleep 34: 1299-1307.

13. Kuczmarski RJ, Ogden CL, Guo SS, Grummer-Strawn LM, Flegal KM, et al. (2002) 2000 CDC Growth Charts for the United States: methods and development. Vital Health Stat 11 : 1-190.

14. The Airlie (VA) Consensus Conference (1988) In: Lohman TG, Roche AF, Martorell R, eds. Standardization of anthropometric measurements. Champaign, IL, Human Kinetics Publishers, pp. 39-80.

15. Lockley SW, Skene DJ, Arendt J (1999) Comparison between subjective and actigraphic measurement of sleep and sleep rhythms. J Sleep Res 8: 175-183.

16. Centers for Disease Control and Prevention (2010) Sleep and sleep disorders. CDC features website (accessed June 25, 2013).

17. Ambrosini GL, O'Sullivan TA, de Klerk NII, Mori TA, Beilln LJ, et al. (2011) Relative validity of adolescent dietary patterns: a comparison of a FFQ and 3 d food record. Br J Nutr 105: 625-633.

18. Colley R, Connor Gorber S, Tremblay MS (2010) Quality control and data reduction procedures for accelerometry-derived measures of physical activity. Health Rep 21: 63-69.

19. Wong SL, Colley R, Connor Gorber S, Tremblay M (2011) Actical accelerometer sedentary activity thresholds for adults. J Phys Act Health 8: 587-591.

20. Puyau MR, Adolph AL, Vohra FA, Zakeri I, Butte NF (2004) Prediction of activity energy expenditure using accelerometers in children. Med Sci Sports Exerc 36: 1625-1631.

21. Colley RC, Garriguet D, Janssen I, Craig CL, Clarke J, Tremblay MS (2009) Physical activity of Canadian children and youth: accelerometer results from the 2007 to 2009 Canadian Health Measures Survey. Health Rep 22: 12-20.

22. Lubans DR, Hesketh K, Cliff DP, Barnett LM, Salmon J, et al. (2011) A systematic review of the validity and reliability of sedentary behaviour measures used with children and adolescents. Obes Rev 12: 781-799.

23. Klingenberg L, Sjödin A, Holmbäck U, Astrup A, Chaput JP (2012) Short sleep duration and its association with energy metabolism. Obes Rev 13: 565-577.

24. Brondel L, Romer MA, Nougues PM, Touyarou P, Davenne D (2010) Acute partial sleep deprivation increases food intake in healthy men. Am J Clin Nutr 91: 1550-1559.

25. Hursel R, Rutters F, Gonnissen HK, Martens EA, Westerterp-Plantenga MS (2011) Effects of sleep fragmentation in healthy men on energy expenditure, substrate oxidation, physical activity, and exhaustion measured over 48 h in a respiratory chamber. Am J Clin Nutr 94: 804-808.

26. St-Onge MP (2013) The role of sleep duration in the regulation of energy balance: effects on energy intakes and expenditure. J Clin Sleep Med 9: 73-80.

27. Bosy-Westphal A, Hinrichs S, Jauch-Chara K, Hitze B, Later W, et al. (2008) Influence of partial sleep deprivation on energy balance and insulin sensitivity in healthy women. Obes Facts 1: 266-273.

28. St-Onge MP, Roberts AL, Chen J, Kelleman M, O'Keeffe M, et al. (2011) Short sleep duration increases energy intakes but does not change energy expenditure in normal-weight individuals. Am J Clin Nutr 94: 410-416.

CHAPTER 4

INFREQUENT BREAKFAST CONSUMPTION IS ASSOCIATED WITH HIGHER BODY ADIPOSITY AND ABDOMINAL OBESITY IN MALAYSIAN SCHOOL-AGED ADOLESCENTS

ABDULLAH NURUL-FADHILAH, PEY SZE TEO, INGE HUYBRECHTS, and LENG HUAT FOO

4.1 INTRODUCTION

An increasing worldwide prevalence of childhood obesity is a major public health challenge. Excessive weight gain and obesity during childhood and adolescence not only increase the risk of a range of health problems in youth, but also of developing chronic diseases in later life [1], [2]. Although it has been shown that genetic factors play a major role in the risk of developing obesity, modifiable environmental factors such as dietary and lifestyle practices are also important in the increasing rates of childhood obesity [2]. Furthermore, many studies have identified the determinants and correlates of excessive weight gain and obesity during childhood and adolescence. Unhealthy diets such as high intakes of energy-dense foods, along with low levels of physical activity have been shown to significantly increase the risk of weight gain and obesity in children and adolescents [3], [4], [5]. However, there is little information about the relationship between specific dietary behaviors such as habitual breakfast consumption practices and adiposity among children and adolescents.

There is evidence suggesting that daily consumption of breakfast is associated with better foods choice, such as more fruit and vegetables, with consequently also better intakes of essential nutrients [6], [7]. However, studies on the influence of infrequent breakfast consumption on obesity or other health problems in growing children and adolescents have been inconclusive. Some have found that children who frequently skip breakfast have a higher risk of being obese compared to those who regularly consumed breakfast [8], [9], [10]. For example, Harding and colleagues found an association between breakfast skipping and obesity among adolescents in the United Kingdom [8]. On the other hand, studies in children and adolescents from Australia, Portugal and Saudi Arabia have reported no such positive association between infrequent breakfast consumption, and body composition and obesity risk [11], [12], [13]. Such inconsistency between studies may possibly be explained by differences in the definition used for breakfast skipping and also in the choice of dietary and lifestyle factors that were used as confounding variables.

Although it is generally agreed that breakfast is the most important meal of the day [14], there has been a gradual increase in the proportion of children and adolescents who reported that they regularly skipped breakfast [15]. A decline in regular breakfast consumption by children has also been reported in Asia [16], [17]. For instance, approximately 10% of school-aged children and adolescents in Hong Kong were reported to be skipping breakfast at least 4 times a week [16]. In Malaysia, it has been found that breakfast is the most frequently missed meal [17]. Because of this trend towards breakfast skipping in children and adolescents, and because of the possible health effects, it is important to determine whether this dietary pattern might affect body adiposity and abdominal obesity of Malaysian children and adolescents.

There is little published information on any relationship between infrequent breakfast consumption and body composition profiles in growing children in Asian countries. Therefore, the aim of the present study was to determine the influence of breakfast consumption patterns on body composition measurements among apparently healthy Malaysian school-aged male and female adolescents.

4.2 PARTICIPANTS AND METHODS

4.2.1 ETHICS STATEMENT

This study was approved by the Research Human Ethics Committees of the Universiti Sains Malaysia (USM) for human studies. In addition, written informed consent was also obtained prior to the study from both the participants and their parents or guardians.

4.2.2 STUDY DESIGN

The present population-based study was carried-out in Kota Bharu, Kelantan, which is located in the Northeastern region of the Peninsular Malaysia. A convenience sample of 237 school-aged Malay adolescents aged 12 to 19 years of age were recruited for the study. Several recruitment approaches were used, including advertisement in schools and community settings and peer-to-peer referral in different communities in the district of Kota Bharu. Participants were selected on the basis that they were apparently healthy, without any clinical signs of bone-related disorders or other health problems that might inhibit physical activity, and if they were not currently taking any medications known to influence bone metabolism. One girl was excluded in the final study, because her body dimensions exceeded the bone scanning area. A total of 236 Malay adolescents, comprising 104 boys and 132 girls were finally included in the study.

4.2.3 MEASUREMENTS

4.2.3.1 GENERAL CHARACTERISTICS AND DIETARY BEHAVIOUR ASSESSMENTS.

A pre-piloted self-administered questionnaire was used to determine socio-demographic and dietary behaviour such as daily breakfast consumption, snacking practices, eating-out practices, and consumption of carbonated and sweetened beverages. This questionnaire, comprised some structured questions and an unstructured open-ended response, where the participants were asked to provide detailed information about their dietary behaviour such as the frequency and place of consumption of common foods and beverages. Frequency of daily breakfast consumption was assessed using an open-ended questionnaire response format, in which participants were asked to report the actual frequency of their usual breakfast consumption. Data were recorded as a continuous variable in the raw form and were then categorized into two breakfast groups namely, frequent breakfast eaters as ≥ 5 times/week and infrequent breakfast eaters as less than 5 times a week. In addition, the reasons of not taking breakfast daily were also obtained from those adolescents who did not consume breakfast daily. A new quantitative food frequency questionnaire (FFQ) was developed and validated for the present study [18] and was used to assess daily energy intake and other nutrient profiles. In brief, participants were asked to recall the foods consumed during the past year and they then recorded their usual frequency of intake as well as portion size usually served for each food item listed in the FFQ.

4.2.3.2 BODY COMPOSITION PROFILE MEASUREMENTS.

Anthropometric measurements such as body weight, height, waist and hip circumferences were assessed according to the standard procedures of the World Health Organization [19]. Each participant was asked to wear light clothing and no shoes during the measurements. Body weight and height were measured to the nearest 0.1 kg and 0.1 cm, respectively, using an electronic scale with attached stadiometer (SECA 220, Germany). Waist and hip circumferences were measured to the nearest 0.1 cm with a measuring tape. Waist circumference was measured at the narrowest point between the lower costal border and the iliac crest at the end of normal expiration, while hip circumference was measured at the maximum circumference of the buttocks in a horizontal plane. All the measurements were taken twice. However if the measurements differed by more than 1.0 cm and 1.0 kg, respectively, a third measurement was taken. The measurements recorded for each participant were the mean values of the two closest measurements.

Body adiposity was assessed using a dual-energy X-ray absorptiometry (DXA) device (GE Lunar Prodigy, USA) at the Department of Medical Radiology at the Hospital Universiti Sains Malaysia. All body scans were performed by one of two trained radiology technicians throughout the study. Quality control for the body scan was performed on a daily basis. The participants were required to wear specific clothing for the DXA scan and removed all metal objects prior to the body scan. Measurements were taken with the participants positioned supine on the scanning table and they were instructed to stay motionless while the ram of the DXA machine passed over the body beginning at the top of the head moving down to the feet. DXA-derived body adiposity levels were expressed as total fat mass in kilograms (kg) and percent of body mass as adipose tissue.

4.2.3.3 ASSESSMENT OF PUBERTAL TANNER STAGE.

Pubertal growth status was determined by self-reported assessment of breast and pubic hair development for girls and genital hair development for boys according to Tanner pubertal stage classifications [20]. The participant was requested to select the stage that most accurately reflected their current appearance, based on the questionnaire containing illustrations and written description of 5 different Tanner pubertal stages. A random subsample of 20% participants (40 male and 40 female participants) was further examined by the trained personnel of same gender to determine the validity of the self-reported pubertal Tanner assessment tool among these participants. These results showed a high correlation between self-reports of pubertal Tanner assessment and direct physical examination by trained personnel ($r = 0.971$; $P<0.001$), indicating that the self-reported pubertal

Tanner stages tool used is able to provide accurate and reliable information on the current sexual maturity of the participants.

4.2.3.4 ASSESSMENTS OF OTHER LIFESTYLE PRACTICES.

A validated computer-based physical activity (PA) questionnaire to assess the total physical activity levels for the past year was completed by the participants [21]. This questionnaire covers three different physical activity domain namely, activity spent during school time, leisure time and household-based activity. Detailed information on frequency, duration and intensity of each activity for the past year was collected.

4.2.4 STATISTICAL ANALYSIS

Body mass index (BMI) was calculated as weight (kg) divided by height (m) squared and converted to age- and sex-specific BMI z-scores using the LMS method with the UK 1990 growth reference data [22]. Classification of BMI was based on the new revised WHO reference chart for BMI-for-age [23]. All the variables were tested for normality by the Kolmogorov-Smirnov test and test of homogeneity of variance before any statistical comparisons were made. Descriptive statistics were reported as mean values±SD for numerical variables and frequency and percentage for categorical variables, unless otherwise indicated. An independent t-test was used to assess the differences between sexes for continuous variables, whereas the Chi-square tests were used for categorical variables. A gender-specific analysis of covariance (ANCOVA) was used to determine the differences in body composition and total adiposity levels according to two breakfast groups, after taking into account other known potential confounding factors such as age, household income, Tanner pubertal status, daily energy intakes, eating-out and snacking frequency and total physical activity levels. Gender-specific analysis was done in order to see any differences of breakfast frequency on body composition between boys and girls. Data analyses were performed using the SPSS for Windows version 18.0 (SPSS Inc. Chicago, IL). A P value of less than 0.05 was considered to be significant.

TABLE 1: General characteristics and body composition profiles of school-aged adolescent boys and girls.

	Boys (n = 104)	Girls (n = 132)	Total (n = 236)
	Mean ± SD		
Age (years)	15.4 ± 1.9	15.2 ± 1.9	15.3 ± 1.9
Household (RM)	2692 ± 3148	1797 ± 1883[b]	2191 ± 2553
Pubertal growth status % (N)			
Pre-pubertal (Tanner 1)	5.8 (6)	0.8 (1)[b]	3.0 (7)
Pubertal (Tanner 2–4)	78.8 (82)	(89)	72.5 (171)
Post-pubertal (Tanner 5)	15.4 (16)	31.8 (42)	24.6 (58)
Daily energy intakes (kcal)	2346 ± 468	2152 ± 547[b]	2238 ± 522)
Eating out practices % (N)			
Daily	7.7 (8)	5.3 (7)	6.4 (15)
4–6 times/week	21.2 (22)	24.2 (32)	(54)
1–3 times/week	71.2 (74)	70.5 (93)	70.8 (167)
Snacking frequency (times/day)	1.8 ± 1.0	2.4 ± 1.1[c]	2.1 ± 1.1
Physical activity (hours/day)	2.1 ± 1.7	1.3 ± 0.9[c]	1.7 ± 1.4
Body Composition Profile			
Body weight (kg)	52.5 ± 14.1	48.6 ± 13.4[a]	50.3 ± 13.8
Height (m)	1.6 ± 0.1	1.5 ± 0.1[c]	1.6 ± 0.1
BMI (kg/m²)	20.4 ± 4.3	20.6 ± 4.8	20.5 ± 4.6
BMI classification % (N)			
Underweight	9.6 (10)	10.6 (14)	10.2 (24)
Normal weight	70.2 (73)	72.0 (95)	71.2 (168)
Overweight	20.1 (21)	17.4 (23)	18.6 (44)
Waist circumference	68.0 ± 11.3	65.1 ± 10.3[a]	66.4 ± 10.8
WHR	0.8 ± 0.1	0.7 ± 0.1[c]	0.8 ± 0.1
TFM (kg)	9.9 ± 8.7	16.3 ± 8.9[c]	13.5 ± 9.4
Percentage of BF (%)	17.1 ± 10.0	31.7 ± 8.4[c]	25.3 ± 11.6

BMI = body mass index, WHR = waist hip ratio, TFM = total fat mass, BF = body fat, RM = ringgit Malaysia. Classification of the BMI was based on the new revised WHO reference chart for BMI-for-age [25]. Significant difference from boys at [a]$p<0.05$, [b]$p<0.01$, and [c]$p<0.001$.

4.3 RESULTS

4.3.1 GENERAL CHARACTERISTICS OF STUDY PARTICIPANTS

Table 1 shows the general characteristics and breakfast consumption status of the participants. Mean age of the participants was 15.3±1.9 years. The majority (71.2%) were within the normal range for body mass index (BMI). In general, boys tended to have significantly higher levels of body weight, height, and waist circumference compared to their female counterparts. In contrast, adolescent girls had significantly higher DXA-derived body adiposity indices, expressed as total body fat and percent body fat (%BF). Daily energy intake was significantly higher among boys compared to girls with mean intakes of 2346±468 kcal and 2152±547 kcal, respectively (p<0.01). The majority of the adolescents reported that they ate food outside of home less than four times a week, while mean snacking frequency was about 2.1±1.1 times a day. Meanwhile, they spent about 1.7±1.4 hours per day in physical activity. A significant difference between boys and girls was in snacking frequency (p<0.001) and physical activity (p<0.001) with girls reporting higher snacking frequency compared to boys. In contrast, adolescent boys had significantly higher daily physical activity levels.

4.3.2 BREAKFAST CONSUMPTION STATUS

Table 2 shows the general breakfast consumption status of participants. About half of the participants (56.4%) reported that they consumed breakfast at least 5 times per week. There was no significant difference found between breakfast consumption frequency by gender (P = 0.154). The majority of these participants took their breakfast at home (72%) while about a quarter of them tended to have breakfast at school (21.6%), with girls more likely to have breakfast at home while boys more likely to have breakfast at a school canteen or stall.

TABLE 2. Breakfast consumption of male and female adolescents.

	Boys (n = 104)	Girls (n = 132)	Total (n = 236)
	% (N)		
Frequency of breakfast consumption per week			
≥ 5 times a week	61.5 (64)	(69)	56.4 (133)
< 5 times a week	38.5 (40)	47.7 (63)	43.6 (103)
Common breakfast foods[1]			
bread	63.5 (66)	78.8 (104)	72.0 (170)
rice dishes	(75)	65.2 (86)	68.2 (161)
noodle dishes	25.0 (26)	36.4 (48)	31.4 (74)
sweet and fried traditional cakes	27.9 (29)	27.3 (36)	27.5 (65)
biscuits	7.7 (8)	21.2 (28)	15.3 (36)
Common breakfast beverages[1]			
chocolate malt drinks	72.1 (75)	72.7 (96)	72.5 (171)
tea	57.7 (60)	60.6 (80)	59.3 (140)
coffee	14.4 (15)	18.2 (24)	16.5 (39)
milk	9.6 (10)	15.9 (21)	13.1 (31)
fruit juices	10.6 (11)	7.6 (10)	8.9 (21)
Place of breakfast[a]			
home	56.7 (59)	83.3 (110)	71.6 (169)
school cafeteria	28.8 (300	15.9 (21)	21.6 (51)
other places (food stalls)	8.7 (9)	0.0 (0)	3.8 (9)

[1]*Participants may report more than one kind of food.*

4.3.3 RELATIONSHIPS BETWEEN BREAKFAST CONSUMPTION AND BODY COMPOSITION PROFILES

A gender-specific multivariate analysis was used to determine the relationships between breakfast consumption practices and body composition profiles (Table 3). In both genders, frequent breakfast eaters had significantly lower levels of body weight ($P<0.05$), BMI ($P<0.05$), BMI z-score

(P<0.05), waist circumference (WC) (P<0.01), DXA-derived body adiposity measures for total body fat (boys P<0.01, girls P<0.05) and%BF (boys P<0.01, girls P<0.05) compared to those of infrequent breakfast practice. These influences persisted even after adjusting for other potential confounders such as socio-demographic status, pubertal growth status, dietary and lifestyle physical activity factors.

TABLE 3: Gender-specific multivariate analysis of the relationships between breakfast consumption status and body composition profiles in male and female adolescents[1].

	≥ 5 times a week	<5 times a week	P-trend
	Mean ± SE		
Boys			
n	64	40	
Body weight (kg)	50.0 ± 1.5	56.4 ± 1.9	0.010
Height (m)	1.59 ± 0.01	1.59 ± 0.01	0.990
BMI (kg/m²)	19.5 ± 0.5	21.8 ± 0.6	0.004
BMI z-score	−0.19 ± 0.15	0.40 ± 0.19	0.021
WC (cm)	66.3 ± 1.3	70.6 ± 1.6	0.006
WHR	0.79 ± 0.01	0.80 ± 0.01	0.256
TBF (kg)	7.8 ± 1.0	13.1 ± 1.3	0.002
BF (%)	15.1 ± 1.2	20.4 ± 1.5	0.006
Girls			
n	69	63	
Body weight (kg)	46.3 ± 1.5	51.0 ± 1.6	0.039
Height (m)	1.52 ± 0.01	1.54 ± 0.01	0.261
BMI (kg/m²)	19.8 ± 0.6	21.5 ± 0.6	0.032
BMI z-score	−0.39 ± 0.17	0.21 ± 0.18	0.017
WC (cm)	62.8 ± 1.2	67.6 ± 1.3	0.008
WHR	0.73 ± 0.01	0.75 ± 0.01	0.155
TBF (kg)	14.9 ± 1.0	17.9 ± 1.1	0.048
BF (%)	30.4 ± 0.9	33.0 ± 1.0	0.045

[1]*adjusted for age (years), household income (RM), pubertal growth status, eatout out status (times/week), snacking practices (times/day), daily energy intakes and daily physical activity levels (hours/day).*

4.4 DISCUSSION

The main findings of this study indicated that breakfast skipping or infrequent breakfast consumption amongst adolescents was significantly associated with higher DXA-determined total body adiposity, abdominal obesity, assessed by WC and body weight, compared to those who habitually ate breakfast, after taking into account other potential confounding factors. This finding is in line with studies in children and adolescents in Hong Kong and in the United States [16],[24]. An analysis of cross-sectional data in 693 Minnesota adolescents at the end of a 2-year follow-up study showed that adolescents who consumed breakfast more frequently tended to have lower BMI and%BF than those consuming breakfast less frequently [24]. In addition, a recent cross-sectional study in Hong Kong also found that Chinese children and adolescents aged from 9- to 18 years, who were breakfast skippers or only ate breakfast twice or less in a week had higher BMI levels compared to those who were non-breakfast skippers [16]. Furthermore, infrequent breakfast consumption during childhood is associated with higher obesity risk in adulthood as shown in previous studies [25], [26]. The National Longitudinal Study of Adolescent Health carried-out by Niemeier and his co-workers showed that adolescents who skipped breakfast each day during adolescence had a significantly greater risk of developing obesity during the transition into adulthood [25]. Similarly, a recent longitudinal study of children aged 9 to 15 years at the start of the study, when followed over 24 years also found that breakfast skipping in both childhood and current adulthood life were significantly associated with higher levels of BMI, waist circumference and blood markers of insulin and low-density lipoprotein-cholesterol compared to those who were taking breakfast at both time points, suggesting that infrequent breakfast consumption over a long period may have detrimental effects on body weight and cardio-metabolic health [26].

In contrast, several studies with Australian, Portuguese and Saudi Arabian children and adolescents found that there was no significant association between daily breakfast eaters and body weight levels in male and female adolescents [11], [12], [13]. These discrepancies may be partly due to differences in definitions of breakfast skipping and confounding variables used in the final analysis model [27]. However, in the present study, a significant inverse association was found between infrequent breakfast eaters and body composition and body adiposity and this remained statistically significant, even after adjustment for potential dietary and lifestyle confounding factors. The lack of a universal definition for breakfast skipping practices and assessment of the breakfast meal may further complicate the interpretation of the influence of breakfast consumption on health-related outcomes. The definition of breakfast skipping may have a direct impact on the responses given by the participants. For instance, in the previous study, breakfast skipping status was defined as 'seldom' or 'never' eating breakfast in a week [11], whereas in the present study it was defined as taking breakfast less than 5 times a week. The use of quantitative classifications, as in the present study, seems to be more helpful in determining the association between breakfast consumption and body composition because self-perception assessment of patterns of eating breakfast in qualitative terms may not be as accurate in reporting actual meal consumption frequency.

Although the mechanisms that explain the influence of infrequent breakfast consumption on body composition are still unknown, there are several plausible theories that could explain such phenomena in adolescents. The habitual skipping of breakfast was associated with poor food choices and unfavorable nutrient intakes [6], [7], [14]. Several studies have shown that children who frequently consumed breakfast tended to consume more fruits and vegetables [6], [7]. Furthermore, breakfast skippers tend to have diets that are high in energy-dense foods and have an increased tendency of overeating at other meals during the day [7], [28], [29]. Several studies have also reported that breakfast skipping was closely associated with dieting practices in girls, because of concerns about body weight and dissatisfaction with their body shape [30], [31], [32]. In the present study, almost half of the adolescent girls reported skipping breakfast because of concerns about becoming fat (data not shown). A similar observation was reported in school-aged adolescent girls in the United Kingdom [8]. It was generally found that adolescents, especially girls, believed that skipping breakfast was an effective method of dieting to lose weight and reduced daily energy intakes [33]. However, our findings show that infrequent breakfast eating was significantly associated with higher body adiposity levels compared regular breakfast consumption.

As the trend towards breakfast skipping has been increasing in children and adolescents, the detrimental effects of breakfast skipping on their health have become increasingly recognised [32]. Therefore, more effort should be made to encourage healthy daily breakfast consumption practices in growing children and adolescents, when behavioural patterns are becoming established during this critical stage of life. One approach could be to introduce healthy breakfast intervention programs at school, as most growing children and adolescents spend much of their time at school. Therefore, active involvement of school authorities, food providers and health personnel would be important to ensure that a successful school breakfast intervention program could be implemented. Continuous monitoring and evaluation would also be needed to ensure that such a program was successful. Healthy eating campaigns at school would not only benefit the students, but may also help their parents in choosing healthy dietary habits at home. Nutrition education by teachers is important for encouraging regular and healthful food choices during breakfast among schoolchildren. Thus, more effort should be directed towards increasing the opportunities for children and adolescents to consume a nutritious breakfast by providing a greater variety of healthy foods for breakfast at school. The government should consider subsidizing the provision of healthy breakfast meals for students from socioeconomically disadvantaged groups.

Some limitations of the present study need to be acknowledged. Due to the cross-sectional design of this study, causality for the positive association between infrequent breakfast consumption and body adiposity and abdominal obesity in adolescents cannot be established. Secondly, for this particular study, we did not look at the nutritional quality of the breakfasts consumed. For instance, the nutrients from breakfast consumption could not be calculated as portion sizes of breakfast foods were not recorded. This finding in apparently healthy adolescents should serve as the basis for future longitudinal studies with large populations to investigate the interaction between infrequent breakfast consumption and obesity and risks of metabolic disorders in growing children. However, a particular strength of this study was to determine body composition and body adiposity accurately by dual energy X-ray absorptiometry (DXA), which is now regarded as the reference method to assess the total body soft tissue composition in children and adolescents. It exposes subjects to only low level of ionizing radiation, is easy to operate and is less expensive compared to CT and MRI procedures [34]. In addition, the inclusion of important biological, dietary and lifestyle confounders such as pubertal growth status, energy intake, snacking and total PA levels in the multivariate analysis model are strengths of this study. Lastly, it is important to note that there is little published information on the breakfast habits of Malaysian adolescents. The large sample size with a power of >70% for detecting differences in body composition status between the habitual and infrequent breakfast eaters over a wide age range, therefore gives confidence for the conclusion that breakfast skipping in this population is a significant influence on health.

4.5 CONCLUSIONS

The main findings of this study show that adolescents who ate breakfast infrequently had significantly higher levels of total adiposity and abdominal obesity than adolescents who consumed breakfast regularly each day. This indicated that breakfast skipping may increase the risk of excessive body adiposity and as a result, may contribute to the risk of obesity and related metabolic consequences. Therefore, daily breakfast consumption with healthy food choices should be encouraged among children and adolescents in order to prevent excessive body weight gain during their critical years of growth. However, longitudinal studies with large sample sizes would be needed to determine the precise mechanism linking daily breakfast consumption with body adiposity, and health and metabolic-related outcomes in growing children and adolescents.

REFERENCES

1. Kopelman P (2007) Health risks associated with overweight and obesity. Obes Rev 8: 13S–17S.
2. Daniels SR, Arnett DK, Eckel RH, Gidding SS, Hayman LL, et al. (2005) Overweight in children and adolescents: pathophysiology, consequences,

prevention, and treatment. Circulation 111: 1999–2012. doi: 10.1161/01. cir.0000161369.71722.10

3. Hill JO, Peters JC (1998) Environmental contributions to the obesity epidemic. Science 280: 1371–1374. doi: 10.1126/science.280.5368.1371

4. Phillips SM, Bandini LG, Naumova EN, Cyr H, Colclough S, et al. (2004) Energy-dense snack food intake in adolescence: longitudinal relationship to weight and fatness. Obes Res 12: 461–472. doi: 10.1038/oby.2004.52

5. Rey-López JP, Vicente-Rodríguez G, Biosca M, Moreno LA (2008) Sedentary behaviour and obesity development in children and adolescents. Nutr Metab Cardio Dis 18: 242–251. doi: 10.1016/j.numecd.2007.07.008

6. Sugiyama S, Okuda M, Sasaki S, Kunitsugu I, Hobara T (2012) Breakfast habits among adolescents and their association with daily energy and fish, vegetable, and fruit intake: a community-based cross-sectional study. Environ Health Prev Med 17: 408–414. doi: 10.1007/s12199-012-0270-1

7. Utter J, Scragg R, Mhurchu CN, Schaaf D (2007) At-home breakfast consumption among New Zealand children: associations with body mass index and related nutrition behaviors. J Am Diet Assoc 107: 570–576. doi: 10.1016/j.jada.2007.01.010

8. Harding S, Teyhan A, Maynard MJ, Cruickshank JK (2008) Ethnic differences in overweight and obesity in early adolescence in the MRC DASH study: the role of adolescent and parental lifestyle. Int J Epidemiol 37: 162–172. doi: 10.1093/ije/dym252

9. Tin SP, Ho SY, Mak KH, Wan KL, Lam TH (2011) Breakfast skipping and change in body mass index in young children. Int J Obesity 35: 899–906. doi: 10.1038/ijo.2011.58

10. Dubois L, Girard M, Potvin Kent M, Farmer A, Tatone-Tokuda F (2009) Breakfast skipping is associated with differences in meal patterns,macronutrient intakes and overweight among pre-schoolchildren. Public Health Nutr 12: 19–28. doi: 10.1017/s1368980008001894

11. William P (2007) Breakfast and the diets of Australian children and adolescents: an analysis of data from the 1995 National Nutrition Survey. Int J Food Sci Nutr 58: 201–216. doi: 10.1080/09637480701198075

12. Mota J, Fidalgo F, Silva R, Ribeiro JC, Santos R, et al. (2008) Relationship between physical activity, obesity and meal frequency in adolescents. Ann Hum Biol 35: 1–10. doi: 10.1080/03014460701779617

13. Abalkhail B, Shawky S (2002) Prevalence of daily breakfast intake, iron deficiency anaemia and awareness of being anaemic among Saudi school students. Int J Food Sci Nutr 53: 519–28. doi: 10.1080/09637480220164370

14. Nicklas TA, O'Neil CO, Myers L (2004) The importance of breakfast consumption to nutrition of children, adolescents, and young adults. Nutr Today 1: 30–39. doi: 10.1097/00017285-200401000-00009

15. Siega-Riz AM, Popkin BM, Carson T (1998) Trends in breakfast consumption for children in the United State from 1965 to 1991. Am J ClinNutr 67: 748S–756S.

16. So HK, Nelson EAS, Li AM, Guldan GS, Yin J, et al. (2011) Breakfast frequency inversely associated with BMI and body fatness in Hong Kong Chinese children aged 9–18 years. Br J Nutr 106: 742–751. doi: 10.1017/s0007114511000754

17. Moy FM, Can CY, Siti Zaleha MK (2006) Eating patterns of school children and adolescents in Kuala Lumpur. Mal J Nutr 12: 1–10.

18. Nurul-Fadhilah A, Teo PS, Foo LH (2012) Validity and reproducibility of a food frequency questionnaire (FFQ) for dietary assessment in Malay adolescents in Malaysia. Asia Pac J Clin Nutr 21: 97–103.

19. World Health Organization (WHO) (1995) Physical Status: the use and interpretation of anthropometry. Technical Report Series. Report of a WHO Expert Committee No. 854. World Health Organization, Geneva.

20. 20. Tanner JM (1986) Normal growth and techniques of growth assessment. Clin Endocrinol Metab 15: 411–451. doi: 10.1016/s0300-595x(86)80005-6

21. Teo PS, Nurul-Fadhilah A, Foo LH (2012) Development and validation of newly computerised-based physical activity questionnaire to estimate habitual physical activity level in Malaysian adolescents. J Sci Med Sport In Press. doi: 10.1016/j. jsams.2012.06.012

22. Cole TJ, Flegal KM, Nicholls D, Jackson AA (2007) Body mass index cut offs to define thinness in children and adolescents: international survey. BMJ 335: 194. doi: 10.1136/bmj.39238.399444.55

23. de Onis M, Onyango AW, Borghi E, Siyam A, Nishida C, et al. (2007) Development of a WHO growth reference for school-aged children and adolescents. Bull World Health Organ 85: 660–667. doi: 10.2471/blt.07.043497

24. Laska MN, Murray DM, Lytle LA, Harnack LJ (2012) Longitudinal associations between key dietary behaviors and weight gain over time: transitions through the adolescent years. Obesity 20: 118–125. doi: 10.1038/oby.2011.179

25. Niemeier HM, Raynor HA, Lloyd-Richardson EE, Rogers ML, Wing RR (2006) Fast food consumption and breakfast skipping: predictors of weight gain from adolescence to adulthood in a nationally representative sample. J Adolesc Health 39: 842–849. doi: 10.1016/j.jadohealth.2006.07.001

26. Smith KJ, Gall SL, McNaughton SA, Blizzard L, Dwyer T, et al. (2010) Skipping breakfast: longitudinal associations with cardio-metabolic factors in the Childhood Determinants of Adult Health Study. Am J Clin Nutr 92: 1316–1325. doi: 10.3945/ ajcn.2010.30101

27. Dialektakou KD, Vranas PBM (2008) Breakfast skipping and body mass index among adolescents in Greece: whether an association exists depends on how breakfast skipping is defined. J Am Diet Assoc 108 ((9)) 1517–1525. doi: 10.1016/j. jada.2008.06.435

28. Keski-Rahkonen A, Kaprio J, Rissanen A, Virkkunen M, Rose RJ (2003) Breakfast skipping and health-compromising behaviours in adolescents and adults. Eur J Clin Nutr 57: 842–853. doi: 10.1038/sj.ejcn.1601618

29. Astbury NM, Taylor MA, Macdonald IA (2011) Breakfast consumption affects appetite, energy intake, and the metabolic and endocrine responses to foods consumed later in the day in male habitual breakfast eaters. J Nutr 141: 1381–1389. doi: 10.3945/jn.110.128645

30. Barker M, Robinson S, Wilman C, Barker DJ (2000) Behaviour, body composition and diet in adolescent girls. Appetite 35: 161–170. doi: 10.1006/appe.2000.0345

31. Shaw ME (1998) Adolescent breakfast skipping: an Australian study. Adolescence 33: 851–861.

32. Rampersaud GC, Pereira MA, Girard BL, Adams J, Metzl JD (2005) Breakfast habits, nutritional status, body weight and academic performance in children and adolescents. J Am Diet Assoc 105: 743–760. doi: 10.1016/j.jada.2005.02.007
33. Cheung PC, Ip PL, Lam ST, Bibby H (2007) A study on body weight perception and weight control behaviours among adolescents in Hong Kong. Hong Kong Med J 13: 16–21.
34. Pietrobelli A, Boner AL, Tatò L (2005) Adipose tissue and metabolic effects: new insight into measurements. Int J Obes 29: S97–100. doi: 10.1038/sj.ijo.0803079

CHAPTER 5

RELATIONSHIP OF MILK INTAKE AND PHYSICAL ACTIVITY TO ABDOMINAL OBESITY AMONG ADOLESCENTS

S. ABREU, R. SANTOS, C. MOREIRA, P. C. SANTOS, S. VALE, L. SOARES-MIRANDA, R. AUTRAN, J. MOTA, AND P. MOREIRA

5.1 INTRODUCTION

In recent decades, the prevalence of obesity, including abdominal obesity (AO), has significantly increased among adolescents [1]. These findings are alarming, in view of the fact that AO is an independent risk factor for insulin resistance, hyperinsulinaemia, dyslipidemia and hypertension in youth [2]. Despite the upward trend in obesity, there is still a lack of knowledge of the factors associated with AO in adolescents. It has been reported that diet and physical activity (PA) play an important role in the prevention of AO [3, 4]. Several observational and prospective studies have suggested that milk or milk product intake is associated with lower risk of excessive adiposity in children, adolescents and adults [5-7]. The weight of evidence suggests that milk intake is more likely to be associated with beneficial weight and body fat than other milk products such as

Printed with permission from Abreu S, Santos R, Moreira C, Santos PC, Vale S, Soares-Miranda L, Autran R, Mota J, and Moreira P. Relationship of Milk Intake and Physical Activity to Abdominal Obesity Among Adolescents. Pediatric Obesity, **9**,1 (2014), DOI: 10.1111/j.2047-6310.2012.00130.x.

yogurt or cheese [8]. It has been suggested that milk is rich in bioactive peptides (whereas other milk products contain little or no such substances) that may modulate body fat accumulation [9, 10]. On the other hand, other studies have found a positive [11] or null association [12] of milk intake with adiposity.

The emergence of the prevalence of AO and related conditions parallels with the decreasing levels of PA, and increasing levels of time spent on sedentary activities (television watching, video game playing and computer use) has increased among adolescents [13, 14]. As recently noted, the practice of structured and vigorous PA is inversely associated with excess central adiposity [3]. Despite the overwhelming evidence of the association between PA and body composition, PA levels are also linked to other health-related factors, lifestyle patterns and psychosocial well-being [15].

Although evidences suggest that milk intake and PA have an independent role in AO, gaps remain in the literature on the combined effects. Moreover, these two lifestyle habits are not mutually exclusive and often co-exist in the same individual [16]. In a recent review, it is suggested that more research is needed in order to compare the combined effects of milk products consumption and PA on body composition [17]. To the best of our knowledge, no study has examined this combined association in adolescents. In this context, the aim of this study was to identify the association of milk intake and PA on AO in a sample of Portuguese adolescents.

5.2 MATERIALS AND METHODS

5.2.1 SAMPLING

Data for the present cross-sectional study were derived from a school-based study—The Azorean Physical Activity and Health Study II—which aimed to evaluate PA, physical fitness, overweight/obesity prevalence, dietary intake, health-related quality of life and other factors in 15–18-year-old adolescents in 2008. This study was carried out in six of the nine Azorean Islands (S. Miguel, Terceira, Faial, Pico, S. Jorge and Graciosa), where 95% of the Azorean population lives.

All participants in this study were informed of its goals, and the parent or guardian of each participant provided written informed consent for his/ her child to participate. The study was approved by the Faculty of Sport, University of Porto, and the Portuguese Foundation for Science and Technology Ethics Committee; it was conducted in accordance with the World Medical Association's Helsinki Declaration for Human Studies.

The population was selected by means of proportionate stratified random sampling, taking into account the location (island) and number of students, by age and sex, in each school. The estimated number of subjects for the representativeness of adolescent population was 1422, but in order to prevent incomplete information, data were collected from 1515 adolescents. Some adolescents were not included in our analysis (n=306), because information was missing on their dietary intake (n=286) and waist circumference (WC; n=20). This resulted in the collection of data for a total of 1209 participants (503 boys). The subjects who were excluded from this study did not significantly differ from those who were included, with regard to age (16.2 ± 1.0 years vs. 16.1 ± 1.0 years, P=0.158), parental education (9.1 ± 4.5 years vs. 9.1 ± 4.4 years, P=0.890) and gender (girls: 61.1% vs. 58.4% and boys: 38.9% vs. 41.6%, P=0.388). Finally, the sample was weighted in accordance with the distribution of the Azorean population in schools and so as to guarantee the real representativeness of each group (by age and gender).

5.2.2 ANTHROPOMETRIC MEASURES

5.2.2.1 BODY HEIGHT AND BODY WEIGHT

Body height and body weight were determined using standard anthropometric methods. Height was measured to the nearest millimetre in bare or stocking feet, with adolescents standing upright against a Holtain portable stadiometer (Crymych, Pembrokeshire, UK). Weight was measured to the nearest 0.10 kg, with participants lightly dressed (underwear and T-shirt) and with the use of a portable digital beam scale (Tanita Inner Scan BC 532, Tanita, Tokyo, Japan).

Body mass index (BMI) was calculated using the ratio of weight/ height^2 (kg m^{-2}). Subjects were classified as normal weight, overweight or obese, according to age- and sex-specific cut-off points specified by the International Obesity Task Force [18, 19]. Underweight subjects (2.6%) were combined with subjects in the normal-weight category because of the fact that they represented a small proportion of the sample. Percentage of body fat (% BF) was assessed using bioelectric impedance analysis (Tanita Inner Scan BC 532).

5.2.2.2 WAIST CIRCUMFERENCE

WC measurements were taken midway between the 10th rib and the iliac crest and recorded to 0.1 cm. A non-elastic flexible tape measure was used, with subjects standing erect—arms by sides, feet together and abdomen relaxed—as well as without clothing covering the waist area. Subjects were divided into two categories (<90th and ≥90th percentiles), according to age- and sex-specific cut-off points specified by Sardinha et al. [20]. Subjects who were in the 90th percentile or above were considered to have AO [21].

5.2.2.3 PUBERTAL STAGE

To determine pubertal stage (which ranged from 1 to 5), each subject was asked to self-assess his/her stage of development of secondary sex characteristics. Breast development in girls and genital development in boys was evaluated according to criteria outlined by Tanner and Whitehouse [22]. Adolescents in Tanner stage 1 (0.4%) were combined with subjects in the Tanner stage 2 because of the fact that they represented a small proportion of the sample.

5.2.3 SOCIO-DEMOGRAPHIC AND LIFESTYLE VARIABLES

Participants answered a questionnaire that assessed several socio-demographic and lifestyle variables.

5.2.3.1 SMOKING

Participants were classified as non-smokers, former smokers (individuals who had stopped smoking for at least 6 months), occasional smokers (individuals who smoked, on average, less than one cigarette per day) and current smokers (individuals who smoked at least one cigarette per day) [23]. Occasional smokers were recoded and combined with current smokers because of the fact that they represented a small proportion of the sample.

5.2.3.2 PARENTAL EDUCATION

For the present study, highest level of parental education (measured by number of school years completed) was used as a proxy measure of socio-economic status. Participants were divided into three categories, reflecting divisions within the Portuguese educational system: mandatory or less (≤ 9 school years), secondary (10–12 school years) and college/university (>12 school years).

5.3.4 DIETARY INTAKE

Dietary intake was measured via a self-administered semi-quantitative food frequency questionnaire (FFQ), validated for the Portuguese adults [24]. This semi-quantitative FFQ was designed in accordance with criteria laid out by Willett [25] and adapted to include a variety of typical Portuguese food items. The FFQ was adapted for adolescents by including foods more frequently eaten by this age group [26]; the adolescent version covered the previous 12 months and comprised 91 food items or beverage categories. For each item, the questionnaire offered nine frequency response options, ranging from 'never' to 'six or more times per day', and standard portion size and seasonality. Any foods not listed in the questionnaire could be listed by participants in a free-response section. Energy and nutritional intake were estimated with regard to respondents' ratings of the frequency, portion and seasonality of each item, using the software Food

Processor Plus (ESHA Research Inc., Salem, OR, USA). This programme uses nutritional information from the United States that has been adapted for use with typical Portuguese foods and beverages. In order to verify the inter-item consistency, the Cronbach's alpha test was applied to the dimensions of the FFQ and the score obtained ($\alpha = 0.892$) was high, which indicated a good internal consistency.

The amount of milk (whole, semi-skimmed and skimmed) that counted as a single serving was considered to be 250 mL. We included all types of milk in one variable because the majority of adolescents were consuming semi-skimmed (83.7%) or skimmed milk (8.6%). Participants were categorized according to the new Portuguese Food Wheel guide [27] and adolescents who consumed two or more servings of milk per day were included in the 'high milk intake group', while those who consumed less than two servings per day comprised the 'low milk intake group'.

5.3.5 PHYSICAL ACTIVITY

PA was assessed via a self-report questionnaire that evaluated leisure-time PAs [28]. This questionnaire has been shown to have good test–retest reliability among Portuguese adolescents (intraclass correlation coefficient: 0.92–0.96) [29]. It consists of five questions with four answer choices (each rated on a 4-point scale): (i) outside school, do you take part in organized sports/PAs?; (ii) outside school, do you take part in non-organized sports/PAs?; (iii) outside school hours, how many times a week do you take part in sports or PAs for at least 20 min?; (iv) outside school hours, how many hours a week do you usually take part in PAs, so much that you get out of breath or sweat?; and (v) do you take part in competitive sports? The maximum number of points possible was 20. A PA index (PAI) was obtained for each respondent by totalling his/her points, which corresponded to activity level rankings that ranged from 'sedentary' to 'vigorous'. Participants whose PAIs were greater than 10 points were classified as 'active', while those whose PAIs were 10 points or less were classified as 'low active' [29]; this procedure has been validated [30].

5.3.6 STATISTICAL ANALYSIS

For the purposes of this study, participants were divided into four groups, according to their milk intake (high or low) and PA (active or low active): (i) low milk intake/low active; (ii) low milk intake/active; (iii) high milk intake/low active and (iv) high milk intake/active.

The Kolmogorov–Smirnov test was used to assess the assumption of normality. One-way analysis of variance, with the Bonferroni post hoc test, was performed to compare continuous variables, and the chi-square test was used to test for categorical variables across groups. When the continuous variables were found to not be normally distributed, the Kruskal–Wallis test was used to determine differences between groups, and the Mann–Whitney test was used to examine unique pairs. In this report, descriptive analysis is presented in terms of means and standard deviations, unless otherwise stated.

A multivariate logistic regression model was constructed to verify the relationship between AO and the combined associations of milk intake and PA, adjusting for age (in years), gender (reference—boys), parental education (reference—mandatory or less), BMI (reference—obese), pubertal stage, energy intake (in kcal), total calcium intake (in mg), protein intake ($g\,kg^{-1}$), total fat intake (% of energy) and dietary fiber (in $g\,1000\,kcal^{-1}$). Age and dietary variables were entered as continuous variables. Furthermore, we adjusted the logistical model by under-reporting energy intake, which was estimated using the ratio between reported energy intake and predicted basal metabolic rate [31, 32]. The thresholds that defined low-energy reporters (under-reporters) were 1.70 and 1.71 for girls and boys between 15 and 17 years old, and 1.67 and 1.81 for girls and boys aged 18. 'Low-energy reporter' (a categorical variable) was included in the model as a confounding factor.

Odds ratios (OR) and 95% confidence intervals (CI) were computed across groups, with the 'low milk intake/low-active' group as the reference group. A P-value of < 0.05 was regarded as significant. All analyses were performed using PASW Statistics v.18 (SPSS, Chicago, IL, USA).

TABLE 1: Characteristics of the study sample, by milk intake and physical activity groups

	Total (n = 1209)	Milk intake/physical activity level				P
		Low milk intake/low active (n = 260)	Low milk intake/active (n = 417)	High milk intake/ low active (n = 167)	High milk intake/active (n = 365)	
Age‡¶ (years)	16.0 (2.0)	16.0 (2.0)	16.0 (2.0)	16.0 (2.0)	16.0 (2.0)	0.215
Weight‡¶ (kg)	60.5 (15.0)	58.5 (13.6)	62.2 (15.2)*	58.6 (14.6)†	61.4 (14.4)*†§	<0.001
Height‡¶ (m)	1.65 (0.12)	1.61 (0.12)	1.66 (0.14)*	1.63 (0.10)†	1.67 (0.14)*†§	<0.001
BMI‡¶ (kg m⁻²)	22.1 (4.3)	22.3 (4.6)	22.1 (4.2)	21.6 (4.8)	21.9 (4.0)	0.160
Weight status (%)‡‡						0.881
Normal	69.1	66.2	68.8	68.9	71.8	
Overweight	23.2	25.8	23.3	23.4	21.4	
Obese	7.6	8.1	7.9	7.8	6.8	
Body fat**†† (%)	21.6 (8.8)	25.0 (8.0)	20.3 (9.1)*	23.9 (8.9)†	19.6 (8.3)*§	<0.001
Waist circumference‡¶ (cm)	78.0 (13.0)	80.0 (14.0)	78.0 (13.0)	77.0 (14.0)*	76.0 (12.0)*†	0.017
Gender‡‡ (%)						<0.001
Girls	58.4	83.1	47.0	80.2	43.8	
Boys	41.6	16.9	53.0	19.8	56.2	
Pubertal stage‡‡ (%)						0.191
Tanner stage 1 or 2	1.0	1.5	0.5	1.2	1.1	
Tanner stage 3	15.7	16.2	13.2	23.4	14.8	
Tanner stage 4	59.1	58.1	61.9	51.5	60.0	

TABLE 1: *Cont.*

	Total (n=1209)	Milk intake/physical activity level				
		Low milk intake/low active (n=260)	Low milk intake/active (n=417)	High milk intake/low active (n=167)	High milk intake/active (n=365)	P
Tanner stage 5	24.2	24.2	24.5	23.9	24.1	
Parental education‡‡ (%)						
Mandatory or less	48.6	61.6	47.1	47.6	41.2	<0.001
Secondary	36.5	32.3	37.1	39.2	37.6	
College/university	14.9	6.0	15.8	13.2	21.2	
Smoking status‡‡ (%)						
Non-smoker	87.0	89.6	86.6	86.2	86.0	0.384
Former smoker	5.7	3.5	6.5	4.2	7.1	
Occasional/current smoker	7.3	6.9	7.0	9.6	6.8	
PAI‡¶	13 (8)	8 (3)	15 (5)*	8 (3)†	16 (5)*§	<0.001

*P < 0.05, compared with the low milk intake/low-active group; †P < 0.05, compared with the low milk intake/active group; §P < 0.05, compared with the high milk intake/low-active group. ‡Data are median (interquartile range) ¶Analysis by Kruskal–Wallis for continuous variables. **Data are mean (standard deviation). ††Analysis by analysis of variance for continuous variables. ‡‡Analysis by chi-square for categorical variables. BMI, body mass index; PAI, physical activity index.

TABLE 2. Dietary characteristics of the study sample, by milk intake and physical activity groups

	Total (n = 1209)	Milk intake/physical activity level				
		Low milk intake/low active (n = 260)	Low milk intake/active (n = 417)	High milk intake/low active (n = 167)	High milk intake/active (n = 365)	P
Energy intake‡§ (kcal d⁻¹)	2301.2 (1431.1)	2070.9 (1343.3)	2044.3 (1458.3)	2544.3 (1358.4)*†	2621.9 (1513.4)*†	<0.001
Protein¶,** (% of energy)	17.8 (3.8)	16.7 (3.5)	17.7 (4.2)*	18.3 (3.6)*	18.4 (3.8)*	<0.001
Protein‡§ (g kg−1 body weight)	1.6 (1.0)	1.4 (1.0)	1.4 (1.0)	2.0 (1.0)*†	1.9 (1.2)*†	<0.001
Carbohydrate¶,** (% of energy)	49.3 (7.9)	50.4 (8.3)	48.8 (8.4)	49.2 (7.4)	49.1 (7.1)	0.082
Total fat¶,** (% of energy)	32.3 (5.7)	32.4 (5.7)	32.7 (5.7)	32.1 (5.4)	31.9 (5.3)	0.329
Dietary fibre‡§ (g 1000 kcal⁻¹)	9.4 (4.2)	9.9 (4.2)	9.6 (4.6)	9.1 (3.8)†	9.1 (3.8)*†	0.004
Total calcium intake‡§ (mg d⁻¹)	1120.6 (419.0)	767.7 (230.3)	818.5 (251.6)	1579.9 (434.0)*†	1560.1 (456.8)*†	<0.001
Milk intake‡§ (servings per day)	1.0 (0.8)	0.9 (0.3)	1.0 (0.3)	2.4 (0.1)*†	2.4 (0.1)*†	<0.001

*$P < 0.05$, compared with the low milk intake/low-active group; †$P < 0.05$, compared with the low milk intake/active group. ‡Data are median (interquartile range). §Analysis by Kruskal–Wallis. ¶Data are mean (standard deviation). **Analysis by analysis of variance.

5.4 RESULTS

Descriptive characteristics of the adolescents in the sample are shown in Table 1. The higher proportion of girls was seen in the low-activity groups, regardless of milk intake (P<0.001). Adolescents in the high milk intake/active group had higher body weight compared with adolescents in the high milk intake/low-active group (61.4 [14.4] vs. 58.6 [14.6], P=0.001, respectively), and higher body height and lower % BF compared with adolescents in the high milk intake/low active and in the low milk intake/low-active groups (P<0.001, for all). Active adolescents had lower % BF compared with low-active adolescents, regardless of milk intake (P<0.001, for all). The higher proportion of parents with mandatory or less education was seen in the low milk intake/low-active group (P<0.001). No significant differences were seen in age, BMI, pubertal stage and smoking across groups.

Adolescents with high milk intakes had lower proportions of AO, compared with those who had low milk intakes (23.1% vs. 29.7%, P=0.006, respectively). Active adolescents also had lower proportions of AO than low-active adolescents (24.6% vs. 30.9%, P=0.011, respectively).

The energy intakes and dietary characteristics of each group are presented in Table 2. Regardless of whether they were active or low active, adolescents whose milk intakes were high had higher levels of energy and total calcium and protein intake, compared with those who had low milk intake (P<0.05). There was no significant difference across groups with regard to carbohydrate and total fat intake.

The proportion of AO across milk intake and PA groups, as indicated in Fig. 1, showed that adolescents with high levels of milk intake and activity had lower proportions of AO, compared with other groups (low milk intake/low active: 34.2%, vs. low milk intake/active: 26.9%, vs. high milk intake/low active: 25.7%, vs. high milk intake/active: 21.9%, P=0.008).e

The results of the multivariate logistic regression analysis, predicting AO from a combination of milk intake and PA, are shown in Table 3. After adjusting for demographic and dietary variables, low-active and active adolescents with high milk intakes were less likely to have AO than were low-active adolescents with low milk intakes (low milk intake/low active, OR=0.928, 95% CI: 0.562–1.531; high milk intake/low active, OR=0.412, 95% CI: 0.201–0.845; high milk intake/active, OR=0.445, 95% CI: 0.235–0.845). To demonstrate whether it is really milk intake making the difference, we made an additional multivariate logistic regression analysis with low milk intake/active group as the reference group. Low-active and active adolescents with high levels of milk intake remain to be less likely to have AO even after compared with active adolescents with low milk intake (low milk intake/low active, OR=1.078, 95% CI: 0.653–1.779; high milk intake/low active, OR=0.444, 95% CI: 0.217–0.909; high milk intake/active adolescents, OR=0.480, 95% CI: 0.263–0.876).

TABLE 3: Odds ratio for abdominal obesity by milk intake and physical activity groups

		Model 1			Model 2		
		OR	95% CI	P*	OR	95% CI	P*
Low milk intake	Low active	1	Reference	0.008	1	Reference	0.027
	Active	0.706	0.501–0.987		0.928	0.562–1.531	
High milk intake	Low active	0.666	0.433–1.025		0.412	0.201–0.845	
	Active	0.539	0.378–0.770		0.445	0.235–0.845	

*P-value for heterogeneity; Model 1—unadjusted model. Model 2—adjusted for age (years), gender (reference—boys), parental education (reference—mandatory or less), body mass index (reference—obese), pubertal stage, low-energy reporter, energy intake (kcal), total fat intake (% of energy), total calcium intake (mg), protein intake (g kg body weight) and density fibre (g 1000 kcal−1). 1, reference category; CI, confidence interval, OR, odds ratio.

5.5 DISCUSSION

The present study explored the combined association of milk intake and PA on AO in adolescents. The results suggested that adolescents with high milk intakes, regardless of whether they were active or low active, were less likely to have AO, compared with those who had low milk intakes. This association was not confounded by other lifestyle factors or nutritional variables, as it remained significant after adjustments.

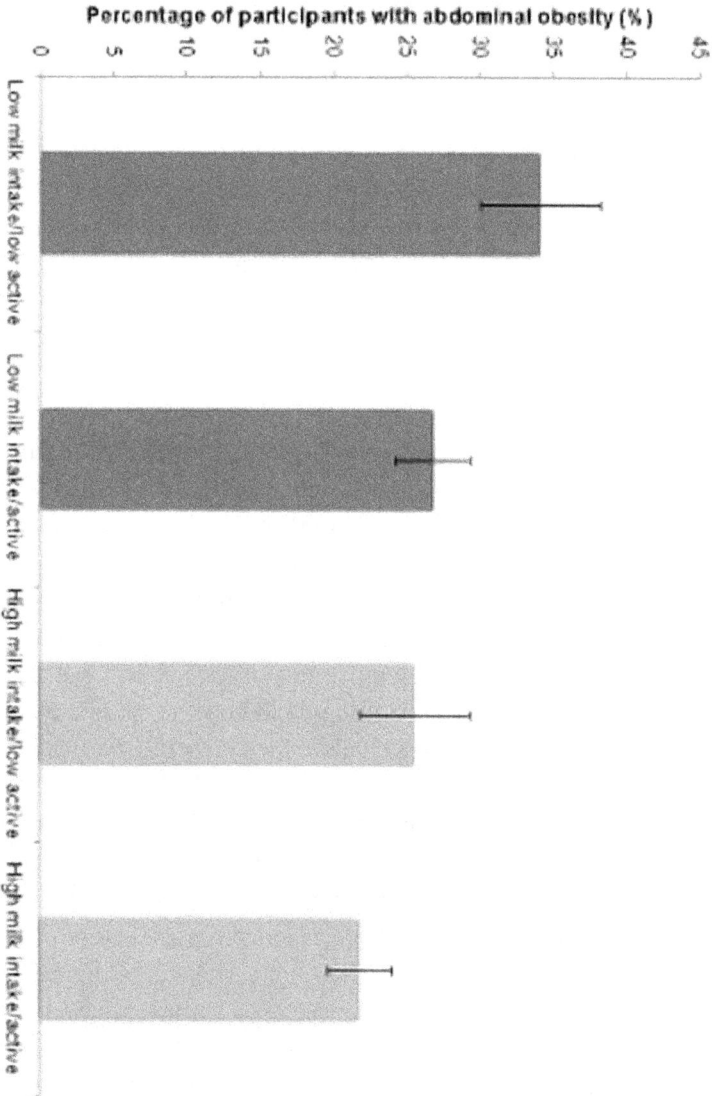

FIGURE 1: Proportion of subjects with abdominal obesity across milk intake and physical activity groups.

Most cross-sectional and prospective studies have found an inverse relationship between milk intake or milk products and BMI, body weight and/or body fat in children and adolescents [5, 7, 33]. Furthermore, evidence shows that the consumption of milk and milk products does not negatively affect weight and body composition [34]. However, studies examining the association between milk intake or milk products and AO are limited. In one study with children, increased milk consumption was associated with lower WC [35]. Bradlee et al. [36] analyzed data from the Third National Health and Nutrition Examination Survey and also found that mean dairy intake was inversely associated with central obesity in adolescents. Previous results, derived from the same sample, had shown that dairy product intake had a protective association with AO in boys [37]. A randomized controlled trial on the effects of a dairy-rich diet on AO with obese children showed that those with isocaloric dairy-rich diets (>800 mg calcium d^{-1}) had lower WC than other groups (i.e. controls with and without energy restrictions) at the end of the study [38]. It is noteworthy that, in addition to its possible 'anti-obesity' effect, milk is an excellent source of nutrients (such as calcium) for adolescents, who experience a period characterized by dynamic changes that occur in response to growth and puberty. Hence, consumption of recommended amounts of milk may help adolescents meet their nutrient requirements and improve their diets' quality [34, 39]. Moreover, moderate evidence shows that intake of milk and milks products is linked to improved bone health in children and adolescents and is also associated with reduced risk of cardiovascular disease, type 2 diabetes and blood pressure in adults [40].

In this study, we also found that active adolescents had a lower proportion of AO. PA also protects against central adiposity by increasing immediate energy requirements, which causes important changes in fuel utilization and mobilization [41]. Evidence suggests that low levels of leisure-time PA are associated with AO in youth [3]. Klein-Platat et al. [42] reported that, in an adolescent sample, AO was negatively associated with structured PA (outside school, >140 min week^{-1}) and positively associated with sedentary activities (e.g. television watching). By the same token, Ortega et al. [43] found that children and adolescents in the lowest tertile of vigorous PA had higher odds of having high WC, when compared with those in the highest tertile.

Concerning dietary habits and PA levels, some studies have found that the consumption of food by more active and less active adolescents differs [16, 44]. In a study by Ottevaere et al. [16], the most active adolescents consumed more milk products than did their less active counterparts. However, previous research indicates that spending more time on PA does not exclusively result in healthier eating habits [16, 44]. Although, in our study, the majority of active adolescents showed low milk intake, active adolescents with high milk intake, when compared with other groups, had lower proportions of AO, which shows the relevance of exploring both dietary patterns and PA simultaneously when assessing AO in adolescents.

When interpreting the results of the combined association between milk intake and PA, we observed that adolescents with high milk intake showed lower odds of expressing AO, regardless of their PA levels. These results are further enhanced by the lack of significance between groups with low milk intake where there was no significant differences between be active or low active. Thus, this finding suggests that the consumption of milk may overcome the potentially negative effects of low PA levels on the likelihood of having AO. Furthermore, milk compounds may also be involved in body fat distribution. Visceral adipose tissue has greater amounts of 11-β-hidroxysteroid dehydrogenase type 1 [45], which is over-expressed in vitro in those with central adiposity [46]. It has been suggested that a high-calcium and high-dairy diet down-regulates 11-β-hidroxysteroid dehydrogenase type 1 expression and decreases the concentration of glucocorticoid, which consequently decreases the size of adipose fat deposits [45]. However, we cannot exclude the hypothesis that milk consumption may also be associated with other healthy eating habits and healthier lifestyles, which may protect against AO.

In addition, we found that adolescents with higher milk intake and activity levels were taller and heavier but had lower % BF than adolescents who were less active and had higher high milk intake. It is well established that increased PA is associated with lower fatness [47] and thus the combined effect of PA and milk intake may enhance beneficial total body fat outcomes. Moreover, milk consumption and PA, along with other factors (i.e. genetics, age, gender, endocrine balance and overall diet) may influence growth. It has been described that children who do not drink milk have a shorter stature than those who do consume milk regularly [48,

49]. On the other hand, PA (i.e. sport participation) has been associated with bone accretion showing an important osteogenic effect, mainly when high-impact and weight-bearing PA occurs [50, 51].

We also found that although energy intake is higher in adolescents with high milk consumption, the additional energy intake does not result in higher odds of AO. In a study to determine the effects of a calcium-rich diet on weight gain during 2 years, 9-year-old girls were randomly assigned to supplying at least 1500 mg (primarily from dairy food) of calcium d^{-1} or their usual diet [52]. Although girls in the calcium-rich diet group consumed approximately 150 more calories d^{-1}, they did not have greater increases in body weight, BMI or fat or lean mass compared with the usual diet group. Furthermore, girls who consumed calcium-rich diet also significantly increased their intake of essential nutrients including calcium, protein, vitamins A and D, phosphorus and magnesium compared with girls on their usual diets. In adults, Zemel et al. [53] conducted 9-month randomized trials to compare the effects of low- (<1 serving per day) and high-dairy diet (>3 servings per day) on weight maintenance. Although the results showed that the high-dairy diet group had a higher energy intake than the low-dairy group, there were no differences in weight and body composition between the two groups after the intervention. Thus, the author suggested that the high-dairy diet group exhibited evidence of greater fat oxidation and was able to consume greater energy without greater weight gain compared with the low-dairy group.

Some limitations to our study should be addressed. First, it should be noted that, as in other cross-sectional studies, conclusions related to cause and effect cannot be drawn. Second, the measure of AO used in this study is an indirect estimate of abdominal fat and there are some sophisticated methods to accurately measure abdominal fat, such as magnetic resonance imagining or dual-energy X-ray absorptiometry. However, such techniques are not feasible to apply in large epidemiological studies because they are complex, time consuming and expensive. Furthermore, it has been suggested that WC is one of the most common proxy measures of AO [1] and is strongly associated with visceral adipose tissue [54]. Third, because in our sample the majority of adolescents (92.7%) consumed semi-skimmed and skimmed milk, we cannot state that any kind of milk is protective against AO. Moreover, we did not include in our analysis all milk products. However, the analysis with total milk product intake (i.e. milk, cheese and yogurt) was done but no significant association was found with AO. The lack of association between total dairy product and AO may be due to the nutritional differences between yogurt, cheese and milk. Cheese is characterized by its fat content and yogurt has frequently more sugar (added in industrial process) than other milk product. Finally, with the use of self-reported PA and dietary intake data, one cannot rule out some reporting bias. Yet, both questionnaires have been previously tested [24, 29], and analysis was controlled to prevent the misreporting of energy intake.

In conclusion, we found that high milk intake seems to have a protective effect on AO, regardless of PA levels in adolescents. Future prospective and randomized clinical investigations, with more accurate measures, are needed on the combined effects of milk intake and/or milk products and PA on AO.

REFERENCES

1. Li C, Ford ES, Mokdad AH, Cook S. Recent trends in waist circumference and waist-height ratio among US children and adolescents. Pediatrics 2006; 118: e1390–e1398.
2. Bacha F, Saad R, Gungor N, Janosky J, Arslanian SA. Obesity, regional fat distribution, and syndrome X in obese black versus white adolescents: race differential in diabetogenic and atherogenic risk factors. J Clin Endocrinol Metab 2003; 88: 2534–2540.
3. Kim Y, Lee S. Physical activity and abdominal obesity in youth. Appl Physiol Nutr Metab 2009; 34: 571–581.
4. Suliga E. Visceral adipose tissue in children and adolescents: a review. Nutr Res Rev 2009; 22: 137–147.
5. Barba G, Troiano E, Russo P, Venezia A, Siani A. Inverse association between body mass and frequency of milk consumption in children. Br J Nutr 2005; 93: 15–19.
6. Marques-Vidal P, Goncalves A, Dias CM. Milk intake is inversely related to obesity in men and in young women: data from the Portuguese Health Interview Survey 1998–1999. Int J Obes (Lond) 2006; 30: 88–93.
7. Novotny R, Acharya S, Grove JS, Daida YG, Vogt TM. Higher dairy intake is associated with lower body fat during adolescence. FASEB J 2003; 18: A2277. [Abstract].
8. Louie JC, Flood VM, Hector DJ, Rangan AM, Gill TP. Dairy consumption and overweight and obesity: a systematic review of prospective cohort studies. Obes Rev 2011; 12: e582–e592.

9. Shah NP. Effects of milk-derived bioactives: an overview. Br J Nutr 2000; 84(Suppl. 1): S3–S10.

10. Zemel MB. Role of dietary calcium and dairy products in modulating adiposity. Lipids 2003; 38: 139–146.

11. Berkey CS, Rockett HR, Willett WC, Colditz GA. Milk, dairy fat, dietary calcium, and weight gain: a longitudinal study of adolescents. Arch Pediatr Adolesc Med 2005; 159: 543–550.

12. Noel SE, Ness AR, Northstone K, Emmett P, Newby PK. Milk intakes are not associated with percent body fat in children from ages 10 to 13 years. J Nutr 2011; 141: 2035–2041.

13. Eaton DK, Kann L, Kinchen S, et al. Youth risk behavior surveillance—United States, 2009. MMWR Surveill Summ 2010; 59: 1–142.

14. Pate RR, Mitchell JA, Byun W, Dowda M. Sedentary behaviour in youth. Br J Sports Med 2011; 45: 906–913.

15. World Health Organization. Global Recommendations on Physical Activity for Health. World Health Organization: Geneva, 2010.

16. Ottevaere C, Huybrechts I, Beghin L, et al. Relationship between self-reported dietary intake and physical activity levels among adolescents: the HELENA study. Int J Behav Nutr Phys Act 2011; 8: 8.

17. Dougkas A, Reynolds CK, Givens ID, Elwood PC, Minihane AM. Associations between dairy consumption and body weight: a review of the evidence and underlying mechanisms. Nutr Res Rev 2011; 15: 1–24.

18. Cole TJ, Bellizzi MC, Flegal KM, Dietz WH. Establishing a standard definition for child overweight and obesity worldwide: international survey. BMJ 2000; 320: 1240–1243.

19. Cole TJ, Flegal KM, Nicholls D, Jackson AA. Body mass index cut offs to define thinness in children and adolescents: international survey. BMJ 2007; 335: 194.

20. Sardinha LB, Santos R, Vale S, et al. Waist circumference percentiles for Portuguese children and adolescents aged 10 to 18 years. Eur J Pediatr 2011; 171: 499–505.

21. Zimmet P, Alberti KG, Kaufman F, et al. The metabolic syndrome in children and adolescents - an IDF consensus report. Pediatr Diabetes 2007; 8: 299–306.

22. Tanner JM, Whitehouse RH. Clinical longitudinal standards for height, weight, height velocity, weight velocity, and stages of puberty. Arch Dis Child 1976; 51: 170–179.

23. World Health Organization. Guidelines for Controlling and Monitoring the Tobacco Epidemic. WHO: Geneva, 1998.

24. Ramos E. Health Determinants in Porto Adolescents—The Epiteen Cohort. University of Porto: Porto, 2006.

25. Willett W. Food Frequency Methods Nutritional Epidemiology, 2nd edn. Oxford University Press: New York, 1998, 74–100.

26. Silva D, Rego C, Guerra A. Characterization of food habits and comparative study between two methods of food assessment in adolescents. Rev Aliment Humana 2004; 10: 33–40.

27. Rodrigues SS, Franchini B, Graca P, de Almeida MD. A new food guide for the Portuguese population: development and technical considerations. J Nutr Educ Behav 2006; 38: 189–195.

28. Telama R, Yang X, Laakso L, Viikari J. Physical activity in childhood and adolescence as predictor of physical activity in young adulthood. Am J Prev Med 1997; 13: 317–323.

29. Mota J, Esculcas C. Leisure-time physical activity behavior: structured and unstructured choices according to sex, age, and level of physical activity. Int J Behav Med 2002; 9: 111–121.

30. Raitakari OT, Porkka KV, Taimela S, Telama R, Rasanen L, Viikari JS. Effects of persistent physical activity and inactivity on coronary risk factors in children and young adults. The Cardiovascular Risk in Young Finns Study. Am J Epidemiol 1994; 140: 195–205.

31. Goldberg GR, Black AE, Jebb SA, et al. Critical evaluation of energy intake data using fundamental principles of energy physiology: 1. Derivation of cut-off limits to identify under-recording. Eur J Clin Nutr 1991; 45: 569–581.

32. Black AE. Critical evaluation of energy intake using the Goldberg cut-off for energy intake:basal metabolic rate. A practical guide to its calculation, use and limitations. Int J Obes Relat Metab Disord 2000; 24: 1119–1130.

33. Novotny R, Daida YG, Acharya S, Grove JS, Vogt TM. Dairy intake is associated with lower body fat and soda intake with greater weight in adolescent girls. J Nutr 2004; 134: 1905–1909.

34. Spence LA, Cifelli CJ, Miller GD. The role of dairy products in healthy weight and body composition in children and adolescents. Curr Nutr Food Sci. 2011; 7: 40–49.

35. Hirschler V, Oestreicher K, Beccaria M, Hidalgo M, Maccallini G. Inverse association between insulin resistance and frequency of milk consumption in low-income Argentinean school children. J Pediatr 2009; 154: 101–105.

36. Bradlee ML, Singer MR, Qureshi MM, Moore LL. Food group intake and central obesity among children and adolescents in the Third National Health and Nutrition Examination Survey (NHANES III). Public Health Nutr 2010; 13: 797–805.

37. Abreu S, Santos R, Moreira C, et al. Association between dairy product intake and abdominal obesity in Azorean adolescents. Eur J Clin Nutr 2012; 66. 830–835.

38. Kelishadi R, Zemel MB, Hashemipour M, Hosseini M, Mohammadifard N, Poursafa P. Can a dairy-rich diet be effective in long-term weight control of young children? J Am Coll Nutr 2009; 28: 601–610.

39. Marshall TA, Eichenberger Gilmore JM, Broffitt B, Stumbo PJ, Levy SM. Diet quality in young children is influenced by beverage consumption. J Am Coll Nutr 2005; 24: 65–75.

40. U.S. Department of Agriculture, U.S. Department of Health and Human Services. Dietary Guidelines for Americans, 2010. US Government Printing Office: Washington, DC, 2010.

41. Samaras K, Campbell LV. The non-genetic determinants of central adiposity. Int J Obes Relat Metab Disord 1997; 21: 839–845.

42. Klein-Platat C, Oujaa M, Wagner A, et al. Physical activity is inversely related to waist circumference in 12-y-old French adolescents. Int J Obes (Lond) 2005; 29: 9–14.

43. Ortega FB, Ruiz JR, Sjostrom M. Physical activity, overweight and central adiposity in Swedish children and adolescents: the European Youth Heart Study. Int J Behav Nutr Phys Act 2007; 4: 61.

44. Cavadini C, Decarli B, Grin J, Narring F, Michaud PA. Food habits and sport activity during adolescence: differences between athletic and non-athletic teenagers in Switzerland. Eur J Clin Nutr 2000; 54(Suppl 1):S16–S20.

45. Morris KL, Zemel MB. 1,25-dihydroxyvitamin D3 modulation of adipocyte glucocorticoid function. Obes Res 2005; 13: 670–677.

46. Masuzaki H, Paterson J, Shinyama H, et al. A transgenic model of visceral obesity and the metabolic syndrome. Science 2001; 294: 2166–2170.

47. Must A, Tybor DJ. Physical activity and sedentary behavior: a review of longitudinal studies of weight and adiposity in youth. Int J Obes (Lond) 2005; 29(Suppl. 2): S84–S96.

48. Black RE, Williams SM, Jones IE, Goulding A. Children who avoid drinking cow milk have low dietary calcium intakes and poor bone health. Am J Clin Nutr 2002; 76: 675–680.

49. Stallings VA, Oddleifson NW, Negrini BY, Zemel BS, Wellens R. Bone mineral content and dietary calcium intake in children prescribed a low-lactose diet. J Pediatr Gastroenterol Nutr 1994; 18: 440–445.

50. Vicente-Rodriguez G. How does exercise affect bone development during growth? Sports Med 2006; 36: 561–569.

51. Gracia-Marco L, Moreno LA, Ortega FB, et al. Levels of physical activity that predict optimal bone mass in adolescents: the HELENA study. Am J Prev Med 2011; 40: 599–607.

52. Lappe JM, Rafferty KA, Davies KM, Lypaczewski G. Girls on a high-calcium diet gain weight at the same rate as girls on a normal diet: a pilot study. J Am Diet Assoc 2004; 104: 1361–1367.

53. Zemel MB, Donnelly JE, Smith BK, et al. Effects of dairy intake on weight maintenance. Nutr Metab (Lond) 2008; 5: 28.

54. de Koning L, Merchant AT, Pogue J, Anand SS. Waist circumference and waist-to-hip ratio as predictors of cardiovascular events: meta-regression analysis of prospective studies. Eur Heart J 2007; 28: 850–856.

CHAPTER 6

THE EFFECT OF "SLEEP HIGH AND TRAIN LOW" ON WEIGHT LOSS IN OVERWEIGHT CHINESE ADOLESCENTS: STUDY PROTOCOL FOR A RANDOMIZED CONTROLLED TRIAL

RU WANG, DONGMEI LIU, XUEQIANG WANG, WEIHUA XIAO, NANA WU, BINGHONG GAO, AND PEIJIE CHEN

6.1 BACKGROUND

Obesity is a global pandemic and its prevalence among children and adolescents has also increased worldwide, becoming a serious public health problem [1]. In China, nearly 215 million people are overweight or obese, and 12% of these are children (<17-years-old), as estimated by the 2002 China National Nutrition and Health Survey [2]. Obesity in childhood has been associated with an increased risk of diabetes, hypertension, cardiovascular disease and various cancers in adulthood [3,4]. Therefore, preventing and treating obesity in children and adolescents is crucial.

The causes of childhood obesity are complex and multifaceted involving genetic factors, environmental, and behavioral factors. The current world-wide epidemic of obesity is believed to be attributable to the modern living environment which promotes a sedentary lifestyle and excessive consumption of calorie-dense food. Accordingly, a lifestyle modification including a healthy diet and increased physical activity has been recommended as the cornerstone of prevention and treatment of obesity. Physical activity increases energy expenditure and, in combination with a healthy diet, is effective in inducing weight loss. However, the reduced weight achieved through weight loss programs is hard to maintain over the longterm. The failure to achieve longterm weight loss is believed to be caused by compensatory changes in appetite and energy expenditure elicited by exercise and dieting. Currently, a complete understanding of the relationship between exercise, appetite regulation, and weight management is lacking.

Recent research has revealed that appetite-regulating hormones might play an important role in moderating the interrelationship between exercise and dieting, appetite, and weight regain. Among various potential appetite-regulating hormones, the gastrointestinal hormones, ghrelin, peptide YY (PYY), cholecystokinin (CCK) and glucagon-like peptide-1 (GLP-1) are well studied. Ghrelin is the only hormone that has been shown to be orexigenic, while PYY, CCK, and GLP-1 are satiety regulatory hormones [5,6]. These hormones are episodic hormonal signals occurring in unison with episodes of eating. They signal satiation and satiety either via the vagus nerve (which connects the gut to the brain) or via blood perfusing the hypothalamus.

It is accepted that in response to weight loss, counter-regulatory adaptations develop in the appetite regulatory system, including the gastrointestinal hormones, defending impositions that promote a negative energy balance. Different weight loss intervention approaches are likely to cause different counter-regulatory adaptations in terms of the content and the magnitude of the response. There is some evidence suggesting that diet-induced weight loss is associated with a compensatory increase in total ghrelin (GT) plasma levels and a blunted postprandial release of PYY and GLP-1 [7,8]. Exercise-induced weight loss may increase the drive to eat, as shown by increased levels of acylated ghrelin (AG) and subjective feelings of hunger in fasting, but it may also improve satiety as evidenced by an increase in the late postprandial release of GLP-1 after exercise training [9].

Few studies have investigated the combined effect of exercise and dieting on appetite in children and adolescents. Based on the limited data, it appears that ghrelin levels increase after a weight reduction program, with no change in PYY levels [10-13]. Similarly, we have observed an increase in ghrelin concentrations after weight loss in adolescents who participated in an exercise and diet intervention for four weeks in a summer camp program in a previous study (unpublished data).

Recently, the effect of high altitude on appetite regulation has attracted researchers' interest. It is a widely observed phenomenon that a high altitude can induce loss of appetite [14-16]. In many studies, loss of appetite and the resulting decrease in energy intake have been attributed to acute mountain sickness (AMS), symptoms of which include headache and anorexia. However, loss of appetite cannot merely be a by-product of AMS because anorexia and weight loss still persist when symptoms of AMS have subsided [17]. Furthermore, studies conducted in normobaric hypoxia chambers, where other environmental stressors associated with high altitude are eliminated (extreme cold and physical exertion), have demonstrated that hypoxia per se can cause reduced appetite and energy intake, and loss of body weight [18]. It has been suggested that the effect of hypoxia on appetite is mediated by the changes in gastrointestinal hormones [19-22].

It is perceivable that to promote success in longterm weight loss, hypoxia can be implemented in a traditional diet and exercise weight loss program, because the negative effect of hypoxia on appetite might be able to balance the positive effect of diet and exercise. Exercise and hypoxia have been used in combination in sports to induce maximal increase in aerobic endurance in athletes, but have rarely been used in weight loss, especially in children and adolescents. We have run several sessions of weight loss summer camps designed for obese adolescents in Shanghai, China. The effect of exercise and hypoxia on weight loss has been explored in our preliminary studies and interesting results have been generated [23,24]. As such, we are now designing a randomly controlled trial to systematically investigate the longterm weight loss effect of exercise with hypoxia in obese adolescents and determine the mediating effect of the gastrointestinal hormones. We hypothesize that: 1) exercise and hypoxia will have an additive effect on weight loss via increasing energy expenditure and suppressing appetite; 2) hypoxia use will lead to less rebound of weight loss after intervention due to its potential negating effects on compensatory changes in appetite elicited by exercise and diet in a traditional weight loss program; and 3) changes in gastrointestinal hormones (including ghrelin, PYY, CCK, and GLP-1), as well as in cytokine interleukin (IL)-6, will be associated with changes in body weight after the intervention and during follow-up.

6.1.1 AIMS

The aims of this randomized controlled trial (RCT) are to evaluate the effectiveness of intermittent hypoxia and exercise, in combination with a balanced diet, on inducing short- and long-term fat loss in Chinese children and adolescents, and to determine the molecular mechanisms behind the benefits of hypoxia in enhancing weight loss.

6.2 METHODS/DESIGN

6.2.1 DESIGN

This study is a randomized controlled clinical trial with two parallel arms involving 40 obese adolescents. To assess the effectiveness of four weeks of intermittent hypoxia added to a traditional exercise and diet intervention on inducing short (after the four-week intervention) and longterm (at two months follow-up) weight loss in obese adolescents, we will recruit 20 adolescent boys and 20 adolescent girls (aged 11 to 15 years) from our summer weight loss camp. They will be stratified according to gender and randomly assigned to two groups: the control group who will exercise, eat a balanced diet, and sleep in a normobaric condition, and the hypoxia group, who will exercise, eat a balanced diet, and sleep in normobaric hypoxia chambers ('sleep high and train low'). Outcome assessment and data analysis will be performed by trained professionals who will be blinded to the group assignment of subjects. The flow of participants through the trial is shown in Figure 1.

6.2.2 SAMPLE SIZE ESTIMATION

Sample size estimation in this RCT is based on the expected fat loss following four weeks of hypoxia exposure plus exercise and dieting. The data of our preliminary experiment showed that the means of fat percentage decrease in the normoxia and hypoxia groups were 3.1 and 6.0% respectively, and the standard deviation of the change was about 3%. It is estimated that a sample size of 17 participants per group will be required to observe a similar result with a power of 80%. Considering a 15% dropout and exit rate, we will recruit 40 subjects with 20 in each group.

6.2.3 ETHICAL APPROVAL AND CONSENT

The study will be conducted according to the principles expressed in the Declaration of Helsinki. The study protocol has been approved by the institutional review board at the Shanghai University of Sport (reference number: 2014 Ethics Approval Note 1). Participants in this study are volunteers. None of the measurements or the intervention are known to entail any significant health risk. The study has its own physician to ensure the eligibility and safety of all participants. All data will be handled and archived confidentially. The benefits and associated risks of the study will be carefully explained and the voluntary nature of participation will be emphasized. Informed consent and assent will be obtained from all participants and their parents or legal guardians. Participants and their parents or legal guardianswill have the option to end the participation at any stage if they so wish. If the physician and the principal investigator believe that there are risks of serious adverse events in the study the trial will be stopped. The trial is registered with Chinese Clinical Trial Registry as ChiCTR-TRC-14004106.

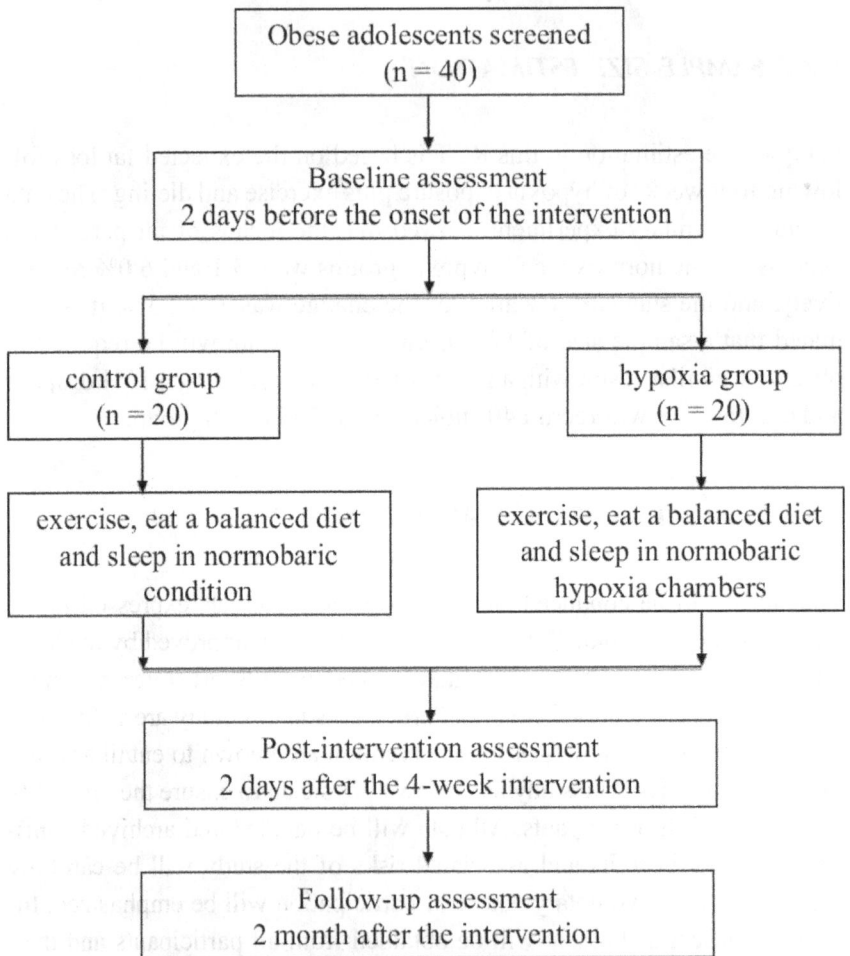

FIGURE 1: Flow of participants through the trial.

6.2.4 SUBJECT RECRUITMENT

Obese adolescents aged 11 to 15 years will be recruited from the children registered for the 2014 summer weight loss camp at the Shanghai University of Sport. A public health nurse will assess the Tanner stage of each subject using the Tanner grading system [25,26]. Obesity will be defined based on body-mass index (BMI), calculated as weight in kilograms divided by height in meters squared (kg/m^2). Although a BMI of ≥ 25 kg/m^2 and ≥ 30 kg/m^2 are international cutoff points for overweight and obesity, for many Asian populations individuals with a BMI of ≥ 23 kg/m^2 are considered to be at increased risk and those with a BMI of ≥ 27.5 kg/m^2 at high risk [27]. Thus, we chose a BMI of ≥ 25 kg/m^2 as the criterion to recruit obese adolescents. Adolescents will be excluded if they have concomitant renal, hepatic, or cardiac disease, and/or are being treated with drugs that could affect body weight and appetite (such as orlistat, lorcaserin, and phentermine-topiramate, as well as appetite suppressants).

6.2.5 RANDOMIZATION AND BLINDING

After a participant is confirmed to be eligible and written informed consent has been obtained, she/he will be randomly assigned to the hypoxia or normoxia group. The randomization procedure, stratified according to gender, will be conducted by an independent statistician using a computerized randomization program. In order to minimize the potential bias, the exercise physiologist and the dietitian who manage the exercise training and the diet intervention will be blinded as to whether a subject will sleep in the hypoxia chamber or not. The hypoxia chamber will be prepared by an independent researcher. The researcher performing outcome assessments will be blinded to the subjects' intervention allocation.

6.2.6 INTERVENTION

All the subjects, including both the normoxia (control) and the hypoxia groups, will undergo four weeks of aerobic exercise training and dieting (eating a balanced diet). In addition, the normoxia group will sleep in normal conditions while the hypoxia group will sleep in a normobaric hypoxic chamber every night. All the measurements will be conducted two days prior to, and post-intervention, and repeated two months later after the intervention (two months follow-up). Fasting blood samples will be collected in the morning of the testing day. In order to maximize the compliance and avoid the occurrence of any accident the intervention will be closely supervised by a physician, a dietitian, and an exercise physiologist.

6.2.7 EXERCISE TRAINING

The same aerobic exercise training will be applied to both the normoxia and the hypoxia groups. Participants will exercise for six days per week, twice daily, for one hour per session. The intensity of the exercise will be estimated using the Metabolic Equivalent of Task (MET) score. MET, the unit of energy expenditure, will be obtained by dividing oxygen uptake values (ml $\cdot$ kg^{-1} $\cdot$ min^{-1}) by 3.5 (1 MET is defined as resting metabolic rate that is 3.5 ml $\cdot$ kg^{-1} $\cdot$ min^{-1}). VO$_2$ will be measured using Cosmed K4b2 Portable Metabolic Measurement System (Cosmed, S.r.l., Rome, Italy) according to the manufacturer's instructions. To promote participants' interest, the exercise training will consist of three different activities including swimming (intensity: 6 MET), aerobic exercise (intensity: 7.5 MET), and basketball (intensity: 6 MET).

6.2.8 DIET MODIFICATION

All participants will receive well-defined and balanced daily meals during the four-week intervention. Dietary recommendations will be individualized based on the individual's basal metabolic rate and will range from 1,600 to 2,000 kcal/day. The basal metabolic rate will be calculated using the Mifflin equation [28]. The caloric intake will be calculated based on the Chinese food chart. Each day, three well-balanced meals will be provided with the following calorie allocations: breakfast 35%, lunch 40%, and dinner 25%. Each meal comprises 30% protein, 20% fat, and 50%

carbohydrate by energy. Animal and vegetable oil and starch-rich food will be minimized, while the intake of vegetables, fruits, bean products, rabbit meat, beef, pork, and cellulose will be increased. This prescribed diet includes pivotal nutrients such as vitamins, minerals, essential amino acids, fiber, and polyunsaturated fatty acids.

6.2.9 HYPOXIA EXPOSURE

To test the hypothesis that hypoxia exposure would ameliorate the compensatory increase in appetite elicited by exercise and diet, the experimental group (hypoxia group) will sleep in a normobaric hypoxia environmental chamber every night during the four- week intervention. The advantage of using an environmental chamber compared to real altitude situations is that the effects of hypoxia can be isolated from the influence of other confounding factors present in a real altitude situation, such as the influence of temperature, humidity, and physical activity levels. The normobaric hypoxia will be designed to mimic an altitude of 2700 m. We will use the large hypoxic training system (Low Oxygen System, Dubai, Germany)) of the hypoxia test laboratory of Shanghai Oriental Oasis Training Base to simulate a hypoxic environment (14.7% O_2; approximately 2700 m). After a one-day hypoxia acclimation period, participants of the hypoxia group will sleep in the hypoxia training laboratory for 10 hours every night (from 21:00 to approximately 7:00 the next day), seven times per week, for four weeks.

6.2.10 ATTRITION AND COMPLIANCE

Due to the voluntary nature of the enrollment of the summer weight loss camp, attrition rates will be very low. In a pilot trial involving 50 overweight male Chinese adolescents, 47 children completed a four-week diet and exercise intervention, and only three children (6%) dropped out of the study due to loss of interest. Considering the addition of a two-month follow-up, we expect a higher attrition rate (15%) in this study. Our recruitment plan was made based on this consideration.

6.2.11 OUTCOME ASSESSMENTS

Baseline assessments will be conducted two days before the onset of the four-week intervention. Post-intervention and two month follow-up assessments will be conducted two days and two months after completion of the intervention, respectively. The primary outcome of the study will be body composition and the secondary outcome measures will include appetite score and blood levels of gastrointestinal hormones including leptin, ghrelin, PYY, CCK and GLP-1, as well as circulating levels of IL-6. All the assessments will be performed in the laboratory of exercise physiology at the Shanghai University of Sport.

6.2.12 PRIMARY OUTCOME

6.2.12.1 BODY COMPOSITION

Body mass and height will be measured using a digital scale (Yaohua Weighing System Co., Shanghai, China) and a wall-mounted stadiometer (TANITA, Tokyo, Japan), respectively. Body composition and fat distribution will be measured using dual energy X-ray absorptiometry (DXA) (GE Lunar Prodigy, Madison, Wisconsin, United States)). The software (ENCORE, version 10.50.086, GE, Madison, Wisconsin, United States)) will be used to analyze total lean mass (TLM), total fat mass (TFM), total body fat percentage (%TBF), android fat percentage (%AF), and gynoid fat percentage (%GF).

6.2.13 SECONDARY OUTCOMES

6.2.13.1 CARDIORESPIRATORY FITNESS

Peak oxygen consumption (VO_{2peak}) for all participants will be measured using the Cosmed (K4b2) portable metabolic system. Expired respiratory gases will be collected on a breath-by-breath basis during a submaximal treadmill (H/P/Cosmos Pulsar 4.0, Cosmos Sports & Medical Ltd., Nussdorf- Traunstein, Germany) test. Exercise will start at a speed of 2 km/h, which will be increased every 2.5 minutes by 1 km/h until 8 km/h is reached. The criterion of exercise termination will be 80% of the maximum heart rate (HR_{max}). Trained research assistants will record heart rate and power output data at the end of each stage. Heart rate will be measured using a polar heart rate monitor (Polar Electro, Kempele, Finland).

6.2.14 BLOOD ANALYSES

Fasting blood samples (2 mL, 12-hour fasting) will be obtained at baseline, post-intervention, and at two months follow-up. Serum levels of gastrointestinal hormones including leptin, ghrelin, PYY, CCK and GLP-1, as well as cytokine IL-6, will be measured using commercially available ELISA kits (R&D Systems, Minneapolis, Minnesota, United States). As reported, the lower limit of sensitivity of the assays will range between 0.8 pg/mL and 10 pg/ml. The intra-assay coefficient of variation (CV) will be less than 5% and the inter-assay CV will be less than 10%. Absorbance will be read at 450 nm wavelength using a microplate reader (Bio-Rad 550, Bio-Rad, Hercules, California, United States).

6.2.15 APPETITE ASSESSMENT

Children's appetite at baseline, during, and post-intervention, and during follow-up will be assessed via a simple eight-item appetite questionnaire (Additional file 1). The questionnaire was developed by modifying the eight-item Council on Nutrition Appetite Questionnaire (CNAQ). The CNAQ is a short, simple, appetite assessment tool, which has been validated and proved to be able to predict weight loss in community-dwelling adults and nursing home residents [29]. We modified the CNAQ to reflect the nature of our intervention.

6.2.16 DATA MANAGEMENT AND STATISTICAL ANALYSIS

Data generated in the study will be collected and summarized using mean (standard deviation) values. Group differences in demographical and clinical characteristics at baseline will be tested using a two-sample t-test for quantitative data and chi-square test for qualitative data. Repeated measures analysis of variance (RM ANOVA) will be used to analyze the main effect of treatment and potential time-by-treatment interactions. For these analyses, parametric assumptions of the normality and homoscedasticity will be checked using standard tests and graphical methods. If those assumptions are violated, data transformation and non-parametric procedures will be considered sequentially. Multivariate regression analysis will be performed to analyze the relationship between changes in body composition, appetite score, and gastrointestinal hormones following intervention and during follow-up. Multiple models will be developed and tested for different sets of outcome measures and regressor variables. All statistical analyses will be performed using the Statistical Package for the Social Sciences (SPSS, Inc., Chicago, Illinois, United States) for Windows version 18.0, and a significance level of 0.05 will be used.

6.3 DISCUSSION

To the best of our knowledge, our study will be the first to evaluate the effectiveness of 'sleep high and train low' on short- and long-term weight loss among obese adolescents. The study will focus on obese adolescents due to the rising prevalence of obese children in China and the adverse impact of childhood obesity on adult health. Adolescent obesity has been attributed mainly to a sedentary lifestyle and an unhealthy diet. In China, a great effort has been made to use exercise and dietary intervention to treat obesity and metabolic disorders in children. However, the weight rebound following most of the weight loss programs has made such an effort fruitless. The weight rebound is believed to be caused by the compensatory increase in appetite induced by exercise and diet. Conceivably, the agent that can counteract this compensatory effect will benefit obese patients in achieving longterm weight loss. Hypoxia is potentially one of such agents:

the anorexia effect of hypoxia has been widely observed and might be utilized to dampen the appetite compensatory effect of exercise and diet, thereby promoting the success of weight loss in the longterm. Due to the profound benefits of exercise training and diet in the obese population, we do not expect to use hypoxia as a replacement, but rather as a supplement to exercise and diet intervention. Therefore, children in the control group will undergo the same exercise training and diet as the hypoxic group in order to evaluate the value of hypoxia in promoting weight loss, and minimizing weight rebound after intervention.

Instead of using continuous hypoxic exposure such as high altitude, we choose to use intermittent hypoxic exposure, which has been recommended as an option for the free-living obese population [30]. The effect of intermittent hypoxia exposure on weight reduction has been reported previously. In a model of diet-induced obese mice, it has been shown that intermittent hypoxic exposure induced decreases in body mass, blood glucose levels, and cholesterol erythropoietin concentrations [27,31]. In a few human studies, the synergistic effect of exercise and hypoxia in treating obesity and associated metabolic disorders has been demonstrated, where low intensity exercise training at normobaric hypoxic condition (15% O2) led to more weight loss and greater improvement in metabolic health compared to training at ambient conditions (21% O_2) [32-34]. However, further evidence-based studies are needed to carefully evaluate the therapeutic value of hypoxia and the model of utilization in treating obesity, especially in children. Intermittent hypoxia exposure, as used in the 'sleep high and train low' paradigm has been proposed for endurance athletes to maximally enhance their endurance exercise capabilities, however the clinical use of intermittent hypoxia in the management of cardiometabolic diseases has rarely been tested. Our study will be the first to evaluate the effect of 'sleep high and train low' on weight loss in obese adolescents. Through monitoring a wide spectrum of health indices including blood pressure, heart rate, vital capacity, blood glucose and insulin levels, blood lipid profile, and immune function we will careful monitor any possible side effects associated with hypoxia exposure.

Furthermore, we will investigate the mechanism for the effect of hypoxia on weight management. We will focus on the regulatory effect of 'sleep high and train low' on gastrointestinal hormones levels. In addition, we hypothesize that the cytokine IL-6 might also play a role in mediating the appetite regulatory effect of exercise (positive effect) and hypoxia (negative effect). The clarification of mechanisms leading to weight loss in 'sleep high and train low' might provide information for the development of new strategies in combating obesity in the future.

6.3.1 TRIAL STATUS

A pilot study involving a small group of overweight children has been completed based on the summer weight loss camp at our institution in 2013. The intervention modality has proven to be tolerated very well among children and has been effective in inducing significant weight loss. For the official trial, participant recruitment will start in April 2014. Baseline measurements will be taken in June 2014, and the four-week intervention will be completed by August 2014, which will be followed by a two month follow-up. Feedback on the preliminary results of participants' health status will be provided to the participants upon completion of the study.

REFERENCES

1. Wang Y, Lobstein T: Worldwide trends in childhood overweight and obesity. Int J Pediatr Obes 2006, 1:11-25.
2. Wu YF, Ma GS, Hu YH, Li YP, Li X, Cui ZH, Chen CM, Kong LZ: The current prevalence status of body overweight and obesity in China: data from the China national nutrition and health survey. Zhonghua Yu Fang Yi Xue Za Zhi 2005, 39:316-320.
3. Cruz ML, Goran MI: The metabolic syndrome in children and adolescents. Curr Diab Rep 2004, 4:53-62.
4. Dietz WH: Health consequences of obesity in youth: childhood predictors of adult disease. Pediatrics 1998, 101:518-525.
5. King PJ: The hypothalamus and obesity. Curr Drug Targets 2005, 6:225-240.
6. Wynne K, Stanley S, Bloom S: The gut and regulation of body weight. J Clin Endocrinol Metab 2004, 89:2576-2582.
7. Doucet E, Cameron J: Appetite control after weight loss: what is the role of blood-borne peptides? Appl Physiol Nutr Metab 2007, 32:523-532.
8. Adam TC, Jocken J, Westerterp-Plantenga MS: Decreased glucagon-like peptide 1 release after weight loss in overweight/obese subjects. Obes Res 2005, 13:710-716.

9. Martins C, Kulseng B, King NA, Holst JJ, Blundell JE: The effects of exercise-induced weight loss on appetite-related peptides and motivation to eat. J Clin Endocrinol Metab 2010, 95:1609-1616.

10. Pedrosa C, Oliveira BM, Albuquerque I, Simoes-Pereira C, Vaz-de-Almeida MD, Correia F: Metabolic syndrome, adipokines and ghrelin in overweight and obese schoolchildren: results of a 1-year lifestyle intervention programme. Eur J Pediatr 2011, 170:483-492.

11. Zou CC, Liang L, Wang CL, Fu JF, Zhao ZY: The change in ghrelin and obestatin levels in obese children after weight reduction. Acta Paediatr 2009, 98:159-165.

12. Krohn K, Boczan C, Otto B, Heldwein W, Landgraf R, Bauer CP, Koletzko B: Regulation of ghrelin is related to estimated insulin sensitivity in obese children. Int J Obes (Lond) 2006, 30:1482-1487.

13. Gueugnon C, Mougin F, Nguyen NU, Bouhaddi M, Nicolet-Guenat M, Dumoulin G: Ghrelin and PYY levels in adolescents with severe obesity: effects of weight loss induced by long-term exercise training and modified food habits. Eur J Appl Physiol 2012, 112:1797-1805.

14. Pugh LG: Physiological and medical aspects of the Himalayan scientific and mountaineering expedition, 1960–61. 1962. Wilderness Environ Med 2002, 13:57.

15. Westerterp-Plantenga MS, Westerterp KR, Rubbens M, Verwegen CR, Richelet JP, Gardette B: Appetite at "high altitude" [operation Everest III (Comex-'97)]: a simulated ascent of Mount Everest. J Appl Physiol (1985) 1999, 87:391-399.

16. Kalson NS, Hext F, Davies AJ, Chan CWM, Wright AD, Imray CHE, Expeditionary BMR: Do changes in gastro-intestinal blood flow explain high-altitude anorexia? Eur J Clin Invest 2010, 40:735-741.

17. Tschop M, Morrison KM: Weight loss at high altitude. Adv Exp Med Biol 2001, 502:237-247.

18. Rose MS, Houston CS, Fulco CS, Coates G, Sutton JR, Cymerman A: Operation Everest. II: nutrition and body composition. J Appl Physiol (1985) 1988, 65:2545-2551.

19. Shukla V, Singh SN, Vats P, Singh VK, Singh SB, Banerjee PK: Ghrelin and leptin levels of sojourners and acclimatized lowlanders at high altitude. Nutr Neurosci 2005, 8:161-165.

20. Tschop M, Strasburger CJ, Topfer M, Hautmann H, Riepl R, Fischer R, Hartmann G, Morrison K, Appenzeller M, Hildebrandt W, Biollaz J, Bärtsch P: Influence of hypobaric hypoxia on leptin levels in men. Int J Obes Relat Metab Disord 2000, 24(Suppl 2):S151.

21. Singh SN, Vats P, Shyam R, Suri S, Kumria MM, Ranganathan S, Sridharan K, Selvamurthy W: Role of neuropeptide Y and galanin in high altitude induced anorexia in rats. Nutr Neurosci 2001, 4:323-331.

22. Bailey DM: Acute mountain sickness: the "poison of the pass". West J Med 2000, 172:399-400.

23. Wang R, Chen PJ, Chen WH: Effect of diet and exercise-induced weight reduction on complement regulatory proteins Cd55 and Cd59 levels in overweight Chinese adolescents. J Exerc Sci Fit 2011, 9:46-51.

24. Wang R, Chen PJ, Chen WH: Diet and exercise improve neutrophil to lymphocyte ratio in overweight adolescents. Int J Sports Med 2011, 32:982-986.

25. Marshall WA, Tanner JM: Variations in the pattern of pubertal changes in boys. Arch Dis Child 1970, 45:13-23.
26. Marshall WA, Tanner JM: Variations in pattern of pubertal changes in girls. Arch Dis Child 1969, 44:291-303.
27. Ling Q, Sailan W, Ran J, Zhi S, Cen L, Yang X, Xiaoqun Q: The effect of intermittent hypoxia on bodyweight, serum glucose and cholesterol in obesity mice. Pak J Biol Sci 2008, 11:869-875.
28. Mifflin MD, St Jeor ST, Hill LA, Scott BJ, Daugherty SA, Koh YO: A new predictive equation for resting energy expenditure in healthy individuals. Am J Clin Nutr 1990, 51:241-247.
29. Wilson MM, Thomas DR, Rubenstein LZ, Chibnall JT, Anderson S, Baxi A, Diebold MR, Morley JE: Appetite assessment: simple appetite questionnaire predicts weight loss in community-dwelling adults and nursing home residents. Am J Clin Nutr 2005, 82:1074-1081.
30. Urdampilleta A, Gonzalez-Muniesa P, Portillo MP, Martinez JA: Usefulness of combining intermittent hypoxia and physical exercise in the treatment of obesity. J Physiol Biochem 2012, 68:289-304.
31. Qin L, Xiang Y, Song Z, Jing R, Hu CP, Howard ST: Erythropoietin as a possible mechanism for the effects of intermittent hypoxia on bodyweight, serum glucose and leptin in mice. Regul Pept 2010, 165:168-173.
32. Netzer NC, Chytra R, Kupper T: Low intense physical exercise in normobaric hypoxia leads to more weight loss in obese people than low intense physical exercise in normobaric sham hypoxia. Sleep Breath 2008, 12:129-134.
33. Wiesner S, Haufe S, Engeli S, Mutschler H, Haas U, Luft FC, Jordan J: Influences of normobaric hypoxia training on physical fitness and metabolic risk markers in overweight to obese subjects. Obesity (Silver Spring) 2010, 18:116-120.
34. Haufe S, Wiesner S, Engeli S, Luft FC, Jordan J: Influences of normobaric hypoxia training on metabolic risk markers in human subjects. Med Sci Sports Exerc 2008, 40:1939-1944.

CHAPTER 7

WAIST-TO-HEIGHT RATIO AND CARDIOMETABOLIC RISK FACTORS IN ADOLESCENCE: FINDINGS FROM A PROSPECTIVE BIRTH COHORT

L. GRAVES, S. P. GARNETT, C. T. COWELL, L. A. BAUR, A. NESS, N. SATTAR, AND A. LAWLOR

7.1 INTRODUCTION

Obesity in childhood is associated with adverse levels of cardiometabolic risk factors, including higher blood pressure (BP), triglycerides, total and low density lipoprotein cholesterol (LDLc) and insulin, and lower high density lipoprotein cholesterol (HDLc) [1-3]. Furthermore, childhood obesity is positively and linearly associated with obesity and related cardiovascular disease in adulthood [4]. It is important to identify children who are at increased risk of developing comorbidities associated with obesity, to potentially intervene and prevent the development of chronic disease including type 2 diabetes.

Waist-to-Height Ratio and Cardiometabolic Risk Factors in Adolescence: Findings from a Prospective Birth Cohort. © Graves L, Garnett SP, Cowell CT, Baur LA, Ness A, Sattar N, and Lawlor DA. Pediatric Obesity (2013), DOI: 10.1111/j.2047-6310.2013.00192.x. Licensed under Creative Commons Attribution 3.0 Unported License, http://creativecommons.org/licenses/by/3.0/.

We have previously reported, using data from the Avon Longitudinal Study of Parents and Children (ALSPAC), that childhood body mass index (BMI), waist circumference and total fat mass are positively associated with cardiovascular risk factors in adolescence and the magnitudes of these associations are similar for all measures of adiposity [2]. There has been recent interest in the use of the waist-to-height ratio (WHtR) for identifying excessive central adiposity in children and adolescents [5-8]. It has been suggested that a WHtR ≥ 0.5, irrespective of age, sex or ethnicity [5, 7, 9], is a valid predictor of higher cardiometabolic risk [10-12]. WHtR may be a more straightforward anthropometric index to apply in the clinical setting where BMI centile charts may not be readily available.

There have been two systematic reviews in adults examining the associations between BMI and WHtR and cardiometabolic outcomes which have indicated broadly similar associations between the different anthropometric measures and cardiometabolic risk factors [7, 13]. However, the utility of WHtR in identifying young people at cardiometabolic risk is unclear. Results from cross-sectional studies are conflicting some indicate that WHtR is more strongly associated with cardiometabolic risk factors than BMI [10, 12, 14-16], while others have found either a weaker [17] or a similar [18, 19] association. To our knowledge, there is only one prospective study looking at this issue in children and adolescents. That study reported similar correlation between BMI and WHtR assessed in children when they were aged 7 to 15 years and the metabolic syndrome in young adulthood [20].

Therefore the aims of this study were to:

1. Examine the cross-sectional association between WHtR and cardiometabolic risk factors in adolescents.
2. Examine the prospective association between WHtR assessed in childhood and cardiometabolic risk factors assessed in adolescence.
3. Examine these associations in relevance to the respective associations with BMI.

7.2 METHODS

7.2.1 PARTICIPANTS

This study is a secondary analysis of data from the ALSPAC (http://www.bristol.ac.uk/alspac). The design and methods have been published [21]. In brief, ALSPAC is a longitudinal population-based cohort that recruited 14 541 pregnant women who were expected to deliver between 1 April 1991 and 31 December 1992 [21]. All members of the ALSPAC cohort were invited to annual follow-up clinics from the age of 7 to 13 years and then approximately every 2 years thereafter. In addition, when the oldest children were approximately 7 years of age, the sample size was increased by inviting eligible cases who had failed to join the study originally resulting in an additional 713 children being enrolled; 8297, 7725 and 5509 participants attended the 7-, 9- and 15-year clinics, respectively. In the present study, baseline 'childhood' anthropometric data were taken from a combination of the 7- and 9-year clinics. If available, data from the 7-year clinic were used preferentially (n=2540) and data from an additional 168 children were used from the 9-year clinic. Anthropometric and cardiometabolic risk factors were taken from the 15-year clinic (n=2858): the 'adolescent' group. The eligibility criteria for these analyses were adolescents who had their waist circumference, height and serum lipid levels measured at the 15 year clinic. There were no childhood anthropometric measurements for 150 adolescents who had both anthropometric and cardiometabolic risk factors measured at the 15-year clinic; consequently, data are missing for 5% (148 of 2858) of the children. The final sample used in the analyses here were 2858 adolescents (cross-sectional analysis) and 2710 children (prospective analysis). The majority (98%) of the mothers of the participants self-identified their ethnicity as white. Ethical approval for the study was obtained from the ALSPAC Ethics and Law Committee and the Local Research Ethics Committees.

7.2.2 ANTHROPOMETRY

Standard protocols for assessing anthropometry were used, with the participants in light clothing and no shoes. Age was recorded in months. Weight was measured to the nearest 0.1 kg using Tanita THF 300GS (Tanita UK Ltd, Yewsley, Middlesex, UK). Height was measured using a Harpenden stadiometer (Holtain Ltd, Crymych, Pembs, UK) to the nearest 1 mm. Waist circumference was measured at the mid-point between the lower rib and the iliac crest to the nearest 1 mm with a flexible tape measure. Height, weight and BMI z scores were determined using age and sex specific national reference values for the UK [22]. WHtR was determined by dividing waist circumference by height.

7.2.3 CARDIOMETABOLIC RISK FACTORS

The participants were requested to fast before attending the 15-year clinic. For those attending morning clinics they were asked to fast overnight. For those attending afternoon clinics, they were asked to fast for a minimum of 6 h prior to attendance. Blood samples were taken from the cubital fossa and immediately spun and plasma was frozen at −80°C. Approximately 3 to 9 months later, the samples were assayed. Total cholesterol, triglyceride and HDLc concentrations were measured using a modified Lipid Research Clinics Protocol with enzymatic reagents for lipid determination [2]. LDLc was determined with the Friedewald equation [23]. An automated assay was used to measure blood glucose concentration. Insulin was measured using an enzyme-linked immunosorbent assay (Mercodia, Uppsala, Sweden) which does not cross react with proinsulin. BP was measured using a Dinamap 9301 Vital Signs Monitor (Morton Medical, London, UK) with appropriate cuff size. Each participant was at rest and his/her arm was supported. For analysis, the mean of the two measurements that were taken was used.

TABLE 1: Anthropometric characteristics in childhood and adolescence. Results are expressed as median and interquartile range unless otherwise indicated

Childhood	Male		Female		Total	
	n		n		n	
Age (months)	1317	89 [89, 90]	1393	89 [89, 90]	2710	89 [89, 90]
Height (cm)	1315	127.0 [123.1, 130.9]	1393	125.7 [122.0, 130.1]	2708	126.5 [122.5, 130.6]
Height z score	1315	0.38 [-0.36, 1.01]	1393	0.23 [-0.49, 0.90]	2708	0.28 [-0.42, 0.95]
Weight (kg)	1317	25.4 [23.2, 28.6]	1393	25.2 [22.8, 28.8]	2710	25.4 [23.0, 28.6]
Weight z score	1317	0.26 [-0.35, 0.94]	1393	0.15 [-0.45, 0.86]	2710	0.20 [-0.41, 0.90]
BMI	1315	15.77 [14.92, 16.88]	1393	15.94 [14.90, 17.40]	2708	15.87 [14.91, 17.14]
BMI z score	1315	0.08 [-0.54, 0.71]	1393	0.04 [-0.58, 0.76]	2708	0.06 [-0.57, 0.74]
Overweight and obese, n (%)	1315	149 (11.3)	1393	226 (16.2)	2708	375 (13.8)
WHtR*	1314	0.44 [0.43, 0.46]	1392	0.44 [0.42, 0.46]	2706	0.44 [0.42, 0.46]
WHtR* ≥0.5, n (%)	1314	82 (6.2)	1392	103 (7.4)	2706	185 (6.8)
Adolescence	**Male**		**Female**		**Total**	
	n		n		n	
Age (months)	1376	184 [183, 186]	1482	184 [183, 187]	2858	184 [183, 187]
Height (cm)	1376	174.9 [170.0, 180.0]	1482	164.6 [161, 168.7]	2858	169.0 [163.5, 175.5]
Height z score	1376	0.47 [-0.16, 1.10]	1482	0.29 [-0.32, 0.96]	2858	0.37 [-0.22, 1.03]
Weight (kg)	1375	62.6 [56.8, 69.7]	1477	57.4 [52.2, 63.8]	2858	60.1 [53.9, 66.8]
Weight z score	1375	0.46 [-0.10, 1.03]	1477	0.36 [-0.29, 1.04]	2852	0.42 [-0.19, 1.03]
BMI	1375	20.38 [18.90, 22.24]	1477	21.10 [19.41, 23.23]	2852	20.71 [19.12, 22.80]
BMI z score	1375	0.32 [-0.30, 0.98]	1477	0.34 [-0.32, 1.01]	2852	0.33 [-0.31, 0.99]

TABLE 1: *Cont.*

Adolescence	Male	Female	Total
	n	n	n
Overweight or obese, n (%)	223 (16.2)	267 (18.1)	490 (17.2)
WHtR*	1376	1482	2858
	0.43 [0.41, 0.46]	0.46 [0.43, 0.49]	0.44 [0.41, 0.48]
WHtR* ≥0.5, n (%)	152 (11.0)	340 (22.9)	492 (17.2)

Waist-to-height ratio. BMI, body mass index; WHtR, waist-to-height ratio.

7.2.4 STATISTICAL ANALYSIS

Data were analysed using IBM SPSS Statistics 19.0 (IBM, Chicago, IL, USA) and MedCalc version 12.5.0 (Ostend, Belgium). The data were examined cross-sectionally and prospectively and explored as continuous variables and as binary categorical variables. Relationships between continuous variables were examined by Spearman correlation coefficients. χ^2 test was used as a measure of association between categorical variables and odds ratios were used to examine the strength of associations. The cut-points used in this analysis to indicate cardiometabolic risk were $\geq 1.7 \, mmol \, L^{-1}$ for triglycerides, $< 1.03 \, mmol \, L^{-1}$ for HDLc, $\geq 5.6 \, mmol \, L^{-1}$ for plasma glucose, $\geq 130 \, mmHg$ for systolic BP, and $\geq 85 \, mmHg$ for diastolic BP, as recommended by the International Diabetes Federation for children and adolescents (10 to 16 years) [24]. The cut-points for LDLc and insulin were $\geq 2.79 \, mmol \, L^{-1}$ and $\geq 16.95 \, IU \, L^{-1}$, respectively, which is $\geq$90th centile for the cohort [2]. Cardiometabolic risk factor co-occurrence was defined as having three or more cardiometabolic risk factors using the binary outcome thresholds listed above. Participants were classified as overweight or obese based on sex- and age- specific International Obesity Task Force (IOTF) BMI criteria [25] and ≥ 0.5 for WHtR [7]. Receiver operator characteristic (ROC) curves were used to identify the optimal WHtR cut-points, sensitivity and specificity.

7.3 RESULTS

The anthropometric characteristics of participants are shown in Table 1. The prevalence of overweight or obese was lower in childhood (13.8%; n=375) than in adolescence (17.2%; n=490). The correlation between BMI z scores in childhood and adolescence was r=0.72, P<0.001, and 63.6% of overweight and obese children remained overweight or obese at 15 years. The proportion of participants who had a high WHtR (≥ 0.5) was also lower in childhood (6.8%; n=185) compared with adolescence (17.2%; n=492). The correlation between WHtR in childhood and adolescence was r=0.57, P<0.001 and 69.2% of children with a high WHtR had a high WHtR as adolescents.

TABLE 2: Biochemistry and blood pressure in adolescence. Data are expressed as median [interquartile range] and the number (%) above cut-points, or below cut-point for HDLc

	Male		Female		Total		p[b]
	n		n		n		
Triglycerides (mmol L^{-1})	1376	0.73 [0.57, 0.96]	1482	0.77 [0.62, 0.99]	2858	0.75 [0.59, 0.98]	
≥1.7 mmol L^{-1}		43 (3.1)		43 (2.9)		86 (3.0)	0.727
LDLc (mmol L^{-1})	1376	1.94 [1.62, 2.30]	1482	2.12 [1.79, 2.52]	2858	2.03 [1.70, 2.41]	
≥2.79 mmol L^{-1}		104 (7.6)		221 (14.9)		325 (11.4)	<0.001
HDLc (mmol L^{-1})	1376	1.20 [1.01, 1.38]	1482	1.33 [1.16, 1.54]	2858	1.27 [1.09, 1.47]	
<1.03 mmol L^{-1}		347 (25.2)		178 (12.0)		525 (18.4)	<0.001
Glucose (mmol L^{-1})	1376	5.3 [5.0, 5.5]	1482	5.1 [4.9, 5.3]	2858	5.2 [5.0, 5.4]	
≥5.6 mmol L^{-1}		313 (22.7)		159 (10.7)		472 (16.5)	0.004
Insulin (IU L^{-1})	1374	8.17 [6.00, 11.16]	1480	9.65 [7.25, 12.76]	2854	8.97 [6.63, 12.05]	
≥16.95 IU L^{-1}		102 (7.4)		155 (10.5)		257 (9.0)	<0.001
Systolic BP (mmHg)	1335	126.5 [119.0, 133.5]	1444	120.5 [113.0, 127.5]	2779	123.5 [115.5, 131.0]	
≥130 mmHg		517 (38.7)		289 (20.0)		806 (29.0)	<0.001
Diastolic BP (mmHg)	1335	66.5 [60.5, 73.5]	1444	66.0 [60.5, 71.0]	2779	66.0 [60.5, 72.0]	
≥85 mmHg		40 (3.0)		22 (1.5)		62 (2.2)	0.009
Risk co-occurrence[a]		104 (7.6)		64 (4.3)		168 (5.9)	<0.001

[a]Risk co-occurrence is the presence of ≥3 of the following: triglycerides ≥1.7 mmol L^{-1}, LDLc ≥2.79 mmol L^{-1}, HDLc <1.03 mmol L^{-1}, plasma glucose ≥5.6 mmol L^{-1}, insulin ≥16.95 IU L^{-1}, systolic blood pressure ≥130 mmHg, or diastolic blood pressure ≥85 mmHg. [b] Pearson χ^2. BP, blood pressure; HDLc, high density lipoprotein cholesterol; LDLc, low density lipoprotein cholesterol

BMI z scores and WHtR were highly correlated in both childhood and adolescence: $r=0.80$ and $r=0.78$ (both $P<0.001$), respectively. The majority (91.9%) of children with a high WHtR were also overweight or obese. Conversely, only 45.1% of overweight or obese children had a high WHtR. In adolescence 72.0% of adolescents with a high WHtR were overweight or obese, and 71.8% of overweight or obese adolescents had a high WHtR.

The prevalence of elevated cardiometabolic risk factors in the adolescents varied from 2.2% ($n=62$) for high diastolic BP, to 29.0% ($n=806$) with high systolic BP, Table 2. In general, elevated cardiometabolic risk factors were more common in males than females, with approximately twice as many males having low HDLc, high glucose levels or high systolic BP compared to females. Co-occurrence of three or more cardiometabolic risk factors was more common in males than females. Correlations were stronger between cardiometabolic risk factors and anthropometric outcomes measured in adolescence compared to those measured in childhood, Table 3.

The proportions of overweight and obese adolescents, or adolescents with a WHtR ≥0.5, that had elevated LDLc, reduced HDLc, elevated glucose, elevated insulin and/or high BP are shown in Table 4. The odds ratios between measures of adiposity and risk factors are shown in Fig. 1. Adolescent males with WHtR ≥0.5 had an increased odds of elevated triglycerides, LDLc, glucose, insulin and systolic BP and low HDLc compared to males with a WHtR <0.5. Furthermore, males with WHtR ≥0.5 had an increased odds ratio of co-occurrence of cardiometabolic risk factors compared to males with a WHtR <0.5 (odds ratio=6.8 [95% confidence interval {CI} 4.4 to 10.6]). Overweight and obese males had correspondingly increased odds of a similar magnitude, compared with males who were not overweight or obese. Females with a high WHtR had increased odds ratio for elevated triglycerides, LDLc, insulin and systolic BP and low HDLc, and were approximately four times more likely (3.8 [2.3 to 6.3]) to have co-occurrence of cardiometabolic risk factors than females with a WHtR <0.5. Overweight and obese females had correspondingly increased odds of the same cardiometabolic risk factors and co-occurrence of these, (Fig. 1).

TABLE 3. Spearman correlations (P value) between BMI z score and waist-to-height ratio measured in childhood and adolescence and cardiometabolic risk factors measured in adolescence

Cardiometabolic risk factors	Childhood				Adolescence			
	BMI z score		WHtR		BMI z score		WHtR	
	Male	Female	Male	Female	Male	Female	Male	Female
Triglycerides (mmol L⁻¹)	0.083 (0.003)	0.052 (0.055)	0.077 (0.005)	0.079 (0.003)	0.270 (<0.001)	0.145 (<0.001)	0.321 (<0.001)	0.185 (<0.001)
LDLc (mmol L⁻¹)	0.073 (0.008)	0.102 (<0.001)	0.096 (<0.001)	0.120 (<0.001)	0.119 (<0.001)	0.158 (<0.001)	0.148 (<0.001)	0.161 (<0.001)
HDLc (mmol L⁻¹)	−0.137 (<0.001)	−0.101 (<0.001)	−0.143 (<0.001)	−0.096 (<0.001)	−0.271 (<0.001)	−0.242 (<0.001)	−0.211 (<0.001)	−0.260 (<0.001)
Glucose (mmol l⁻¹)	0.001 (0.964)	−0.015 (0.570)	0.012 (0.661)	−0.014 (0.597)	0.077 (0.004)	−0.004 (0.888)	0.092 (0.001)	−0.116 (0.542)
Insulin (IU L⁻¹)	0.119 (<0.001)	0.111 (<0.001)	0.099 (<0.001)	0.105 (<0.001)	0.284 (<0.001)	0.192 (<0.001)	0.352 (<0.001)	0.189 (<0.001)
Systolic BP (mmHg)	0.129 (<0.001)	0.139 (<0.001)	0.060 (0.033)	0.103 (<0.001)	0.228 (<0.001)	0.228 (<0.001)	0.148 (<0.001)	0.183 (<0.001)
Diastolic BP (mmHg)	0.025 (0.368)	0.003 (0.912)	−0.044 (0.119)	−0.063 (0.021)	0.031 (0.257)	0.21 (0.417)	−0.022 (0.429)	0.015 (0.576)

BMI, body mass index; BP, blood pressure; HDLc, high density lipoprotein cholesterol; LDLc, low density lipoprotein cholesterol; WHtR, waist-to-height ratio.

Male

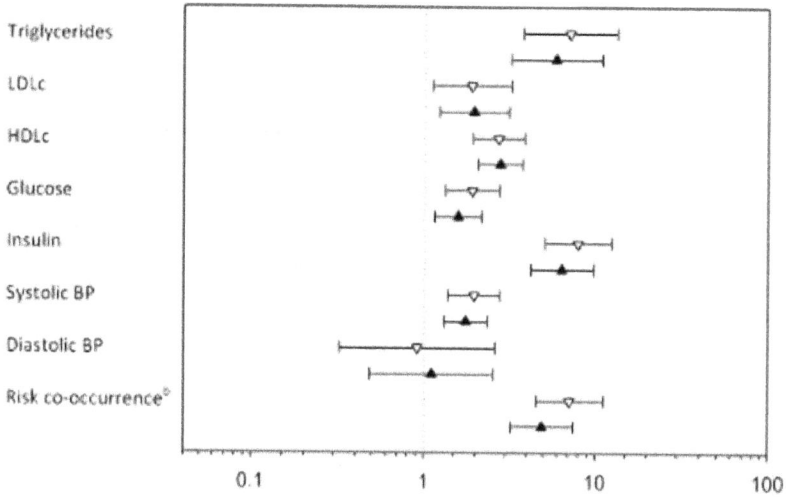

Female

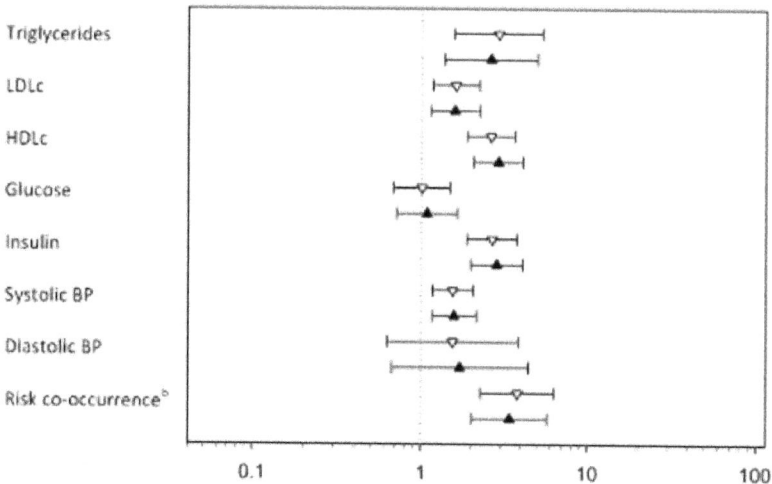

FIGURE 1: Odds ratio (95%CI) for risk factors associated with overweight and obesity defined by BMI (symbol: black triangle) and WHtR of ≥0.5 (symbol: white triangle) in adolescents (cross-sectional analysis). Risk factors were defined as follows: triglycerides ≥1.7 mmol/L, LDLc ≥2.79 mmol/L, HDLc < 1.03 mmol/L, plasma glucose ≥5.6 mmol/L, insulin ≥16.95 IU/L, systolic blood pressure ≥130 mmHg, or diastolic blood pressure ≥85 mmHg. bRisk co-occurrence was defined as ≥3 of the above.

The Complexity of Adolescent Obesity

TABLE 4: The proportion of adolescents with cardiometabolic risk factors, stratified by sex and anthropometric status (cross sectional analysis)

Outcome and exposure	Male			Female		
	% with increased adiposity* and risk factor/s	% without increased adiposity* and with risk factor/s	P[b]	% with increased adiposity* and risk factor/s	% without increased adiposity* and with risk factor/s	P†
Triglycerides (≥1.7 mmol L⁻¹)						
BMI	9.9	1.8	<0.001	5.6	2.2	0.003
WHtR	12.5	2.0	<0.001	2.9	2.0	0.001
LDLc (≥2.79 mmol L⁻¹)						
BMI	12.1	6.6	0.004	20.2	13.7	0.007
WHtR	12.5	6.9	0.013	20.3	13.3	0.002
HDLc (<1.03 mmol L⁻¹)						
BMI	43.5	21.7	<0.001	23.2	9.4	<0.001
WHtR	44.1	22.9	<0.001	21.2	9.3	<0.001
Glucose (≥5.6 mmol L⁻¹)						
BMI	30.0	21.4	0.005	11.2	10.5	0.72
WHtR	34.2	21.3	<0.001	10.9	10.7	0.97
Insulin (≥16.95 IU L⁻¹)						
BMI	22.9	4.4	<0.001	8.2	7.4	<0.001
WHtR	28.3	4.8	<0.001	18.9	8.0	<0.001
Systolic BP (≥130 mmHg)						
BMI	50.2	36.6	<0.001	26.5	18.6	0.003
WHtR	52.7	37.0	<0.001	25.6	18.3	0.004
Diastolic BP (≥85 mmHg)						
BMI	3.3	2.9	0.81	2.3	1.4	0.26
WHtR	2.7	3.0	0.85	2.1	1.3	0.31
Risk co-occurrence‡						
BMI	20.6	5.0	<0.001	9.7	3.1	<0.001
WHtR	27.0	5.1	<0.001	9.7	2.7	<0.001

*BMI was categorized as overweight/obese or not overweight/obese and WHtR was categorized as <0.5 or ≥0.5. †Pearson χ². ‡Risk co-occurrence is the presence of ≥3 of the following: triglycerides ≥1.7 mmol L⁻¹, LDLc ≥2.79 mmol L⁻¹, HDLc <1.03 mmol L⁻¹, plasma glucose ≥5.6 mmol L⁻¹, insulin ≥16.95 IU L⁻¹, systolic blood pressure ≥130 mmHg, or diastolic blood pressure ≥85 mmHg. BMI, body mass index; BP, blood pressure; HDLc, high density lipoprotein cholesterol; LDLc, low density lipoprotein cholesterol; WHtR, waist-to-height ratio.

TABLE 5: The proportion of adolescents with cardiometabolic risk factors, stratified by sex and anthropometric status in childhood (prospective analysis)

Outcome and exposure	Male			Female		
	% with increased adiposity* and risk factor/s	% without increased adiposity* and with risk factor/s	P†	% with increased adiposity* and risk factor/s	% without increased adiposity* and with risk factor/s	P†
Triglycerides ($\geq$1.7 mmol L^{-1})						
BMI	6.7	2.3	0.002	1.3	2.9	0.17
WHtR	11.0	2.3	<0.001	1.0	2.8	0.27
LDLc ($\geq$2.79 mmol L^{-1})						
BMI	10.0	7.2	0.22	17.0	14.2	0.58
WHtR	11.0	7.3	0.22	16.5	14.5	0.58
HDLc (<1.03 mmol L^{-1})						
BMI	40.7	23.6	<0.001	16.6	10.8	0.02
WHtR	42.7	24.4	<0.001	16.5	11.4	0.12
Glucose ($\geq$5.6 mmol L^{-1})						
BMI	24.7	22.5	0.50	10.4	9.6	0.92
WHtR	28.0	22.3	0.23	11.7	10.2	0.63
Insulin ($\geq$16.95 IU L^{-1})						
BMI	16.1	5.8	<0.001	14.5	8.3	0.001
WHtR	19.8	6.2	<0.001	13.7	9.0	0.22
Systolic BP ($\geq$130 mmHg)						
BMI	53.1	36.9	<0.001	27.5	18.9	0.006
WHtR	57.0	37.5	0.001	25.3	19.9	0.13
Diastolic BP ($\geq$85 mmHg)						
BMI	3.4	2.9	0.71	1.8	1.4	0.65
WHtR	3.8	2.9	0.66	1.0	1.5	0.69
Risk co-occurrence‡						
BMI	18.1	6.1	<0.001	6.3	3.4	0.04
WHtR	24.4	6.4	<0.001	6.1	3.7	0.27

*BMI was categorized as overweight/obese or not overweight/obese and WHtR was categorized as <0.5 or $\geq$0.5. †χ^2 (Pearson). ‡Risk co-occurrence is the presence of $\geq$3 of the following: triglycerides $\geq$1.7 mmol L^{-1}, LDLc $\geq$2.79 mmol L^{-1}, HDLc <1.03 mmol L^{-1}, plasma glucose $\geq$5.6 mmol L^{-1}, insulin $\geq$16.95 IU L^{-1}, systolic blood pressure $\geq$130 mmHg, or diastolic blood pressure $\geq$85 mmHg. BMI, body mass index; BP, blood pressure; HDLc, high density lipoprotein cholesterol; LDLc, low density lipoprotein cholesterol; WHtR, waist-to-height ratio.

The specificity and sensitivity of a WHtR cut-point of 0.5 in male adolescents for identifying cardiometabolic risk factor co-occurrence was 90.0 (95% CI 88.2 to 91.6) and 41.3 (31.8 to 51.4), respectively. For female adolescents the specificity and sensitivity of a WHtR cut-point of 0.5 was 76.2 (73.7 to 78.2) and 53.1 (40.2 to 65.7). Using ROC analysis the optimal WHtR cut point for identifying co-occurrence of risk factors was 0.47 (specificity 83.5 [81.3 to 85.5]; sensitivity 51.9 [41.9 to 61.8]) for male adolescents and 0.48 (specificity 65.8 [63.3 to 68.3]; sensitivity 67.2 [54.3 to 78.4] for female adolescents.

The proportions of overweight and obese children or those with a WHtR ≥0.5 who had elevated LDLc, reduced HDLc, elevated glucose, elevated insulin and/or high BP during adolescence are shown in Table 5. Like the cross-sectional analysis, male children who had a WHtR ≥ 0.05 or who were overweight or obese had increased odds of cardiometabolic risk factors in adolescence, Fig. 2. However, the CIs around the odds ratio tended to be wider. Male children with WHtR ≥0.5 had approximately five times higher probability (4.6 [2.6 to 8.1]) of co-occurrence of risk factors during adolescence than male children with a WHtR <0.5. Overweight and obese male children had approximately four times higher probability (3.6 [2.2 to 5.8]) of co-occurrence of risk factors during adolescence. Similar associations between both anthropometric measures and cardiometabolic risk factors were also observed in female children, although the odds ratios were generally small, and the lower limits of the CIs below one, Fig. 2.

The specificity and sensitivity of a WHtR cut-point of 0.5 in male children for identifying cardiometabolic risk factor co-occurrence in adolescents was 94.7 (93.3 to 95.9) and 21.1 (13.4 to 30.6), respectively. For female children the specificity and sensitivity of a WHtR cut-point of 0.5 was 91.4 (89.8 to 92.9) and 17.0 (8.1 to 29.8). Using ROC analysis the optimal WHtR cut point for identifying co-occurrence of risk factors in male children was the same as it was in male adolescents 0.47 (specificity 83.3 [81.0 to 85.3]; sensitivity 37.9 [28.1 to 48.4]), but lower in female children compared to female adolescents 0.44 (specificity 54.4 [51.7 to 57.1]; sensitivity 71.7 [57.7 to 83.2]).

7.4 DISCUSSION

To our knowledge this is the first study to demonstrate a prospective association between having a high WHtR in childhood and cardiometabolic risk co-occurrence in adolescent boys. The results demonstrate that the of risk for having a WHtR ≥0.5 was comparable to being overweight or obese as defined by sex- and age- specific IOTF BMI criteria. For example, children with a WHtR ≥0.5, had two to five times higher odds of cardiometabolic risk co-occurrence compared to children who had a WHtR <0.5 and children who were overweight or obese had two to four times higher odds compared to normal weight children. However, there was a sex difference and the association between anthropometric measures in childhood and cardiometabolic risk co-occurrence in adolescence was significantly stronger in boys than girls. In the clinical environment, using a WHtR cutpoint of 0.5 has several advantages over defining a child as overweight or obese by BMI; it is a simpler index to calculate, easily understood by adolescents and families and does not require sex- and age- specific centiles.

The findings of this study are broadly consistent with another prospective study that examined correlations between BMI and WHtR in Australian children and adult cardiometabolic risk factors [20]. While direct comparisons between studies is difficult, it is interesting to note that the correlations between WHtR and BMI measured at 7 to 11 years with triglycerides (rho=0.07 and 0.05 for WHtR and BMI, respectively) and insulin (rho=0.11 for both WHtR and BMI) measured in adulthood were of a similar magnitude to what we report between WHtR and BMI measured at 7 to 9 years and triglycerides and insulin measured in adolescence.

The association between WHtR and cardiometabolic risk, both measured in adolescence, support a number of other cross-sectional studies [26, 27], which have been recently reviewed [7]. In general, all studies showed good agreement in the magnitude and outcome of their analysis between WHtR and BMI and outcomes of cardiometabolic risk. Consistent with our study, both WHtR and BMI had a stronger association with triglycerides and HDLc, than LDLc. The association between anthropometric measures and BP tended to be stronger for systolic BP compared to diastolic BP and both WHtR and BMI were associated with fasting insulin and a 'cardiometabolic risk score', albeit defined differently among the different studies.

There is no consensus on the cross-sectional association of WHtR and BMI and fasting glucose [3, 15, 17]. In part, this may be explained by the differing age of the cohorts (range from 4 to 17 years) and methods of analysing the data. Findings from our study suggest that adolescent males with a high WHtR or who are overweight or obese have an increased risk of an elevated fasting glucose. However, it is of note that in our study a high proportion of adolescents (23% of males; 11% of females) had fasting blood glucose levels $\geq 5.6 \text{mmol L}^{-1}$. In the absence of evidence to indicate that this population has disturbances in glucose metabolism, these findings could reflect the diurnal variation in blood glucose [28], since some adolescents had blood taken in the afternoon after a 6h fast and/or inadequate fasting. The results pertaining to fasting glucose in this study need to be interpreted with caution.

More children were classified as overweight or obese using BMI criteria compared to those classified as having a high WHtR. Children with a WHtR ≥ 0.5 were more severely obese compared to children were defined as overweight or obese using BMI criteria, mean $\pm$ standard deviation BMI z-score was 2.05 ± 0.9 and 1.82 ± 0.9, respectively. The most appropriate cut-point for WHtR to identify children and adolescents at cardiometabolic risk is not clear. In the present study we used ≥ 0.5 which has demonstrated utility in adults [7] and children [10] but other cut-points have been suggested [8]. Our results indicated that a cut-point ≥ 0.5 was highly specific in identifying cardiometabolic risk co-occurrence in male children and adolescents as well as female children (90 to 95%), but had poor sensitivity (17 to 53%); the risk of being wrongly labelled as having co-occurrence of cardiometabolic risk factors was small, but many of those who were at risk were not identified. Statistically optimum cut-points were identified as 0.47 for male children and male adolescents and 0.44 and 0.48 for female children and female adolescents, respectively. However, by increasing the sensitivity, the specificity decreased particularly for female children (from 91 to 54%); using lower cut-points more children and adolescents would be incorrectly labelled as being as having co-occurrence of cardiometabolic risk factors. Given the stigma of being incorrectly labelled and the limited resources for managing children and adolescents at cardiometabolic risk it could be prudent to use a higher but more specific cut-point.

There are a number of limitations to the study including the number of participants which had complete data. Initially over 14 000 pregnant women were recruited, with over 5500 participants attending the 15 years clinic, yet only 2710 met our inclusion criteria for our prospective analysis and 2858 for our cross-sectional analysis. The implications of attrition are not clear and may affect the generalizability of the findings. Nevertheless, this is the largest study in children and adolescents addressing the association between WHtR and cardiometabolic risk factors, as well as the first in the UK.

Another potential limitation relates to measuring waist circumference and applies to both the location of the measurement and sensitivity around measuring waist circumference in heavier children. There is no universally accepted method of measuring waist circumference. In this study the waist circumference was measured at the mid-point between the lowest rib and the iliac crest, which has been demonstrated to be reproducible and highly correlated with total body and trunk adiposity [29]. It is recognized that removal of clothing and placement of the measuring tape may be awkward or embarrassing for the overweight or obese children and needs to be handled sensitively.

In conclusion, we found that BMI z scores and WHtR were highly correlated and that they have similar associations with cross-sectional and prospective cardiometabolic risk factors in adolescence. WHtR is a simple calculation that could be used to identify male children and adolescents for cardiometabolic risk.

REFERENCES

1.   Falaschetti E, Hingorani AD, Jones A, et al. Adiposity and cardiovascular risk factors in a large contemporary population of pre-pubertal children. Eur Heart J 2010; 31: 3063–3072.
2.   Lawlor DA, Benfield L, Logue J, et al. Association between general and central adiposity in childhood, and change in these, with cardiovascular risk factors in adolescence: prospective cohort study. BMJ 2010; 341: c6224–c6224.

3. Botton J, Heude B, Kettaneh A, et al. Cardiovascular risk factor levels and their relationships with overweight and fat distribution in children: the Fleurbaix Laventie Ville Santé II study. Metabolism 2007; 56: 614–622.

4. Venn AJ, Thomson RJ, Schmidt MD, et al. Overweight and obesity from childhood to adulthood: a follow-up of participants in the 1985 Australian Schools Health and Fitness Survey. Med J Aust 2007; 186: 458–460.

5. Goulding A, Taylor RW, Grant AM, Parnell WR, Wilson NC, Williams SM. Waist-to-height ratios in relation to BMI z-scores in three ethnic groups from a representative sample of New Zealand children aged 5–14 years. Int J Obes (Lond) 2010; 34: 1188–1190.

6. Xiong F, Garnett SP, Cowell CT, et al. Waist circumference and waist-to-height ratio in Han Chinese children living in Chongqing, south-west China. Public Health Nutr 2011; 14: 20–26.

7. Browning LM, Hsieh SD, Ashwell M. A systematic review of waist-to-height ratio as a screening tool for the prediction of cardiovascular disease and diabetes: 0.5 could be a suitable global boundary value. Nutr Res Rev 2010; 23: 247–269.

8. Nambiar S, Hughes I, Davies PS. Developing waist-to-height ratio cut-offs to define overweight and obesity in children and adolescents. Public Health Nutr 2010; 13: 1566–1574.

9. Ashwell M, Hsieh SD. Six reasons why the waist-to-height ratio is a rapid and effective global indicator for health risks of obesity and how its use could simplify the international public health message on obesity. Int J Food Sci Nutr 2005; 56: 303–307.

10. Garnett SP, Baur LA, Cowell CT. Waist-to-height ratio: a simple option for determining excess central adiposity in young people. Int J Obes 2008; 32: 1028–1030.

11. Taylor RW, Williams SM, Grant AM, Taylor BJ, Goulding A. Predictive ability of waist-to-height in relation to adiposity in children is not improved with age and sex-specific values. Obesity 2011; 19: 1062–1068.

12. McCarthy HD, Ashwell M. A study of central fatness using waist-to-height ratios in UK children and adolescents over two decades supports the simple message – 'keep your waist circumference to less than half your height. Int J Obes (Lond) 2006; 30: 988–992.

13. Ashwell M, Gunn P, Gibson S. Waist-to-height ratio is a better screening tool than waist circumference and BMI for adult cardiometabolic risk factors: systematic review and meta-analysis. Obes Rev 2012; 13: 275–286.

14. Savva SC, Tornaritis M, Savva ME, et al. Waist circumference and waist-to-height ratio are better predictors of cardiovascular disease risk factors in children than body mass index. Int J Obes Relat Metab Disord 2000; 24: 1453–1458.

15. Kahn H, Imperatore G, Cheng Y. A population-based comparison of BMI percentiles and waist-to-height ratio for identifying cardiovascular risk in youth. J Pediatrics 2005; 146: 482–488.

16. Hara M, Saitou E, Iwata F, Okada T, Harada K. Waist-to-height ratio is the best predictor of cardiovascular disease risk factors in Japanese schoolchildren. J Atheroscler Thromb 2002; 9: 127–132.

17. Sung RYT, Yu CCW, Choi KC, et al. Waist circumference and body mass index in Chinese children: cutoff values for predicting cardiovascular risk factors. Int J Obes (Lond) 2006; 31: 550–558.

18. Freedman DS, Kahn HS, Mei Z, et al. Relation of body mass index and waist-to-height ratio to cardiovascular disease risk factors in children and adolescents: the Bogalusa Heart Study. Am J Clin Nutr 2007; 86: 33–40.

19. Manios Y, Kourlaba G, Kafatos A, Cook TL, Spyridaki A, Fragiadakis GA. Associations of several anthropometric indices with insulin resistance in children: the Children Study. Acta Paediatr 2008; 97: 494–499.

20. Schmidt MD, Dwyer T, Magnussen CG, Venn AJ. Predictive associations between alternative measures of childhood adiposity and adult cardio-metabolic health. Int J Obes (Lond) 2011; 35: 38–45.

21. Boyd A, Golding J, Macleod J, et al. Cohort profile: the 'Children of the 90s' – the index offspring of the Avon Longitudinal Study of Parents and Children. Int J Epidemiol 2013; 42: 111–127.

22. Pan H, Cole TJ. LMS Growth Program. 2010. [WWW document]. URL http://www.healthforallchildren.com/?product=lmsgrowth (accessed January 2011).

23. Friedewald W, Levy R, Fredrickson D. Estimation of the concentration of low-density lipoprotein cholesterol in plasma, without use of the preparative ultracentrifuge. Clin Chem 1972; 18: 499–502.

24. Zimmet P, Alberti G, Kaufman F, et al. The metabolic syndrome in children and adolescents. Lancet 2007; 369: 2059–2061.

25. Cole TJ, Bellizzi MC, Flegal KM, Dietz WH. Establishing a standard definition for child overweight and obesity worldwide: international survey. BMJ 2000; 320: 1240–1243.

26. Kondaki K, Grammatikaki E, Pavón DJ, et al. Comparison of several anthropometric indices with insulin resistance proxy measures among European adolescents: the Helena Study. Eur J Pediatr 2011; 170: 731–739.

27. Androutsos O, Grammatikaki E, Moschonis G, et al. Neck circumference: a useful screening tool of cardiovascular risk in children. Pediatr Obes. 2012; 7: 187–195.

28. Troisi RJ, Cowie CC, Harris MI. Diurnal variation in fasting plasma glucose: implications for diagnosis of diabetes in patients examined in the afternoon. JAMA 2000; 284: 3157–3159.

29. Wang J. Waist circumference: a simple, inexpensive, and reliable tool that should be included as part of physical examinations in the doctor's office. Am J Clin Nutr 2003; 78: 902–903.

Figure 2 is not available in this version of the article. To view this additional information, please use the citation on the first page of this chapter.

CHAPTER 8

NEUROBEHAVIOURAL CORRELATES IN OLDER CHILDREN AND ADOLESCENTS WITH OBESITY AND OBSTRUCTIVE SLEEP APNEA

EVAN TAN, DIONE HEALEY, ELIZABETH SCHAUGHENCY, PATRICK DAWES, AND BARBARA GALLAND

8.1 INTRODUCTION

Sleep-disordered breathing (SDB) is characterised by a total cessation of airflow (apnoea) or substantial reduction of airflow (hypopnoea) in breathing during sleep and encompasses the full spectrum of primary snoring, upper airway resistance syndrome and obstructive sleep apnoea (OSA). Primary snoring is reported in 5–10% of children and OSA in 1–5%.[1] Approximately one-third of children with obesity will have OSA or report symptoms of OSA.[2, 3] Obesity possibly plays a more important role in the pathogenesis of OSA in older children and adolescents than in younger children, in whom adenotonsillar hypertrophy features more strongly.[4] There is no clear definition of the age at which obesity begins to influence OSA risk, but one study reports that increased risk of developing OSA due

Reprinted with permission from Tan E, Healey D, Schaughency E, Dawes P, and Galland B. Neurobehavioural Correlates in Older Children and Adolescents with Obesity and Obstructive Sleep Apnoea. Journal of Paediatrics and Child Health *50,1 (2014), DOI: 10.1111/jpc.12390.*

to being overweight or obese is predominantly found among adolescents age ≥12 years, with little increase in risk noted among children younger than 12 years.[5] Well-established neurobehavioural morbidities associated with OSA in children include daytime sleepiness,[6, 7] lower intelligence and memory scores,[7, 8] increased problem behaviours[7, 9-11] and poorer executive functioning.[4, 9-11] Previous research has also documented improvements in children's overall behaviour and neurocognitive function following treatment of SDB,[12, 13] although research in older children and adolescents is not so well established.

Both physical health risks and psychological distress can be associated with obesity in adolescents.[14-16] Thus, the presence of combined obesity and OSA could exacerbate neurobehavioural morbidities. We are only aware of two studies that have considered this in older children and adolescents with obesity [17, 18] and one in overweight children and adolescents.[11] Rhodes et al., [17] in a small study of 14 children/adolescents with morbid obesity (mean age 13 years), found that those with OSA had poorer general memory, verbal memory, learning and vocabulary compared with their obese but non-OSA counterparts. Recently, Hannon et al. [18] reported on the relationship between OSA and neurocognitive functioning in 37 adolescents (12–18 years) with severe obesity (>97th percentile), showing that OSA was associated with lower maths scores but no other neurocognitive measures. Beebe et al.[11] investigated the associations of SDB with neurobehavioural functioning in 163 overweight children/adolescents (>95th percentile) aged 10–16.9 years. They found no associations with formal cognitive test results of intelligence or memory, but SDB was associated with lowered academic grades and some subscales of parent- and teacher-reported behaviour, and those with OSA were viewed by their teachers as having more learning problems.

The goal of this study was to add to the small evidence base of literature around neurobehavioural correlates of combined OSA and obesity in older children and adolescents suggesting that the combination may be associated with poorer assessments of academic achievement and learning, with a particular emphasis on the emerging evidence from the studies described above[11, 17, 18]; within this, we considered underlying factors that could explain this association.

8.2 METHODS

This study was approved by the Lower South Regional Ethics Committee, Dunedin, New Zealand. Thirty-one participants volunteered by invitation through the local paediatric obesity clinic and in response to advertisements. Participants had to be aged 10–18 years old with obesity. Obesity was defined using the age- and sex-specific Cole cut-off criteria[19] (International Obesity Task Force): a body mass index (BMI) conceptually equivalent to a BMI $\geq 30 \, \text{kg/m}^2$ at age 18 years. Exclusion criteria included craniofacial abnormalities, neuromuscular disease and recognised obesity syndromes. Parents completed a questionnaire about their child's sleep and breathing. [20] Habitual snoring was considered present if parents reported their child snoring '4–6 nights per week' or 'every night' in response to the question 'How often does your child snore?', with four response choices ('never', '1–3 nights a week', '4–6 nights a week' and 'every night'). Height was measured to the nearest 0.1 cm using a wall-mounted stadiometer, and weight was measured to the nearest 0.1 kg. Waist and neck circumference were measured to the nearest 0.1 cm. Tonsil size was graded on the Brodsky scale,[21] and a lateral neck X-ray was taken to grade adenoid hypertrophy. The scoring system for tonsil size and adenoid hypertrophy was based on that described by Goldstein et al.[20] Neighbourhood deprivation scores (New Zealand Deprivation Index 2006; NZDep2006)[22] based on participants' current address were calculated for each domicile using GeoStan NZ (version 2.1.1). The NZDep2006 scores range from 1 (indicating the least deprived domicile) to 10 (most deprived). Meshblocks (small geographical areas containing a median of 87 people) receive deprivation scores between 1 and 10, where 1 indicates an area is one of the least deprived 10% and 10 indicates an area is one of the most deprived 10%, with this classification based on measures of income, employment, education and access to transportation. Participants underwent one night of polysomnography (PSG) in a sleep laboratory. An experienced clinical psychology trainee blind to the participant's OSA status conducted neuropsychological assessments within a dedicated assessment room. These were conducted within a maximum of 2 weeks either side of the PSG study.

8.2.1 POLYSOMNOGRAPHY

The PSG montage included two electroencephalogram (EEG) leads (C4/A1 and C3/A2), two electrooculogram (EOG) leads, submental electromyogram (EMG), electrocardiogram, chest and abdominal wall motion by inductance plethysmography (SleepSense, Scientific Laboratory Products, Elgin, IL, USA), arterial oxygen saturation (Masimo Technology, Irvine, CA, USA) and nasal airflow via a nasal thermistor. Snoring was recorded by digital snorometer incorporated into the Visi-3 software system. EEG, EOG and EMG signals were relayed through the integrated hardware/software system of a PowerLab (AD Instruments Pty Ltd, Bella Vista, NSW, Australia), and the other signals were time-synchronised through a Visi-3 system (Stowood Scientific Instruments, Oxford, UK). Sleep was scored according to the criteria of Rechtschaffen and Kales[23] for total sleep time (TST) (time from sleep onset to sleep waking minus the time awake overnight), sleep efficiency calculated as TST/time in bed (TIB) times 100, sleep latency (time between TIB and sleep onset) and arousal index (defined as the number of arousals per hour). Apnoea was defined as cessation of airflow lasting for more than two respiratory cycles and hypopnoea as a decrease in airflow to less than 50% baseline amplitude with a concurrent desaturation of >3%. The apnoea–hypopnoea index (AHI) was defined as the total number of apnoeas and hypopnoeas per hour of TST. Diagnosis of OSA was based on a cut-off for OSA at an AHI >2, and OSA was further classified as mild (2 > AHI ≤ 5) or moderate to severe (AHI >5).[24, 25] Snoring was scored manually, with events first identified on screen and then confirmed via the audio output, where events were identified as an acoustic vibration presenting as a snorting sound with obvious obstruction.

8.2.2 NEUROBEHAVIOURAL ASSESSMENT BATTERY

General intelligence was measured using the Wechsler Abbreviated Scale of Intelligence (WASI). Verbal, performance and full IQ scores were derived from four subtests: vocabulary, block design, similarities and matrix reasoning. Reliability coefficients range from 0.92 to 0.95 for both verbal and performance IQ and from 0.95 to 0.97 for full IQ.[26]

Memory and learning were assessed using the Wide Range Assessment of Memory and Learning (WRAML-2), which evaluates an individual's memory functioning as well as the acquisition of new learning. The core battery is comprised of two verbal, two visual and two attention–concentration subtests yielding a Verbal Memory Index, a Visual Memory Index and an Attention–Concentration Index. Together these subtests yield a General Memory Index.[27] The test has sound psychometric properties.[27]

Reading and maths skills were assessed using the Wechsler Individual Achievement Test II Australian (WIAT-II Australian). The WIAT-II allows the assessment of problem-solving ability and is adapted for Australian language and metrics. The test consists of four composite scores: reading, mathematics, written language and oral language. Only the reading and mathematics composite scores were used in the current study. Reliability coefficients of the reading and mathematics composites range from 0.95 to 0.97 and from 0.93 to 0.97, respectively.[28]

Behavioural measures were derived from the Behaviour Assessment System for Children 2, which consists of three different response-type questionnaires: the Parent Rating Scale (PRS), the Teacher Rating Scale (TRS) and the Self-Report of Personality (SRP). The PRS consists of four different domains: Externalising Problems, Internalising Problems, the Adaptive Skills Composite and the Behavioural Symptoms Index. The TRS in addition contains the School Problems Composite. The SRP consists of the School Problems Composite, Internalising Problems Composite, Inattention/Hyperactivity Composite, Personal Adjustment Composite and Emotional Symptoms Index.[29]

The Behaviour Rating Inventory of Executive Function (BRIEF) was used to assess executive function. This is an 86-item parent- and teacher-rated questionnaire consisting of three summary measures: the Behavioural Regulation Index (BRI), Metacognition Index (MI) and Global Executive Composite (GEC) scales.[30] The BRI assesses significant others' perceptions of the child's ability to modulate emotions and behaviour via appropriate inhibitory control, while the MI reflects the child's ability to initiate, plan and organise self-managed tasks. Together, they yield the GEC index, which is a summary score of the child's overall performance. [30]

8.2.3 STATISTICAL ANALYSIS

Statistical analyses were performed using STATA version 11.0 (Stata-Corp, College Station, TX, USA). Comparisons of demographic and sleep-related characteristics between the groups were made using unpaired Student's t-tests. Post hoc one-sample Student's t-tests were used to compare the means of the neuropsychological measures obtained against their respective sex- and/or age-standardised mean scores. All tests were two-sided, with $P \leq 0.05$ considered statistically significant. Regression analyses were used to analyse potential associations between AHI category (≤ 2 or >2) and a number of neuropsychological assessment measures, both univariately and then multivariately adjusting for intelligence (WASI full score), age, gender and BMI Z-scores where appropriate. Although all the neuropsychological test t-scores were standardised by age, and some by gender, OSA and non-OSA group comparisons in the multivariate model all incorporated age as a covariate because age met the criteria for inclusion as a candidate variable with a $P < 0.25$.[31] BMI Z-scores were included for the same reason despite being age- and gender-adjusted.

The study was powered at the 80% level to detect a difference of one or more standard deviations between groups in relation to our most important outcome, academic assessment scores. This was based on previous studies, where medium to large group effect sizes were encountered. [17, 18] However, for the comparison of behavioural and other cognitive and executive function measures, the study may not have been powered strongly enough to detect between-group differences. Therefore, we chose to report effect sizes in addition to P values. Cohen's d was calculated to measure the between-group effect sizes using a conventional rule whereby a Cohen's d of 0.2 is considered small, 0.5 medium and 0.8 large.

TABLE 1: Demographic and sleep- and breathing-related characteristics

	All (n = 31)	Non-OSA (n = 16)	OSA (n = 15)	P value
Age (years)	13.7 (2.5)	13.1 (2.3)	14.3 (2.6)	0.186
Sex (n)				0.606
Male	13	6	7	
Female	18	10	8	
Ethnicity (%)				0.920
New Zealand European	68	69	67	
Maori	13	6	20	
Other	19	25	13	
Deprivation index	5.3 (2.0)	4.9 (2.1)	5.7 (1.9)	0.261
Parent-reported habitual snoring (%)	41	33	50	0.362
Body mass index (kg/m²)§	32.6 (4.9)	31.5 (5.6)	33.7 (3.8)	0.520
Body mass index Z-score	3.0 (0.7)	2.9 (0.9)	3.1 (0.4)	0.210
Neck circumference (cm)	38.6 (5.9)	36.8 (2.9)	40.5 (7.5)	0.074
Waist circumference (cm)	105.6 (13.1)	103.5 (13.1)	107.8 (13.3)	0.391
Tonsil size†	2.2 (2.0)	1.8 (1.9)	2.7 (2.0)	0.213
Lateral neck radiograph‡	1.6 (1.8)	1.5 (1.7)	1.7 (1.9)	0.728
Total sleep time (min)	448.3 (45.8)	450.3 (53.5)	446.1 (37.5)	0.802
Sleep efficiency (%)	83.9 (7.6)	87.0 (5.2)	80.5 (8.4)	0.014
Arousal index (No/h)	6.0 (2.4)	4.9 (1.8)	7.3 (2.5)	0.006
Percentage of total sleep time snoring, median (IQR)	5.7 (1.4–20.3)	3.0 (1.4–17.7)	15.6 (1.7 71.0)	0.050
Apnoea–hypopnoea index, median (IQR)	1.9 (0.8–4.7)	0.9 (0.5–1.2)	4.7 (2.4–8.3)	<0.001
Median SaO₂ (%)	98.8 (0.8)	99.1 (0.8)	98.5 (0.6)	0.016
SaO₂ nadir (%)	94.6 (2.8)	95.7 (1.5)	93.4 (3.5)	0.024

Unless otherwise indicated, values are given as mean (standard deviation). †Graded on the Brodsky scale[21] as the reduction in pharyngeal luminal diameter: 0–1+, 0% to 25% (score = 0); 2+, 26% to 50% (2); 3+, 51% to 75% (4); and 4+, 76% to 100% (6). ‡Adenoid hypertrophy: normal adenoid pad (score = 0) or mild (2), moderate (4) or severe adenoid hypertrophy (6). §The International Obesity Task Force approach and Cole criteria[19] were used to define obesity, conceptually equivalent to a body mass index at age 18 years of ≥30 kg/m². OSA, obstructive sleep apnoea.

8.3 RESULTS

Participant characteristics and sleep-related data are given in Table 1. The sample of 31 children (13 boys/18 girls) were predominantly New Zealand European (mean age = 13.7 years). Fifteen fulfilled the criteria for OSA, which was classed as mild ($2 > AHI \leq 5$) in 9 and moderate to severe ($AHI > 5$) in 6. Sixteen children were classed in the non-OSA group ($AHI \leq 2$). The average deprivation index of participants was 5.3 (on a scale from 1, least deprived, to 10, most deprived) with no significant difference between the non-OSA and OSA groups. Habitual snoring was common in both groups. Snoring on the PSG night was higher in the OSA group. Only three participants did not snore any time during the night. Grades for tonsil size and adenoid hypertrophy were not significantly different between groups. BMI Z-scores in the OSA group (mean = 3.1) were slightly but not significantly higher than those in the non-OSA group (mean = 2.9). The OSA group had a higher arousal index, poorer sleep efficiency and significantly lower overnight SaO_2 and SaO_2 nadir than the non-OSA group.

8.3.1 GENERAL COGNITIVE FUNCTIONING, MEMORY, LEARNING AND ACADEMIC ACHIEVEMENT

In the non-OSA group, two subtests fell below the normative data in respect of the WRAML-2 (attention and learning) and WIAT-II (reading); other assessments were comparable to normative data (Table 2). The OSA group performed significantly poorer than normative data on several of the subtests. Comparing OSA and non-OSA groups, significantly lower WIAT-II maths scores were found in the OSA group ($P = 0.034$), producing a large effect size. The association became non-significant when controlling for IQ, age, gender and BMI Z-score. IQ was the strongest predictor in this association. No other statistically significant differences were found between groups, although some measures (but not memory measures) returned medium to large effect sizes.

TABLE 2: Summary of cognitive measures according to OSA group

Assessment	Standard score, mean (95% confidence interval)		Between-group differences		
	Non-OSA	OSA	Unadjusted P value	Adjusted P value†	Cohen's d
WASI					
Verbal	97.5 (89.5–105.4)	89.9 (84.6–95.3)*	0.107	NA	−0.61
Performance	95.4 (85.0–105.9)	95.3 (88.6–101.9)	0.977	NA	−0.01
Full	98.2 (91.5–104.9)	91.5 (85.9–97.2)*	0.118	NA	−0.59
WRAML-2					
Verbal memory	106.1 (99.4–112.8)	105.3 (99.6–110.9)	0.836	0.268	−0.08
Visual memory	93.6 (87.1–100.2)	89.3 (80.2–98.4)	0.414	0.399	−0.30
Attention and learning	88.7 (81.3–96.0)*	91.0 (84.6–97.4)*	0.618	0.066	0.19
Global score	94.8 (86.8–102.8)	93.5 (88.2–98.9)*	0.781	0.377	−0.10
WIAT-II					
Maths	94.6 (87.1–102.2)	84.5 (78.6–90.5)**	0.034	0.234	−0.82
Reading	92.3 (86.3–98.2)*	86.9 (81.3–92.5)**	0.169	0.408	−0.52

*P ≤ 0.05; **P ≤ 0.001; significant difference from standard score normative mean of 100 (standard deviation = 15). All test scores are coded such that higher scores reflect better performance. †Adjusted analyses included IQ (WASI full score), age, gender and body mass index Z-score as covariates. OSA, obstructive sleep apnoea; WASI, Wechsler Abbreviated Scale of Intelligence; WIAT-II, Wechsler Individual Achievement Test II; WRAML-2, Wide Range Assessment of Memory and Learning 2.

TABLE 3: Summary of behaviour measures according to OSA group (Behavioural Assessment System for Children 2)

Assessment	t-Score, mean (95% confidence interval)		Between-group differences		
	Non-OSA	OSA	Unadjusted P value	Adjusted P value†	Cohen's d
Self-report of Personality					
School problems	50.8 (47.0–54.7)	61.4 (54.0–68.5)*	0.010	0.026	1.02
Internalising problems	48.7 (45.1–52.2)	55.5 (47.9–63.1)	0.085	0.343	0.66
Inattention/hyperactivity	54.8 (50.6–58.9)	60.1 (53.7–66.6)*	0.138	0.256	0.57
Emotional Symptom Index	50.2 (45.9–54.5)	56.4 (49.4–63.4)	0.112	0.467	0.61
Personal adjustment	49.2 (44.3–54.1)	42.7 (36.3–49.2)*	0.096	0.403	−0.64
Parent Rating Scale					
Internalising problems	56.3 (50.1–62.5)	62.4 (53.2–71.6)*	0.252	0.384	0.44
Externalising problems	53.1 (48.4–57.7)*	62.1 (50.3–73.9)*	0.139	0.149	0.57
Behavioural Symptoms Index	55.3 (49.8–61.3)	63.7 (53.1–74.4)*	0.157	0.263	0.55
Adaptive skills	47.2 (41.0–53.4)	42.8 (37.6–48.0)*	0.254	0.899	−0.44
Teacher Rating Scale					
Internalising problems	52.9 (46.5–59.2)	56.8 (52.4–61.2)*	0.301	0.957	0.44
Externalising problems	52.6 (44.5–60.7)	58.4 (46.1–70.7)	0.379	0.353	0.37
School problems	55.5 (46.6–64.4)	57.5 (51.1–64.2)*	0.705	0.847	0.16
Behavioural Symptoms Index	55.2 (48.2–62.3)	59.1 (48.9–69.3)	0.486	0.746	0.30
Adaptive skills	45.2 (39.3–51.1)	44.8 (37.7–52.0)	0.926	0.598	−0.04

*$P \leq 0.05$; **$P \leq 0.001$; significant difference from t-score normative mean of 50 (standard deviation = 10). Scores are coded such that lower scores reflect better performance, except for adaptive skills and personal adjustment, where higher scores indicate better adjustment. †Adjusted analyses included IQ (Wechsler Abbreviated Scale of Intelligence full score), age and body mass index Z-score as covariates. OSA, obstructive sleep apnoea.

TABLE 4: Summary of executive function measures according to OSA group (Behaviour Rating Inventory of Executive Function)

Assessment	t-Score, mean (95% confidence interval)		Between-group differences		
	Non-OSA	OSA	Unadjusted P value	Adjusted P value†	Cohen's d
Parent report					
Behaviour Rating Inventory	57.7 (50.6–64.8)*	62.5 (53.9–71.1)*	0.364	0.062	0.35
Metacognition Index	62.1 (56.0–68.2)*	62.4 (55.5–69.3)*	0.940	0.632	0.03
Global	63.0 (56.6–69.4)**	63.3 (55.5–71.1)*	0.944	0.490	0.03
Teacher report					
Behaviour Rating Inventory	59.8 (50.9–66.6)*	65.7 (52.1–79.3)*	0.316	0.361	0.43
Metacognition Index	65.6 (54.0–77.3)*	70.5 (61.0–79.9)**	0.507	0.910	0.28
Global	62.8 (52.0–73.6)*	70.4 (59.1–81.9)*	0.300	0.610	0.44

*P ≤ 0.05; **P ≤ 0.001; significant difference from t-score mean of 50 (standard deviation = 10). All test scores are coded such that lower scores reflect better performance. †Adjusted analyses included IQ (Wechsler Abbreviated Scale of Intelligence full score), age and body mass index Z-score as covariates. OSA, obstructive sleep apnoea.

8.3.2 BEHAVIOUR

For the non-OSA group, the variables of self-report of inattention/hyperactivity scores and parent report of executive functioning were statistically higher (i.e. indicating poorer performance) than the normative data, but still within the average (non-clinical) range (Table 3). The OSA group had poorer ratings relative to normative data for self- and teacher-reported school problems and inattention/hyperactivity, parent- and teacher-reported internalising problems, parent-reported externalising behaviour, adaptive skills and the composite score for behaviour (Behavioural Symptoms Index). The composite score for self-report of problematic schooling was significantly higher in the OSA than in the non-OSA group, and several other self- and parent-reported measures yielded medium effect sizes.

8.3.3 EXECUTIVE FUNCTIONING

Both OSA and non-OSA groups' scores for the three indices of parent and teacher-reported executive functioning difficulties were more than one SD above the normative (age and sex-normed) mean (Table 4). None were in the clinical range. No statistically significant differences were found between the OSA and non-OSA groups in respect of executive function measures, and group effect sizes were small and below the medium cut-off.

8.4 DISCUSSION

This study investigated possible neurobehavioural deficits attributable to OSA in a small sample of children with obesity. In line with previous research,[17, 18] obese children/adolescents with OSA displayed worse performance in relation to achievement assessments compared with those without OSA, with some evidence for general behavioural deficits and less consistent evidence for other cognitive deficits. Within our study, two variables within subscales for academic achievement and behaviour yielded the strongest associations with OSA. These were maths performance and self-report of school problems, although general cognitive functioning as assessed by IQ explained a considerable amount of the relationship with maths performance. Mathematical skills require multiple precursor pathways involving several distinct cognitive systems[32] that could be compromised in OSA, where both sleep disruption and repetitive hypoxaemia are involved.[33] The strong relations between intelligence and academic achievement in maths[34] and between intelligence and executive functioning[35, 36] provide justification for controlling for full IQ in respect of maths skills. Although not statistically significant, effect sizes suggest that the OSA group performed more poorly on a variety of measures, particularly IQ, visual memory (which could be related to poorer maths performance) and reading. A large group effect size (OSA vs. non-

OSA) was found for maths scores, compared with a medium effect size for reading. Reading skills do not rely so much on aspects of working memory as maths skills do and are highly practiced.

Previous studies have found an association between the combination of OSA and obesity/overweight and poorer academic functioning using a variety of measures,[11, 17, 18] including maths scores,[18] but none have considered IQ as a covariate in the analysis. Many studies of younger children (non-obese cohorts) have consistently shown a significant link between poorer school performance, including maths scores, and OSA.[11, 37-39] Some research suggests the underlying mechanism linking OSA to poorer academic achievement is hypoxia,[38] but this remains uncertain, as other research links persistent snoring or OSA to poorer school performance independent of hypoxic status.[37, 39]

We found that self-report of school problems yielded the largest effect size and, within our small sample, was significantly associated with OSA before and after adjusting for covariates. The school problem score is a composite of the participant's subjective experience of teachers and school, including responder ratings to statements such as 'school is boring' and 'teachers make me feel stupid'. This is likely an important influence, as student engagement and connectedness to school are associated with academic performance.[40] However, with this score being self-report, there could be limitations in precision. No other behavioural domains played out in the group comparison data. However, the wide confidence intervals and medium effect sizes for several measures do not rule out the possibility that a larger sample size may expose important differences. In previous studies, habitual snoring has been related to as many or more behaviour and executive function problems than moderate to severe OSA, and sometimes across multiple domains.[9, 10] Thus another possible explanation for deficits across all for executive functioning, irrespective of OSA status, relates to our findings that habitual snoring was common in both OSA and non-OSA groups.

The obesity–OSA combination in respect of behavioural outcomes in children/adolescents is a relatively unexplored field. Owens et al.[41] reported poorer behavioural outcomes, particularly internalising behaviour, related to weight in children with OSA aged 3 to 18 years, and Beebe et al.[11] reported some subscales of parent- and teacher-reported poorer behavioural functioning associated with OSA. In younger children, one study showed behavioural problems were highly prevalent in all children with OSA, but the problems existed independently of whether children were obese or of normal weight.[42] Studies of behaviours associated with OSA specific to the adolescent age group, irrespective of weight status, are sparse.

In the current study, executive functioning as rated by parents and teachers on the BRIEF yielded small to medium effect sizes for OSA groups compared with non-OSA. Although a larger sample size may have produced a statistically significant association between poorer executive functioning and OSA, a null finding is consistent with that reported by Hannon et al.[18] in a comparable study. We observed ratings of poorer performance within the obese cohort (irrespective of OSA status) compared with normative data. Two studies using the BRIEF in mainly normal-weight children[10, 11] did not find a clear relationship with executive functioning across the spectrum of SDB severity, although one did show a high proportion of children with SDB whose executive functioning was impaired compared with normal population estimates, that is, above one standard deviation from the mean.[10] Thus, one possible explanation is that obesity in older children and adolescents may be associated with poorer executive function, which might make establishing significant associations with OSA more difficult (e.g. a larger sample size might be needed). Indeed, there is some evidence that executive dysfunction might be present in obese children and adolescents.[43] Without a concurrent normal-weight control group, we cannot confirm this within the current study, and to the best of our knowledge, no additional studies aside from that of Hannon et al.[18] focus on OSA and executive function in obese children/adolescents. The BRIEF represents informant ratings; therefore, poorer performance ratings could be influenced by other factors that influence adolescents' daily functioning, such as possible disengagement from or disaffection with the learning environment.

Some further limitations require discussion. First, the study was small and cross-sectional and relied on parent- and self-report, militating against strong conclusions being drawn, especially inferences about causality. No control group was included, limiting an assessment of the effect of the severity of OSA on neurobehavioural outcomes and comparisons with normal-weight participants. The study was powered sufficiently for educational assessment measures based on previous reports[17, 18] but perhaps not strongly enough for the other neurobehavioural outcomes, and for this reason, Cohen's d was calculated to demonstrate between-group effect sizes. Anecdotally, we found it very difficult to engage obese children and adolescents within this age range, possibly due to the sensitive nature of the topic of obesity and perhaps linked to the greater risk of adjustment difficulties in obese youths than in non-obese youths in respect of depression, anxiety and lower self-esteem.[44, 45] These difficulties point to the need for enhanced strategies to engage obese children/adolescents in research of this nature. Strengths of the study include the objective assessment of OSA using PSG, considered the gold standard in OSA diagnostics in both adults and children. Participants' BMI eligibility for the study was assessed according to well-established BMI-for-age standards.[19]

To our knowledge, this is the third study within this age group specifically addressing neurobehavioural correlates in combined OSA and obesity. The two other comparable studies were also small[17, 18] but also used robust methods for sleep, respiratory and neuropsychological assessments and yielded analogous findings exposing deficiencies in some educational achievement assessments. The evidence for associations between OSA and other cognitive and behavioural outcomes, including memory, in obese youth remains mixed and requires evidence from larger studies to clarify potential associations. In this study, neither memory nor executive functioning were implicated. Memory has been previously implicated in one study only.[17] In addition, longitudinal studies and comparison studies with normal-weight adolescents suffering OSA are required. Inclusion of measures of neuropsychological covariates in the OSA–obesity combination would be valuable. Current treatment modalities for OSA in obese children and adolescents include weight loss. One study of overweight children reported that over two-thirds with OSA reduced their AHI to ≤ 2 with weight loss.[46] Whether or not improvements in daytime functioning go hand in hand remains to be determined. A causal model to delineate the physiological, neuropsychological and psychosocial pathways whereby OSA affects neurobehavioural functioning in both obese and non-obese cohorts will no doubt be complex but, at some point, may be possible through continued research efforts.

REFERENCES

1. Marcus CL, Brooks LJ, Draper KA et al. Diagnosis and management of childhood obstructive sleep apnea syndrome. Pediatrics 2012; 130: e714–755.
2. Shine NP, Coates HL, Lannigan FJ. Obstructive sleep apnea, morbid obesity, and adenotonsillar surgery: a review of the literature. Int. J. Pediatr. Otorhinolaryngol. 2005; 69: 1475–1482.
3. Wing YK, Hui SH, Pak WM et al. A controlled study of sleep related disordered breathing in obese children. Arch. Dis. Child. 2003; 88: 1043–1047.
4. Beebe D. Neurobehavioral morbidity associated with disordered breathing during sleep in children: a comprehensive review. Sleep 2006; 29: 1115–1134.
5. Arens R, Marcus CL. Pathophysiology of upper airway obstruction: a developmental perspective. Sleep 2004; 27: 997–1019.
6. Kohler MJ, Thormaehlen S, Kennedy JD et al. Differences in the association between obesity and obstructive sleep apnea among children and adolescents. J. Clin. Sleep Med. 2009; 5: 506–511.
7. O'Brien LM. The neurocognitive effects of sleep disruption in children and adolescents. Child Adolesc. Psychiatr. Clin. N. Am. 2009; 18: 813–823.
8. Blunden S, Lushington K, Kennedy D, Martin J, Dawson D. Behaviour and neurocognitive performance in children aged 5–10 years who snore compared to controls. J. Clin. Exp. Neuropsychol. 2000; 22: 554–568.
9. Beebe DW, Wells CT, Jeffries J, Chini B, Kalra M, Amin R. Neuropsychological effects of pediatric obstructive sleep apnea. J. Int. Neuropsychol. Soc. 2004; 10: 962–975.
10. Bourke RS, Anderson V, Yang JS et al. Neurobehavioural function is impaired in children with all severities of sleep disordered breathing. Sleep Med. 2011; 12: 222–229.
11. Beebe DW, Ris MD, Kramer ME, Long E, Amin R. The association between sleep disordered breathing, academic grades, and cognitive and behavioral functioning among overweight subjects during middle to late childhood. Sleep 2010; 33: 1447–1456.
12. Galland BC, Dawes PJ, Tripp EG, Taylor BJ. Changes in behaviour and attentional capacity after adenotonsillectomy. Pediatr. Res. 2006; 59: 711–716.
13. Friedman BC, Hendeles-Amitai A, Kozminsky E et al. Adenotonsillectomy improves neurocognitive function in children with obstructive sleep apnea syndrome. Sleep 2003; 26: 999–1005.
14. Swallen KC, Reither EN, Haas SA, Meier AM. Overweight, obesity, and health-related quality of life among adolescents: the National Longitudinal Study of Adolescent Health. Pediatrics 2005; 115: 340–347.
15. Falkner NH, Neumark-Sztainer D, Story M et al. Social, educational, and psychological correlates of weight status in adolescents. Obes. Res. 2001; 9: 32–42.
16. de Beer M, Hofsteenge GH, Koot HM et al. Health-related-quality-of-life in obese adolescents is decreased and inversely related to BMI. Acta Paediatr. 2007; 96: 710–714.
17. Rhodes SK, Shimoda KC, Waid LR et al. Neurocognitive deficits in morbidly obese children with obstructive sleep apnea. J. Pediatr. 1995; 127: 741–744.

18. Hannon TS, Rofey DL, Ryan CM, Clapper DA, Chakravorty S, Arslanian SA. Relationships among obstructive sleep apnea, anthropometric measures, and neurocognitive functioning in adolescents with severe obesity. J. Pediatr. 2012; 160: 732–735.

19. Cole TJ, Bellizzi MC, Flegal KM, Dietz WH. Establishing a standard definition for child overweight and obesity worldwide: international survey. BMJ 2000; 320: 1240–1243.

20. Goldstein NA, Pugazhendhi V, Rao SM et al. Clinical assessment of pediatric obstructive sleep apnea. Pediatrics 2004; 114: 33–43.

21. Brodsky L. Modern assessment of tonsils and adenoids. Pediatr. Clin. North Am. 1989; 36: 1551–1569.

22. Salmond C, Crampton P, Atkinson J. NZDep2006 Index of Deprivation user's manual. Wellington: Department of Public Health, University of Otago; 2007.

23. Rechtschaffen A, Kales A. A Manual of Standardized Terminology, Techniques, and Scoring Systems for Sleep Stages of Human Subjects. Los Angeles: Brain Information Service/Brain Research Institute , University of California–Los Angeles, 1968.

24. Uliel S, Tauman R, Greenfeld M, Sivan Y. Normal polysomnographic respiratory values in children and adolescents. Chest 2004; 125: 872–878.

25. Verhulst SL, Schrauwen N, Haentjens D, Van Gaal L, De Backer WA, Desager KN. Reference values for sleep-related respiratory variables in asymptomatic European children and adolescents. Pediatr. Pulmonol. 2007; 42: 159–167.

26. The Psychological Corporation. Wechsler Abbreviated Scale of Intelligence (WASI) Manual. San Antonio, TX: Harcourt Assessment, 1999.

27. Sheslow D, Adams W. Wide Range Assessment of Memory and Learning – Second Edition Administration and Technical Manual. Wilmington, DE: Wide Range, Inc., 2003.

28. Wechsler D. Wechsler Individual Achievement Test – Second Edition – Australian Standardised Edition. San Antonio, TX: Harcourt Assessment, 2002.

29. Reynolds CR, Kamphaus RW. Behaviour Assessment System for Children, 2nd edn. Minneapolis, MN: NCS Pearson, 2004.

30. Gioia GA, Isquith PK, Guy SC, Kenworthy L. Behaviour Rating Inventory of Executive Function (BRIEF). Odessa, FL: Psychological Assessment Resources, 2000.

31. Hosmer DW, Lemeshow S. Applied Logistic Regression. New York: John Wiley & Sons, 1989.

32. LeFevre JA, Fast L, Skwarchuk SL et al. Pathways to mathematics: longitudinal predictors of performance. Child Dev. 2010; 81: 1753–1767.

33. Beebe DW, Gozal D. Obstructive sleep apnea and the prefrontal cortex: towards a comprehensive model linking nocturnal upper airway obstruction to daytime cognitive and behavioural deficits. J. Sleep Res. 2002; 11: 1–16.

34. Lynn R, Meisenberg G, Mikk J, Williams A. National IQs predict differences in scholastic achievement in 67 countries. J. Biosoc. Sci. 2007; 39: 861–874.

35. Ardila A, Pineda D, Rosselli M. Correlation between intelligence test scores and executive function measures. Arch. Clin. Neuropsychol. 2000; 15: 31–63.

36. Weyandt LL, Mitzlaff L, Thomas L. The relationship between intelligence and performance on the test of variables of attention (TOVA). J. Learn. Disabil. 2002; 35: 114–120.

37. Uema SF, Pignatari SS, Fujita RR, Moreira GA, Pradella-Hallinan M, Weckx L. Assessment of cognitive learning function in children with obstructive sleep breathing disorders. Braz. J. Otorhinolaryngol. 2007; 73: 315–320.
38. Gozal D. Sleep-disordered breathing and school performance in children. Pediatrics 1998; 102: 616–620.
39. Urschitz MS, Guenther A, Eggebrecht E et al. Snoring, intermittent hypoxia and academic performance in primary school children. Am. J. Respir. Crit. Care Med. 2003; 168: 464–468.
40. Reyes MR, Brackett MA, Rivers SE, White M, Salovey P. Classroom emotional climate, student engagement, and academic achievement. J. Educ. Psychol. 2012; 104: 700–712.
41. Owens JA, Mehlenbeck R, Lee J, King MM. Effect of weight, sleep duration, and comorbid sleep disorders on behavioral outcomes in children with sleep-disordered breathing. Arch. Pediatr. Adolesc. Med. 2008; 162: 313–321.
42. Rudnick EF, Mitchell RB. Behaviour and obstructive sleep apnea in children: is obesity a factor? Laryngoscope 2007; 117: 1463–1466.
43. Lokken KL, Boeka AG, Austin HM, Gunstad J, Harmon CM. Evidence of executive dysfunction in extremely obese adolescents: a pilot study. Surg. Obes. Relat. Dis. 2009; 5: 547–552.
44. Griffiths LJ, Parsons TJ, Hill AJ. Self-esteem and quality of life in obese children and adolescents: a systematic review. Int. J. Pediatr. Obes. 2010; 5: 282–304.
45. Kalarchian MA, Marcus MD. Psychiatric comorbidity of childhood obesity. Int. Rev. Psychiatry 2012; 24: 241–246.
46. Verhulst SL, Franckx H, Van Gaal L, De Backer W, Desager K. The effect of weight loss on sleep-disordered breathing in obese teenagers. Obesity (Silver Spring) 2010; 17: 1178–1183.

PART III

IMPLICATIONS AND CONSEQUENCES

CHAPTER 9

WEIGHT STATUS AND WEIGHT-MANAGEMENT BEHAVIORS AMONG PHILADELPHIA HIGH SCHOOL STUDENTS, 2007–2011

CLARE M. LENHART, KATHERINE W. BAUER, AND FREDA PATTERSON

9.1 INTRODUCTION

Recent data suggest that rates of childhood obesity in the United States are no longer rising (1). This stabilization has provided optimism that clinical and public health efforts to stem the childhood obesity epidemic have begun to take effect (2). Consistent with these national findings, recent data from Philadelphia showed declines in obesity rates among students in grades kindergarten through 12; rates among students in grades kindergarten through 8 and among male students declined significantly. Among students in grades 9 through 12, the prevalence of obesity declined, although not significantly, between 2006–2007 and 2009–2010 (3). The confluence

Reprinted with permission from the Centers for Disease Control and Prevention. Lenhart CM, Bauer KW, Patterson F. Weight Status and Weight-Management Behaviors Among Philadelphia High School Students, 2007–2011. Preventing Chronic Disease: Public Health Research, Practice, and Policy **10** (2013), DOI: *http://dx.doi.org/10.5888/pcd10.130087.*

of national attention to childhood obesity and programmatic and policy-based interventions in Philadelphia may account for these declines (3).

Although obesity rates among youth have reached a plateau or are decreasing among some populations, it remains important to identify the behavioral changes associated with these trends. For example, limiting the intake of sugar-sweetened beverages and time spent watching television are effective ways to help adolescents prevent excessive weight gain (4,5). It is also essential to consider whether the heightened focus on obesity in schools and communities across the United States is prompting adolescents to use weight-loss strategies that are harmful or counterproductive—such as fasting or using diet pills or laxatives—to healthful weight management (6).

The objective of our study was to examine whether the stabilization in obesity prevalence among Philadelphia high school students observed in a previous study (3) was accompanied by changes in weight-management behaviors. Study findings will offer insight into the weight-management behaviors of urban high school students, including those who want to lose weight. Findings may also illuminate whether the sharpened focus on childhood obesity has unintended consequences.

9.2 METHODS

We used data collected in Philadelphia by the Youth Risk Behavior Survey (YRBS). The YRBS is a surveillance system maintained by the Centers for Disease Control and Prevention to monitor youth health behaviors. The survey uses a 2-stage cluster sampling design to produce a representative sample of high school students; it is administered biennially. Standard YRBS procedures require passive parental consent, and nonopposing students are invited to anonymously complete the in-school survey. The survey is provided in a multiple-choice, self-administered, paper-and-pencil format (7). We used data collected for the Philadelphia YRBS in 2007 (N = 2,119), 2009 (N = 1,165) and 2011 (N = 1,239). In each of the data collection years, the school participation rate was 76% or more; within schools, of the students invited to complete the survey, the response rate ranged from 76% in 2007 to 78% in 2011.

TABLE 1: Demographic Characteristics of Participating High School Students, Study on Weight Status and Weight-Management Behaviors, Philadelphia, 2007–2011

Characteristic	2007			2009			2011		
	Unweighted Count	Weighted Estimate (SD)	%	Unweighted Count	Weighted Estimate (SD)	%	Unweighted Count	Weighted Estimate (SD)	%
Total	2,119	39,867 (1,838)	—	1,165	37,982 (1,846)	—	1,239	34,509 (1,292)	—
Sex									
Female	1,194	22,875 (1,222)	57.4	653	19,840 (1,176)	52.2	669	17,645 (901)	51.1
Male	925	16,993 (1,115)	42.6	512	18,141 (1,302)	47.8	570	16,864 (974)	48.9
Age, y									
≤14	170	3,442 (570)	8.6	57	2,562 (471)	6.7	122	3,434 (637)	10.0
15	544	9,644 (1,215)	24.2	260	10,249 (1,255)	27.0	295	8,540 (1,037)	24.7
16	644	11,244 (1,001)	28.2	380	10,489 (973)	27.6	324	9,312 (941)	27.0
17	550	10,996 (1,225)	27.6	332	8,661 (892)	2.8	300	7,597 (845)	22.0
≥18	211	4,542 (734)	11.4	136	6,020 (1,461)	15.8	198	5,626 (816)	16.3
Race/ethnicity									
African American	1,191	214,690 (970)	53.9	643	24,868 (1,434)	65.5	648	20,430 (961)	59.2
Non-Hispanic white	291	5,480 (923)	13.7	143	4,825 (663)	12.7	164	5,080 (643)	14.7
Hispanic	138	3,206 (565)	8.0	98	2,249 (367)	5.9	99	2,407 (315)	7.0
Asian	184	3,377 (601)	8.5	87	1,663 (252)	4.4	122	1,948 (235)	5.6
Mixed race/other	315	6,336 (517)	15.9	194	4,377 (424)	11.5	206	4,636 (429)	13.4

We examined the following demographic variables: sex, age, and race/ethnicity. Body mass index (BMI) was calculated by using self-reported weight (kg) divided by the square of self-reported height (m); age- and sex-specific BMI percentiles were computed (8). Students whose BMI was at or above the 95th percentile were considered obese; students whose BMI was in the 85th through 94th percentile were considered overweight (9).

We also evaluated the following weight-related variables: weight perception, weight-loss intention, soda consumption (≥1 soda per day in past week), fruit and vegetable consumption (≥5 servings per day in past week), physical activity levels, screen time (television viewing and recreational computer use), and extreme weight-management strategies (Appendix). Because only 1.2% of students were classified as underweight during the study period, we classified underweight students as normal-weight students. Weight perception was measured by using a single item that asked students to self-identify as being one of the following: very underweight, slightly underweight, about the right weight, slightly overweight, or very overweight. Accurate weight perception was defined as being overweight or obese per BMI and self-identifying as overweight (either slightly or very) or as being of normal weight per BMI and self-identifying as normal weight. We classified as inaccurate all other combinations of BMI category and perceived weights status.

Physical activity levels were evaluated as a single item that asked students on how many days of the past 7 days they were active for at least 60 minutes; responses were dichotomized to 0 through 4 days and 5 or more days because 5 days or more of activity per week is recommended by the American College of Sports Medicine (10). Screen time was measured as average hours per day of television viewing and recreational computer use (combined); responses were dichotomized as 0 or 1 hour and 2 or more hours (11). Use of extreme weight-management strategies was measured by 3 yes/no questions on the use of fasting; diet pills, powders, or liquids; and vomiting in the past 30 days. Earlier versions of the YRBS have demonstrated appropriate validity and reliability (12,7).

We conducted statistical analyses on weighted data by using SAS, version 9.3, PROC SURVEY procedures (SAS Institute, Inc, Cary, North Carolina) to account for the complex sampling design of the YRBS. Sampling errors were estimated by using the primary sampling units and strata provided in the data and calculated through Taylor series linearization. Sampling weights were used to adjust for nonresponse and oversampling and to allow for generalizability of findings to the population of high school students in Philadelphia. We used descriptive statistics to examine the demographic characteristics of the samples. Individual multivariable regression models were developed to examine the prevalence of each of the study outcomes across the 3 study years. Regression models included students' race/ethnicity and age as covariates to account for differences in these demographic characteristics across the study years. We used the F statistic to identify significant differences in the estimated prevalence rates across survey years and made post-hoc comparisons of prevalence rates for outcomes for which the overall F statistic indicated differences. Similar regression models and corresponding F statistics were developed to examine changes in weight-management behaviors among overweight and obese students who indicated a desire to lose weight.

9.3 RESULTS

The demographic composition of the sample was stable during the study period (Table 1). The proportion of female students ranged from 57% in 2007 to 51% in 2011. In 2007, an estimated 9% of respondents were aged 14 years or younger; 24% were aged 15, 28% were aged 16, 28% were aged 17, and 11% were aged 18 years or older. Approximately 54% were African American, 14% white, 8% Hispanic, 9% Asian, and 16% mixed race/ethnicity or other.

We found no significant differences in the prevalence of obesity or overweight among female students from 2007 to 2011 (Table 2). In 2007, 31.1% of female students reported having at least 1 soda per day; this proportion decreased to 22.5% in 2011 (P = .001). Additionally, the prevalence of female students engaging in 5 or more days of physical activity in the previous week increased from 26.0% in 2007 to 31.9% in 2011 (P = .003). However, the prevalence of female students who reported fasting to lose weight also increased significantly from 12.2% in 2007 to 17.0% in 2011 (P = .02). We observed no other significant differences in weight-management behaviors or weight perceptions among female students.

TABLE 2: Self-Reported Weight Status and Weight-Management Behaviors Among Female and Male High School Students, Philadelphia, 2007–2011[a]

Characteristic	Females				Males			
	2007, % (SE)	2009, % (SE)	2011, % (SE)	$F_{2,101}$ (P)	2007, % (SE)	2009, % (SE)	2011, % (SE)	$F_{2,101}$ (P)
Overweight	18.3 (0.01)	21.8 (0.02)	22.3 (0.02)	2.74 (.07)	18.0 (0.01)	16.5 (0.02)	14.2 (0.01)	1.92 (.15)
Obese	14.5 (0.01)	14.2 (0.02)	13.9 (0.01)	0.06 (.94)	17.2 (0.01)	19.4 (0.02)	19.4 (0.02)	0.64 (.53)
Inaccurate weight perception	63.9 (0.03)	59.0 (0.03)	62.1 (0.03)	1.26 (.29)	52.7 (0.03)	56.8 (0.03)	53.9 (0.03)	0.89 (.41)
Trying to lose weight	50.6 (0.02)	54.8 (0.02)	52.2 (0.02)	0.97 (.38)	31.2 (0.02)	33.6 (0.03)	29.6 (.03)	1.2 (.31)
Consumes ≥1 soda per day	31.1[b] (0.02)	25.5[b,c] (0.02)	22.5[c] (0.02)	7.0 (.001)	29.3 (0.02)	29.2 (0.03)	24.2 (0.02)	1.94 (.15)
Consumes ≥5 servings of fruit and vegetables per day	17.0 (0.01)	15.5 (0.02)	18.7 (0.02)	0.83 (.44)	18.6 (0.01)	19.3 (0.02)	19.7 (0.02)	0.09 (.91)
Performs ≥5 days of physical activity per week	26.0[b] (0.01)	23.6[b] (0.02)	31.9[c] (0.02)	6.14 (.003)	37.5 (0.02)	41.4 (0.03)	40.0 (0.02)	0.95 (.39)
Spends ≥2 hours of screen time per day	72.9 (0.01)	73.9 (0.02)	69.1 (0.02)	2.01 (.14)	67.8[b] (0.02)	77.0[c] (0.02)	68.2[b] (0.02)	6.24 (.003)
Extreme weight-management behavior								
Any extreme weight-management behavior	19.7 (0.01)	22.4 (0.02)	23.6 (0.02)	1.98 (.14)	16.9 (0.01)	14.8 (0.03)	19.3 (0.02)	1.06 (.35)
Fasting	12.2[b] (0.01)	13.1[b,c] (0.02)	17.0[c] (0.02)	4.10 (.02)	9.2 (0.01)	6.9 (0.01)	11.2 (0.01)	2.08 (.13)
Diet pills	4.8 (0.01)	6.6 (0.01)	6.2 (0.01)	1.05 (.35)	4.0 (0.01)	4.8 (0.01)	3.3 (0.01)	0.41 (.67)
Vomiting	4.7 (0.01)	7.0 (0.01)	5.0 (0.01)	1.09 (.34)	5.5 (0.01)	4.8 (0.01)	3.1 (0.02)	2.05 (.13)

[a] Models adjusted for students' age, race/ethnicity, and complex sampling strategy.
[b,c] Within this row, percentages that share a common superscripted letter (b or c) are not statistically different at an a level of .05. Percentages that do not share a common superscripted letter are statistically different.

TABLE 3: Prevalence of Inaccurate Weight Perception and Use of Weight-Management Behaviors Among Overweight and Obese Female and Male Students Who Report Trying to Lose Weight, Philadelphia, 2007–2011[a]

Characteristic	Females				Males			
	2007, % (SE)	2009, % (SE)	2011, % (SE)	F_2 (P)	2007, % (SE)	2009, % (SE)	2011, % (SE)	F_2 (P)
Inaccurate weight perception	48.3 (0.03)	43.0 (0.05)	47.0 (0.05)	0.5 (.61)	34.9 (0.04)	28.5 (0.05)	31.3 (0.04)	0.7 (.50)
Consumes ≥1 soda per day	23.7 (0.02)	19.7 (0.03)	18.6 (0.03)	1.08 (.34)	26.4 (0.03)	27.5 (0.05)	23.3 (0.04)	0.24 (.79)
Consumes ≥5 servings of fruits and vegetables per day	19.5[b] (0.02)	10.4[c] (0.02)	17.2[b,c] (0.03)	4.03 (.02)	22.7 (0.03)	17.1 (0.03)	16.6 (0.04)	0.9 (.40)
Performs ≥5 days of physical activity per week	23.3[b] (0.02)	22.9[b,c] (0.04)	32.6[c] (0.03)	3.69 (.03)	26.1 (0.04)	36.3 (0.06)	32.8 (0.05)	1.14 (.33)
Spends ≥2 hours of screen time per day	75.6 (0.03)	75.1 (0.03)	71.9 (0.04)	0.4 (.67)	75.9 (0.03)	80.1 (0.04)	73.4 (0.04)	0.84 (.43)
Extreme weight-management behavior								
Any extreme weight-management behavior	28.4 (0.03)	32.5 (0.04)	32.7 (0.04)	0.81 (.45)	23.9 (0.03)	17.3 (0.04)	21.7 (0.04)	0.91 (.41)
Fasting	16.4 (0.02)	18.6 (0.03)	24.4 (0.03)	2.7 (.07)	15.7 (0.03)	10.4 (0.03)	16.6 (0.04)	1.62 (.20)
Diet pills	9.4 (0.02)	15.9 (0.04)	11.1 (0.02)	1.62 (.20)	2.7 (0.01)	8.6 (0.04)	3.0 (0.02)	1.37 (.26)
Vomiting	7.9 (0.02)	9.8 (0.03)	7.8 (0.02)	0.24 (.79)	9.1 (0.03)	5.9 (0.02)	2.1 (0.02)	3.10 (.05)

[a] Models adjusted for students' age and race/ethnicity.

[b, c] Within this row, percentages that share a common superscripted letter (b or c) are not statistically different at an α level of .05. Percentages that do not share a common superscripted letter are statistically different.

Among male students, we found no significant differences in the prevalence of overweight or obesity during the study period (Table 2). The percentage of male students reporting 2 or more hours of screen time per day increased significantly from 67.8% in 2007 to 77.0% in 2009 (P = .003). We observed no other significant differences in weight-management behaviors or weight perceptions among male students.

In 2011, the final survey year, 79.0% of overweight or obese female students and 63.9% of overweight or obese male students expressed a desire to lose weight, compared with 25.2% of normal-weight female students and 15.1% of normal-weight male students. Among overweight or obese students who wanted to lose weight, we found a significant increase in physical activity and a significant decrease in fruit and vegetable consumption (Table 3) among female students but no significant changes in weight management behaviors among male students. Among these students in 2011, approximately one-fifth (18.6% of females, 23.3% males) reported having at least 1 soda per day, and three-quarters (71.9% of females, 73.4% males) participated in 2 or more hours of screen time each day. Almost one-third of students engaged in 5 or more days of physical activity in the previous week (32.6% of females, 32.8% males) or had 5 servings of fruits and vegetables each day (17.2% of females, 16.6% males). One-third of female students (32.7%) and one-fifth of male students (21.7%) reported using extreme weight-management behaviors.

9.4 DISCUSSION

The current study examined trends in weight status and weight-management behaviors using a representative sample of high school students in Philadelphia. Among these students, we found no significant differences in the prevalence of overweight or obesity according to self-reported height and weight. These findings align with those of another study (3), which found no significant changes in the prevalence of obesity among high school students in Philadelphia and used measured height and weight. Although these trends are encouraging because they may represent a slowing of the youth obesity epidemic, the continued and consistent high prevalence of overweight and obesity among male and female students is a public health problem. Even with a leveling of obesity rates, an estimated 30% of boys and 40% of girls born in the year 2000 are expected to develop diabetes in their lifetime (13). The burden of childhood obesity across the lifespan—for the individual in terms of physical and psychological co-morbid conditions (14) and for society in terms of elevated health care costs (15)—is considerable. Therefore, reducing youth overweight and obesity rates remains a public health priority.

The weight-management behaviors of a diverse sample of urban youth reported here are sources of concern. Although we observed improvements in the consumption of sugar-sweetened beverages and participation in regular physical activity among female students, levels of participation in many behaviors important for healthful weight management are still low. Similarly, of the obese and overweight students who reported trying to lose weight, most reported high levels of screen time and low levels of regular physical activity and adequate fruit and vegetable consumption. Of special concern, one-quarter of overweight or obese students who reported trying to lose weight used extreme weight-management behaviors such as fasting, diet pills, and vomiting. Together, these data point to a myriad of poor weight-management behaviors that could belie the stabilizing levels of BMI and suggest that public health efforts do not provide adolescents with helpful information on how to address their weight healthfully.

Our data showed that at least one-half of female students and approximately one third of male students reported trying to lose weight. Evidence of such a motivated population could be interpreted as a public health opportunity to replace ineffective weight-management efforts with more healthful behaviors. Population-level efforts that address the individual, social, and environmental determinants of weight- management behaviors in conjunction with public policy initiatives (16,17) may have contributed to the stabilization of youth obesity rates (2). Continued progress may require more intense programming efforts so that healthful weight-loss behaviors are adopted instead of extreme behaviors, particularly in metropolitan areas such as Philadelphia that are characterized by environments that do not offer ready access to healthful foods (18) or adequate and safe facilities for physical activity (19). Another population-level barrier to the promotion of healthful weight-loss behaviors is the reticence of health care professionals to address childhood obesity and prescribe behavior-management strategies for this high-risk population (20,21); thus, a concerted effort is needed to increase the efficacy of health care professionals to address childhood obesity and promote increased physical activity and healthful diets.

Our study had several limitations, including the use of self-reported data instead of objective measures. Additionally, because of the wide range of behaviors assessed by the YRBS during a single class period, we largely used single-item measures to examine weight-management behaviors. Use of single-item measures may have affected the validity and reliability of the study findings. Despite these limitations, data obtained by the YRBS are essential for understanding the behavioral patterns of adolescents in Philadelphia and the United States as a whole, and findings can serve as a basis for further analytical research.

Findings from this descriptive study and other recent studies that show a plateau in the prevalence of overweight and obesity among high school students (3) suggest that continued vigilance in educating high school students about healthful dietary and physical activity practices and promotion of environments that support healthful weight-related behaviors are necessary. Additionally, given the tenacity of overweight and obesity rates among high school students (3), continued research is needed to identify policies and programs that resonate with this age group. Finally, greater access to targeted community-based obesity prevention and treatment programs is needed for the large proportion of young people who desire to achieve a healthful weight; these programs are especially needed because of the propensity of high school students to engage in unhealthy behaviors, such extreme weight-management behaviors and extensive screen time, while trying to lose weight.

APPENDIX: VARIABLES EXAMINED IN STUDY ON OBESITY AND WEIGHT-RELATED BEHAVIORS AMONG HIGH SCHOOL STUDENTS IN PHILADELPHIA, PENNSYLVANIA, AND QUESTIONS USED FROM YOUTH RISK BEHAVIOR SURVEY, 2007, 2009, AND 2011

1. Weight perception
How do you describe your weight?

1. Very underweight
2. Slightly underweight
3. About the right weight
4. Slightly overweight
5. Very overweight

2. Weight-loss intention (yes/no)
Which of the following are you trying to do about your weight?

1. Lose weight
2. Gain weight
3. Stay the same weight
4. I am not trying to do anything about my weight

Participants who chose option a were coded as intending to lose weight.

3. Soda consumption (≥1 per day in last week)
During the past 7 days, how many times did you drink a can, bottle, or glass of soda or pop, such as Coke, Pepsi, or Sprite? (Do not count diet soda or diet pop.)

1. I did not drink soda or pop during the past 7 days
2. 1 to 3 times during the past 7 days
3. 4 to 6 times during the past 7 days
4. 1 time per day
5. 2 times per day
6. 3 times per day
7. 4 or more times per day

Participants who chose any of options d through g were coded as having 1 or more soda drinks in the last week.

4. Fruit and vegetable consumption (≥5 servings per day in the last week)
Composite variable calculated from responses to the following questions:

During the past 7 days, how many times did you drink 100% fruit juices such as orange juice, apple juice, or grape juice? (Do not count punch, Kool-Aid, sports drinks, or other fruit-flavored drinks.)

1. I did not drink 100% fruit juice during the past 7 days
2. 1 to 3 times during the past 7 days
3. 4 to 6 times during the past 7 days
4. 1 time per day
5. 2 times per day
6. 3 times per day
7. 4 or more times per day

During the past 7 days, how many times did you eat fruit? (Do not count fruit juice.)

1. I did not eat fruit during the past 7 days
2. 1 to 3 times during the past 7 days
3. 4 to 6 times during the past 7 days
4. 1 time per day
5. 2 times per day
6. 3 times per day
7. 4 or more times per day

During the past 7 days, how many times did you eat green salad?

1. I did not eat green salad during the past 7 days
2. 1 to 3 times during the past 7 days
3. 4 to 6 times during the past 7 days
4. 1 time per day
5. 2 times per day
6. 3 times per day
7. 4 or more times per day

During the past 7 days, how many times did you eat potatoes? (Do not count french fries, fried potatoes, or potato chips.)

1. I did not eat potatoes during the past 7 days
2. 1 to 3 times during the past 7 days
3. 4 to 6 times during the past 7 days
4. 1 time per day
5. 2 times per day
6. 3 times per day
7. 4 or more times per day

During the past 7 days, how many times did you eat carrots?

1. I did not eat carrots during the past 7 days
2. 1 to 3 times during the past 7 days
3. 4 to 6 times during the past 7 days
4. 1 time per day
5. 2 times per day
6. 3 times per day
7. 4 or more times per day

During the past 7 days, how many times did you eat other vegetables? (Do not count green salad, potatoes, or carrots.)

1. I did not eat other vegetables during the past 7 days
2. 1 to 3 times during the past 7 days
3. 4 to 6 times during the past 7 days
4. 1 time per day
5. 2 times per day
6. 3 times per day
7. 4 or more times per day

Variable computed as directed in the 2011 Youth Risk Behavior Survey Data User's Guide (p. 45). For each contributing question, a was assigned a value of 0, b = 2/7, c = 5/7, d = 1, e = 2, f = 4 and g = 4. Responses were totaled across each contributing question to achieve the total daily servings of fruits and vegetables during the past 7 days.

5. Physical activity levels (active for ≥60 minutes per day on 5 of the last 7 days)

During the past 7 days, on how many days were you physically active for a total of at least 60 minutes per day? (Add up all the time you spent in any kind of physical activity that increased your heart rate and made you breathe hard some of the time.)

1. 0 days
2. 1 day
3. 2 days
4. 3 days
5. 4 days
6. 5 days
7. 6 days
8. 7 days

Participants who chose any of options f, g, or h were coded as being active for at least 60 minutes per day on 5 of the last 7 days.

6. Television viewing

On an average school day, how many hours do you watch TV?

1. I do not watch TV on an average school day
2. Less than 1 hour per day
3. 1 hour per day
4. 2 hours per day
5. 3 hours per day
6. 4 hours per day
7. 5 or more hours per day
8. 7. Recreational computer use

On an average school day, how many hours do you play video or computer games or use a computer for something that is not school work? (Include activities such as Xbox, PlayStation, Nintendo DS, iPod touch, Facebook, and the Internet.)

1. I do not play video or computer games or use a computer for something that is not school work
2. Less than 1 hour per day
3. 1 hour per day
4. 2 hours per day
5. 3 hours per day
6. 4 hours per day
7. 5 or more hours per day
8. 8. Extreme weight-management strategies

During the past 30 days, did you go without eating for 24 hours or more (also called fasting) to lose weight or to keep from gaining weight?

1. Yes
2. No

During the past 30 days, did you take any diet pills, powders, or liquids without a doctor's advice to lose weight or to keep from gaining weight? (Do not include meal replacement products such as Slim Fast.)

1. Yes
2. No

During the past 30 days, did you vomit or take laxatives to lose weight or to keep from gaining weight?

1. Yes
2. No

REFERENCES

1.   Ogden CL, Carroll MD, Kit BK, Flegal KM. Prevalence of obesity and trends in body mass index among US children and adolescents, 1999–2010. JAMA 2012;307(5):483–90.

2. Robert Wood Johnson. Declining childhood obesity rates—where are we seeing the most progress? http://www.rwjf.org/content/dam/farm/reports/issue_briefs/2012/rwjf401163. Accessed August 13, 2013.

3. Robbins JM, Mallya G, Polansky M, Schwarz DF. Prevalence, disparities, and trends in obesity and severe obesity among students in the Philadelphia, Pennsylvania, school district, 2006–2010. Prev Chronic Dis 2012;9:120118.

4. Mitchell JA, Rodriguez D, Schmitz KH, Audrain-McGovern J. Greater screen time is associated with adolescent obesity: a longitudinal study of the BMI distribution from ages 14 to 18. Obesity (Silver Spring) 2013;21(3):572–5.

5. Economos CD, Bakun PJ, Herzog JB, Dolan PR, Lynskey VM, Markow D, et al. Children's perceptions of weight, obesity, nutrition, physical activity and related health and socio-behavioural factors. Public Health Nutr 2012; 1–9.

6. Neumark-Sztainer DR, Wall MM, Haines JI, Story MT, Sherwood NE, van den Berg PA. Shared risk and protective factors for overweight and disordered eating in adolescents. Am J Prev Med 2007;33(5):359–69.

7. Brener ND, Kann L, Kinchen SA, Grunbaum JA, Whalen L, Eaton D, et al. Methodology of the Youth Risk Behavior Surveillance System. MMWR Recomm Rep 2004;53(RR-12):1–13.

8. Kuczmarski RJ, Ogden CL, Guo SS, Grummer-Strawn LM, Flegal KM, Mei Z, et al. 2000 CDC growth charts for the United States: methods and development. Vital Health Stat 11 2002;(246):1–190.

9. Ogden CL, Flegal KM. Changes in terminology for childhood overweight and obesity. Natl Health Stat Report 2010;25(25):1–5.

10. Garber CE, Blissmer B, Deschenes MR, Franklin BA, Lamonte MJ, Lee IM, et al. American College of Sports Medicine position stand. Quantity and quality of exercise for developing and maintaining cardiorespiratory, musculoskeletal, and neuromotor fitness in apparently healthy adults: guidance for prescribing exercise. Med Sci Sports Exerc 2011;43(7):1334–59.

11. American Academy of Pediatrics. American Academy of Pediatrics: children, adolescents, and television. Pediatrics 2001;107(2):423–6.

12. Brener ND, Collins JL, Kann L, Warren CW, Williams BI. Reliability of the Youth Risk Behavior Survey questionnaire. Am J Epidemiol 1995;141(6):575–80.

13. Narayan KM, Boyle JP, Thompson TJ, Sorensen SW, Williamson DF. Lifetime risk for diabetes mellitus in the United States. JAMA 2003;290(14):1884–90.

14. American College of Preventive Medicine. Adolescent obesity—time for a commitment to action. A resource from the American College of Preventive Medicine. 2011. http://c.ymcdn.com/sites/www.acpm.org/resource/resmgr/timetools-files/adolescentobesityclinicalref.pdf. Accessed August 13, 2013.

15. Pelone F, Specchia ML, Veneziano MA, Capizzi S, Bucci S, Mancuso A, et al. Economic impact of childhood obesity on health systems: a systematic review. Obes Rev 2012;13(5):431–40.

16. Spear BA, Barlow SE, Ervin C, Ludwig DS, Saelens BE, Schetzina KE, et al. Recommendations for treatment of child and adolescent overweight and obesity. Pediatrics 2007;120(Suppl 4):S254–88.

17. National Heart, Lung, and Blood Institute. Working group report on future research directions in childhood obesity prevention and treatment 2008. http://www.nhlbi. nih.gov/meetings/workshops/child-obesity/index.htm. Accessed January 17, 2013.
18. Karpyn A, Young C, Weiss S. Reestablishing healthy food retail: changing the landscape of food deserts. Child Obes 2012;8(1):28–30.
19. Chase N, Beets M. Comparison of physical activity of rural and urban youth meta-analysis. Abstract presented at American Alliance for Health, Physical Education, Recreation and Dance National Convention and Exposition. 2010 Mar 16–20; Indianapolis, IN.
20. O'Brien SH, Holubkov R, Reis EC. Identification, evaluation, and management of obesity in an academic primary care center. Pediatrics 2004;114(2):e154–9.
21. Slusser W. Family physicians and the childhood obesity epidemic. Am Fam Physician 2008;78(1):34–7.

CHAPTER 10

FITNESS, FATNESS, AND ACADEMIC PERFORMANCE IN SEVENTH-GRADE ELEMENTARY SCHOOL STUDENTS

LUÍS B. SARDINHA, ADILSON MARQUES, SANDRA MARTINS, ANTÓNIO PALMEIRA, AND CLÁUDIA MINDERICO

10.1 BACKGROUND

Physical fitness is associated with a variety of health benefits in young people and adults. Low cardiorespiratory fitness, as part of the general health-related fitness of children and adolescents, has been associated with a cluster of cardiovascular disease (CVD) risk factors [1], independent of fatness and physical activity [2], and it is well recognized as a relevant marker of cardiovascular health [3]. Low cardiorespiratory fitness is also related to obesity [4], and changes in cardiorespiratory fitness are a significant predictor of changes in fatness that occur from childhood to adolescence, even after controlling for confounding factors such as physical activity, gender, and maturity [5]. Cardiorespiratory fitness may also improve other biological outcomes such as bone mineral density [6], arterial stiffness [7] and mental health outcomes [6].

Fitness, Fatness, and Academic Performance in Seventh-Grade Elementary School Students. © *Sardinha LB, Marques A, Martins S, Palmeira A, and Minderico C. BMC Pediatrics 14,176 (2014); doi:10.1186/1471-2431-14-176.* Licensed under Creative Commons Attribution 4.0 International License, http://creativecommons.org/licenses/by/4.0/.

Additionally, cardiorespiratory fitness has been shown to have positive effects on cognition. The evidence is strengthened by findings from studies that report a positive relationship between cardiorespiratory fitness and academic performance among children and adolescents from elementary up to secondary school [8-12]. Exercise and physical activity have the potential to improve or maintain cardiorespiratory fitness. On the other hand, cardiorespiratory fitness affects brain plasticity [13], and it is associated with cognitive health, better cognitive abilities, larger brain structures, elevated brain function [14-16], and improved memory [17,18] along with neurocognitive functions and cognitive control [19]. Improving neurocognitive functions and the brain plasticity may result in better academic performance, as has been demonstrated in previous studies [11].

The evidence about how weight status might affect students' school outcome is not conclusive. Some studies have not established a clear relationship between weight status and academic performance [9,20-22], while others have shown that overweight status and obesity are inversely associated with academic performance [23-26]. This controversial relationship needs to be further addressed.

There is evidence from analyses of economic outcomes that the quality of education, measured on an outcome basis of students' cognitive skills, has a great effect on the economy [27]. If weight status and cardiorespiratory fitness are related with students' academic achievement, policymakers and society should recognize its importance in order to contribute to better health, education and consequently economic development. However, the importance of health-related fitness directly or indirectly in economics has been neglected by health economists [28,29].

Despite the fact that several studies have found relationships between cardiorespiratory fitness, weight status and academic performance [9,10,22,26], most of these studies did not take into consideration their dynamic changes over time in different cohorts, and the possible relationship between academic achievement and the combined association of cardiorespiratory fitness/weight status. These types of studies are important because they allow establishing a better outcome than studies with one cohort sample. Therefore, the aim of this study was to investigate the relationship between cardiorespiratory fitness, weight status and academic performance among seventh-grade students, using three cohort samples of children and adolescents.

10.2 METHODS

10.2.1 STUDY DESIGN AND PARTICIPANTS

This study used data from the Physical Activity and Family-based Intervention in Paediatric Obesity Prevention in the School Setting (PESSOA Project). This project was applied to grade 5, 6 and 7 students from fourteen Portuguese public schools, in the Oeiras Municipality, between 2009 and 2011, and involved 4468 children and adolescents. The PESSOA program is a school-based cluster randomized controlled trial that addresses mediator variables, such as personal and social factors, and physical and social environmental factors within an ecological model that are related to and, influence physical activity. Schools were randomly allocated to one of three different groups: the first (control) group was intervened with a standard protocol with general information regarding eating and physical activity behaviours; the second group (intervention 1), besides the standard counselling, was provided a 90 min additional weekly session of physical activity; the third group (intervention 2), in addition to the standard counselling was provided a 90 min additional weekly session with health and weight educational program and physical activity, implementing principles (consistent with the tenets of the self-determination theory) and basic knowledge within the components of physical activity, eating behaviour and well-being designed to influence healthier choices.

The study received approval from the Scientific Committee of the Faculty of Human Kinetics at the University of Lisbon, the Portuguese Minister of Education, and the principals of each of the fourteen schools surveyed. The study was conducted according to ethical standards in sport and exercise science research [30]. Data were collected in the school setting after an agreement of participation of all the schools. Participants were informed about the objectives of the study and informed written consent was obtained from them and from their legal guardians.

Participation was voluntary. All healthy students that attended the physical education classes were considered eligible to participate. For the purpose the results presented in this study included 1531 grade 7 students (787 male, 744 female), ranging in age from 12 to 14 years (Mage = 12.3 ± 0.60), from 3 different cohorts. The first cohort started the study in grade 5 and was followed to grade 7. The second cohort started in grade 6 and was followed until grade 8. Finally, the last cohort started in grade 7 and finished the study in grade 9.

10.2.2 MEASURES AND PROCEDURES

Academic performance was assessed using the marks students had, at the end of their academic year, in mathematics, language (Portuguese), foreign language (English), and sciences. These marks were provided by the administrative services of each school at the end of the school year.

In Portuguese elementary schools, student marks range from 1 to 5 (1 = very poor, 2 = poor, 3 = average, 4 = good, and 5 = very good). An index of academic achievement was computed using the sum of the original marks of the four disciplines, ranging from 4 to 20. For data analysis students were grouped into low achievement (if the sum of marks of the four disciplines was between 4 and 11), average achievement (if the sum of marks of the four disciplines was between 12 and 15), and high academic achievement (if the sum of marks of the four disciplines was between 16 and 20).

To assess cardiorespiratory fitness the Progressive Aerobic Cardiovascular Endurance Run (PACER), from the Fitnessgram test battery, was used. The PACER is an incremental running test that uses a 20 metre shuttle run which progressively increases in difficulty. Participants were classified as fit and unfit according to the Fitnessgram cut points for cardiorespiratory fitness. The classification was based on gender- and age-related criterion-referenced standards. The standards are related to minimum levels of fitness that prevent diseases from a sedentary lifestyle [31].

To assess the weight status, participants were weighed to the nearest 0.1 kg wearing minimal clothes, and without shoes, and height was measured to the nearest 0.1 cm. BMI was obtained using the Quetelet index [weight (kg)/height (m)^2]. Participants were classified into normal weight and overweight or obese, according to the gender- and age-related criterion-referenced standards by the International Obesity Task Force (IOTF) [32].

Cardiorespiratory fitness and weight status data were collected during physical education classes over a period of one week. To ensure accurate completion of Fitnessgram administration, researchers and teachers supervised the entire data collection process.

10.2.3 DATA ANALYSIS

Descriptive statistics were performed to characterize the sample. Bivariate relationship between academic performance and gender, and weight status and cardiorespiratory fitness were tested by the chi-square test. Multinomial logistic regression analysis was used to study the relationship between cardiorespiratory fitness, weight status and academic achievement. In the multinomial logistic regression model for academic achievement we considered three groups: (i) students with low achievement, as a reference category, (ii) students with average academic achievement, and (iii) students with high achievement. Unadjusted and adjusted odds ratio (OR) with 95% confidence intervals (CI) were calculated. Adjustments were performed by controlling for gender, weight status, cardiorespiratory fitness, and different cohorts. The OR was calculated against the reference categories of male, obese weight status, and unfit cardiorespiratory fitness. The relationship between academic achievement and the combined association of cardiorespiratory fitness/weight status was also analysed, using multinomial logistic regression. The models were adjusted for gender and cohorts. For the association of cardiorespiratory fitness/weight status, four groups were created: (i) cardiorespiratory fit/normal weight students, (ii) cardiorespiratory fit/overweight or obese students, (iii) cardiorespiratory unfit/normal weight students, and (iv) cardiorespiratory unfit/overweight or obese students. Data analysis was performed using IBM SPSS Statistics version 20 (SPSS, Chicago, IL, USA). For all tests statistical significance was set at $p < 0.05$.

TABLE 1: Characteristics of elementary school students from grade 7 by different cohorts

	Cohort 1	Cohort 2	Cohort 3	Total
	n (%)	n (%)	n (%)	n (%)
Gender				
Male	184 (51.3)	215 (50.7)	388 (51.9)	787 (51.4)
Female	175 (48.7)	209 (49.3)	360 (48.1)	744 (48.6)
Weight status				
Obesity	24 (7.1)	29 (7.1)	57 (7.6)	110 (7.4)
Overweight	71 (21.0)	101 (24.6)	164 (22.3)	336 (22.7)
Normal weight	243 (67.7)	280 (68.3)	513 (69.9)	1036 (69.9)
Cardiorespiratory fitness				
Unfit	101 (28.1)	119 (28.1)	166 (22.2)	386 (19.9)
Fit	258 (71.9)	305 (71.9)	582 (77.8)	1145 (74.8)
Cardiorespiratory fitness/weight status				
Unfit/overweight	46 (12.7)	56 (13.2)	71 (9.5)	173 (11.3)
Unfit/normal weight	56 (15.7)	60 (14.2)	94 (12.5)	210 (13.7)
Fit/overweight	55 (15.4)	78 (18.5)	154 (20.6)	288 (18.8)
Fit/normal weight	202 (56.2)	229 (54.1)	405 (57.4)	860 (56.2)
Mathematics				
Low achievement	70 (19.5)	113 (26.7)	187 (25.0)	370 (24.2)
Average achievement	172 (47.9)	210 (49.5)	289 (38.6)	671 (43.8)
High achievement	117 (32.6)	101 (23.8)	272 (36.4)	490 (32.0)
Portuguese language				
Low achievement	40 (11.1)	52 (12.3)	115 (15.4)	207 (13.5)
Average achievement	208 (57.9)	259 (61.1)	351 (46.9)	818 (53.4)
High achievement	111 (30.9)	113 (26.7)	282 (37.7)	506 (33.1)
Foreign language (English)				
Low achievement	54 (15.0)	76 (17.9)	118 (15.8)	248 (16.2)
Average achievement	159 (44.3)	230 (54.2)	333 (44.5)	722 (47.2)
High achievement	146 (40.7)	118 (27.8)	297 (39.7)	561 (36.6)
Sciences				
Low achievement	31 (8.6)	62 (14.6)	107 (14.3)	200 (13.1)
Average achievement	183 (51.0)	247 (58.3)	339 (45.3)	769 (50.2)
High achievement	145 (40.4)	115 (27.1)	302 (40.4)	562 (36.7)

TABLE 1: *Cont.*

	Cohort 1	Cohort 2	Cohort 3	Total
	n (%)	n (%)	n (%)	n (%)
Overall academic achievement				
Low achievement	60 (16.7)	91 (21.5)	146 (19.5)	297 (19.4)
Average achievement	213 (59.3)	267 (63.0)	392 (52.4)	872 (57.0)
High achievement	86 (24.0)	66 (15.6)	210 (28.1)	362 (23.6)

Cohort 1 started the study in grade 5, and these data were collected in 2011. Cohort 2 started the study in grade 6, and these data were collected in 2010. Cohort 3 started the study in grade 7, and these data were collected in 2009.

10.3 RESULTS

The general sample's characteristics are presented in Table 1. For weight status, the proportion of the participants who were normal weight was 69.9% and 30.3% were overweight or obese. Almost three-fourths (74.8%) of all participants were in the fit category for cardiorespiratory fitness. Overall, the majority of students passed (>2) in mathematics, language, foreign language and science, achieving an average academic performance. For the overall academic achievement 76.4% reached the low and average level while 23.6% achieved the high level.

For the overall sample, students' academic achievement did not differ significantly by gender ($\chi^2(2)=1.040$, p=0.595). However, statistically significant differences were found for weight status ($\chi^2(4)=32.259$, p<0.001), and cardiorespiratory fitness ($\chi^2(2)=19.983$, p<0.001). Those who were normal weight and presented a higher cardiorespiratory fitness had better academic achievement (Table 2). Similar results were observed for each cohort.

Table 3 presents the results of the unadjusted and adjusted multinomial logistic regression. Being male or female was not related to academic achievement in the unadjusted analysis. However, being female was related to high academic achievement when all the variables were adjusted to the model (OR=1.57, 95% CI: 1.09-2.26, p=0.016). For weight status, overweight or normal weight students, compared with obese students, had higher OR for having an average or high academic achievement versus those who had low academic achievement. It is important to highlight that the OR of having high or average academic achievement versus low academic achievement of normal weight students was higher than overweight in both unadjusted (OR=4.98, 95% CI: 2.53-9.81, p<0.001) and adjusted analysis (OR=3.72, 95% CI: 1.85-7.49, p<0.001). Fit students, compared with unfit students, had significantly higher odds for having a high academic achievement, in both the unadjusted (OR=2.27, 95% CI: 1.57-3.26, p<0.001), and adjusted model (OR=2.27, 95% CI: 1.46-3.52, p<0.001). This means that individually or adjusted for other variables, including the effect of the cohorts, cardiorespiratory fitness is an important predictor of high academic achievement. On the other hand, average academic achievement was only related with higher cardiorespiratory fitness in the unadjusted analysis, failing to remain significant after adjusting covariates. This reinforces the importance of cardiorespiratory fitness as a predictor of high academic achievement.

Figure 1 shows the OR of the relationship between academic achievement and the combined association of cardiorespiratory fitness/weight status. Students classified as cardiorespiratory fit/normal weight (OR=5.49, 95% CI: 3.05-9.86, p<0.001), as well as those classified as cardiorespiratory fit/overweight or obese (OR=3.09, 95% CI: 1.57-6.06, p=0.001), and cardiorespiratory unfit/normal weight (OR=2.62, 95% CI: 1.32.5.18, p=0.006) were more likely to have better academic performance, compared with those cardiorespiratory unfit/overweight or obese students.

10.4 DISCUSSION

The main finding of the present study was that cardiorespiratory fitness and weight status were independently and combined related to academic achievement in seventh-grade students independent of the different cohorts, providing further support that aerobically fit and lean students are more likely to have better performance at school regardless of the year that they were born.

TABLE 2: Academic achievement by selected factors (chi-square)

	Cohort 1				Cohort 2				Cohort 3				Total			
	L	A	H	p	L	A	H	p	L	A	H	p	L	A	H	p
Gender				0.141				0.796				0.193				0.595
Male	56.7	46.9	58.1		53.8	49.8	50.0		50.7	55.9	45.2		52.9	51.8	49.2	
Female	43.3	53.1	41.9		46.2	20.2	50.0		49.3	44.1	54.8		47.1	48.2	50.8	
Weight status				0.042				0.029				0.001				<0.001
Normal weight	60.7	67.1	81.5		65.9	66.2	80.0		57.0	71.0	76.7		60.4	69.5	78.4	
Overweight	26.8	19.7	17.3		21.2	28.1	15.4		29.5	21.2	19.4		26.5	23.3	18.2	
Obesity	12.5	7.5	1.2		12.9	5.8	4.6		13.4	7.8	3.9		13.1	7.2	3.4	
Cardiorespiratory fitness				0.003				0.033				0.035				<0.001
Unfit	36.7	31.5	14.0		33.0	29.6	15.2		30.1	20.7	19.5		32.3	26.0	17.4	
Fit	63.3	68.5	86.0		67.0	70.4	84.8		69.9	79.3	80.5		67.7	74.0	82.6	

L — low academic achievement; A — average academic achievement; H — high academic achievement. Cohort 1 started the study in grade 5, and these data were collected in 2011. Cohort 2 started the study in grade 6, and these data were collected in 2010. Cohort 3 started the study in grade 7, and these data were collected in 2009.

TABLE 3: Multivariate multinomial logistic regression predicting average and high overall academic achievement

Characteristic	Unadjusted model		Adjusted model	
	Average academic achievement	High academic achievement	Average academic achievement	High academic achievement
	OR (95% CI)	OR (95% CI)	OR (95% CI)	OR (95% CI)
Gender[a]				
Female	1.04 (0.80-1.36)	1.16 (0.85-1.58)	1.12 (0.86-1.62)	1.57 (1.09-2.26)*
Weight status[b]				
Overweight	1.59 (0.98-2.59)	2.63 (1.27-5.47)**	1.49 (0.91-2.44)	2.22 (1.05-4.66)*
Normal weight	2.09 (1.34-3.25)**	4.98 (2.53-9.81)***	1.88 (1.18-2.98)**	3.72 (1.85-7.49)***
Cardiorespiratory fitness[c]				
Fit	1.36 (1.02-1.81)*	2.27 (1.57-3.26)***	1.31 (0.92-1.88)	2.27 (1.46-3.52)***

*OR – Odds ratio; CI – confidence interval. Multinomial Logistic Regression with maximum-likelihood ratio was tested for selected variables. Low academic achievement is the reference group for outcome. In the unadjusted model each variable was tested independently as a predictor of academic achievement. In the adjusted model, the effect of cohorts was controlled and all the variables were tested in the same model, controlling the effect of each other. [a]Reference category is "male." [b]Reference category is "obese." [c]Reference category is "unfit". *p <0.05, **p < 0.01, ***p < 0.001.*

Although several studies focusing on general physical fitness have established a relationship between academic performance and fitness or physical activity [33-35], we investigated a specific component of physical fitness. The results confirm and extend prior findings relating cardiorespiratory fitness with academic achievement in elementary school, independently of the birth year [9,12,21,36,37].

In a study among school children, Van Dusen et al. [10] have found that, among several physical fitness tests, cardiorespiratory fitness was the strongest fitness component related to academic achievement, which corroborated previous investigations [8,9]. More recently, two other studies with similar aims to the present study, from different countries, have also found that cardiorespiratory fitness was a predictor of academic achievement [22,26]. It has been shown that fit students were less likely to miss school and to do poorly on standardized tests [24,38], which are important risk factors often linked to dropping out of school.

The importance of this particular fitness component on academic achievement was seen in our study in the unadjusted and adjusted analysis, which means that individually or after adjustment for important covariates this variable is a predictor of academic achievement. Fit students had a 127% increased chance of reaching high academic achievement than cardiorespiratory unfit. These results demonstrate the important contribution of fitness, particularly cardiorespiratory capacity in students' cognition; contributing to a growing body of literature about the relationship between physical fitness and academic achievement and supporting that a particular component of fitness is associated with general high academic performance. The findings of the present study are strengthened by the fact that three different cohorts were considered. This is to say that although they were all students from the 7th grade, the sample consisted of students who were born three years apart, demonstrating the consistency of the results with different subsamples.

Causal inferences or explanations for the physical fitness-academic achievement association cannot be made from this study. However, mechanisms (i.e., physiological, psychological and behavioural) have been proposed to explain the link between fitness and academic performance. Studies have demonstrated that physical activity and fitness: 1) stimulate neural development, increasing the density of neuronal synapses [39], 2) increase levels of norepinephrine and endorphins, which are important to reduce stress and improve mood [40]; and 3) might increase the vasculature in the cerebral cortex [41]. At a biochemical level, physical activity and exercise augment the synthesis of brain-derived neurotrophic factor, also known as BDNF, which enhances brain plasticity by changing the structure of the neuron and strengthening its signalling capability [42,43]. Psychologically, physical fitness is positively associated with particular cognitive functioning related to attention and working memory [14,17]. Moreover, physical fitness contributes to accelerated psychomotor development, reduces anxiety and stress, and increases self-esteem, which are related to academic achievement [44]. Besides these suggested physiological and psychological effects, physical activity and physical fitness improve students' behaviour in the learning context, consequently increasing the odds of better concentration and achievement [35].

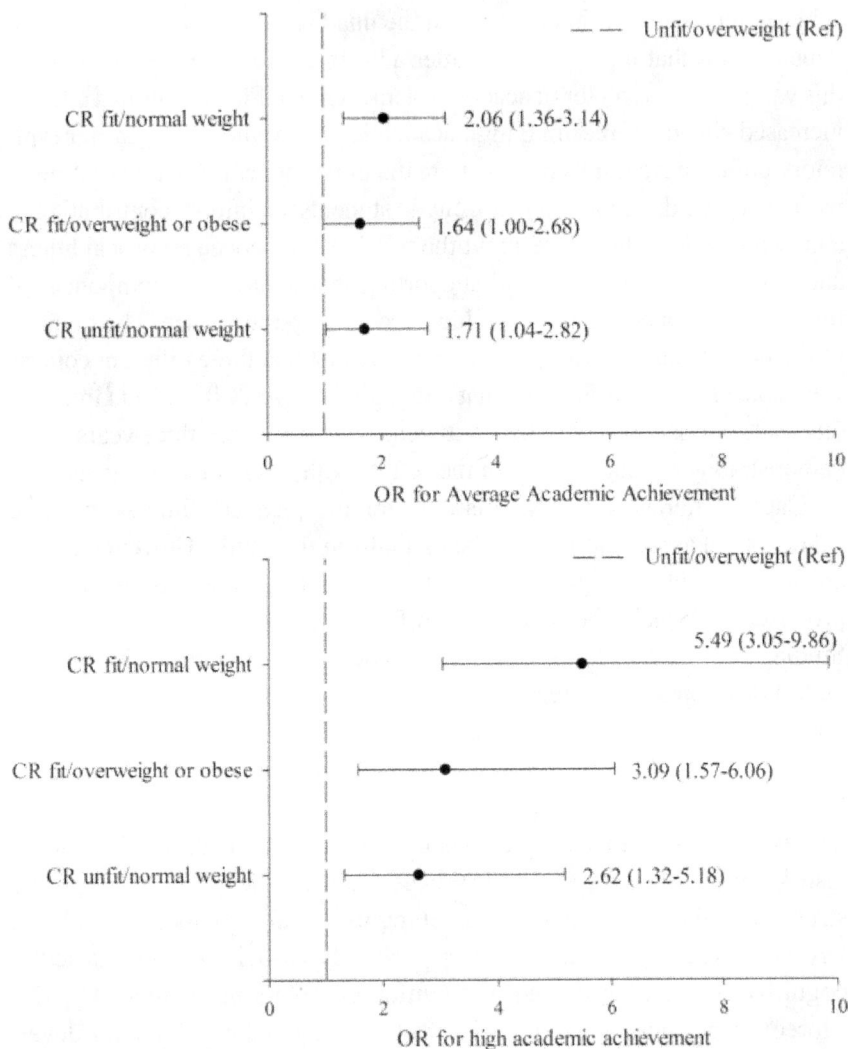

FIGURE 1: Odds ratio of predicting average and high academic achievement by cardiorespiratory fitness/weight status.

Similarly to cardiorespiratory fitness, having normal weight was also associated with high academic achievement. Overweight students were 2.22 times and normal weight students were 3.72 times as likely to have high academic achievement as obese students. The relationship between weight status and academic achievement is congruent with some studies [8,23,24], but departs from other studies on which a relationship was not identified [9,10,12,20,21]. These disruptive findings perhaps are due to differences in BMI was quantified. We used a BMI classification; however in other studies BMI is treated as a continuous variable to prevent loss of information [22]. Further exploration research is required for the understanding of the relationship between academic achievement and weight status.

Although the relationship between academic achievement and weight status is not yet clearly established, two potential pathways have been proposed to associate weight status and academic outcomes. First, psychosocial pathways consider that overweight or obese students have lower self-esteem and body image [45], resulting in internalizing and externalizing behaviour problems that can affect students' performance at school [25]. Second, physiological pathways consider that overweight and obesity are linked with health problems, leading to missed classes or lateness [46], both of which detrimentally affect school performance.

When analysing the combined association of cardiorespiratory fitness and weight status it was observed that for cardiorespiratory fit and normal weight students the odds of reaching high academic achievement increased by 449%. This result reinforced the finding for cardiorespiratory fitness and weight status and suggests that the combination of these two fitness components is a strong predictor of high academic achievement.

Because most children and adolescents are not physically fit [47], and fail to meet physical activity recommendation [48], school-based physical activity is important to offer or increase opportunities for physical activity [49]. Physical activity can be included in the school context in a number of ways without detracting from academic performance [34,49]. Considering that physical activity and physical fitness are related with academic achievement [12,21,37], schools should strive to meet recommendation of daily physical activity and offer students a balanced academic program that includes opportunities for a variety of daily physical activities.

In spite of the contribution of this study to the current understanding of the cardiorespiratory fitness- and weight status-academic achievement relationship, the study is not without some limitations. The cross-sectional design demonstrated an association between the variables, but did not indicate causality. Results need to be interpreted with some caution, because it is possible that the relationship between academic achievement and cardiorespiratory fitness was mediated by variable(s) not included in this study, such as socioeconomic status, parents' education, and home background. Moreover, the used of categorical scholastic achievement instead of standardized academic outcomes could also be a limitation, due the fact that students marks may be related with other factors besides their cognitive performance.

10.5 CONCLUSION AND RECOMMENDATIONS

The present study provides information regarding the independent influence of cardiorespiratory fitness and weight status on academic achievement in seventh-grade students. These findings suggest a synergic effect of cardiorespiratory fitness and weight status on academic achievement. Although other investigations have observed associations between cardiorespiratory fitness and weight status with academic achievement [22,26], the present research innovates by including three different cohorts, enabling to extend previous findings to children that were born in different years. These reinforce that children and adolescents should have more physical activity opportunities that allow improving cardiorespiratory fitness and weight status during school time.

REFERENCES

1. Anderssen SA, Cooper AR, Riddoch C, Sardinha LB, Harro M, Brage S, Andersen LB: Low cardiorespiratory fitness is a strong predictor for clustering of cardiovascular disease risk factors in children independent of country, age and sex. Eur J Cardiovasc Prev Rehabil 2007, 14:526-531.
2. Andersen LB, Sardinha LB, Froberg K, Riddoch CJ, Page AS, Anderssen SA: Fitness, fatness and clustering of cardiovascular risk factors in children from Denmark,

Estonia and Portugal: the European Youth Heart Study. Int J Pediatr Obes 2008, 3(Suppl 1):58-66.

3. Ortega FB, Ruiz JR, Castillo MJ, Sjostrom M: Physical fitness in childhood and adolescence: a powerful marker of health. Int J Obes 2008, 32:1-11.

4. Tanha T, Wollmer P, Thorsson O, Karlsson MK, Linden C, Andersen LB, Dencker M: Lack of physical activity in young children is related to higher composite risk factor score for cardiovascular disease. Acta Paediatr 2011, 100:717-721.

5. Ornelas RT, Silva AM, Minderico CS, Sardinha LB: Changes in cardiorespiratory fitness predict changes in body composition from childhood to adolescence: findings from the European Youth Heart Study. Phys Sportsmed 2011, 39:78-86.

6. Janssen I, Leblanc AG: Systematic review of the health benefits of physical activity and fitness in school-aged children and youth. Int J Behav Nutr Phys Act 2010, 7:40.

7. Ried-Larsen M, Grontved A, Froberg K, Ekelund U, Andersen LB: Physical activity intensity and subclinical atherosclerosis in Danish adolescents: the European Youth Heart Study. Scand J Med Sci Sports 2013, 23:e168-e177.

8. Castelli DM, Hillman CH, Buck SM, Erwin HE: Physical fitness and academic achievement in third- and fifth-grade students. J Sport Exerc Psychol 2007, 29:239-252.

9. Eveland-Sayers BM, Farley RS, Fuller DK, Morgan DW, Caputo JL: Physical fitness and academic achievement in elementary school children. J Phys Act Health 2009, 6:99-104.

10. Van Dusen DP, Kelder SH, Kohl HW 3rd, Ranjit N, Perry CL: Associations of physical fitness and academic performance among schoolchildren. J Sch Health 2011, 81:733-740.

11. Chaddock L, Hillman CH, Pontifex MB, Johnson CR, Raine LB, Kramer AF: Childhood aerobic fitness predicts cognitive performance one year later. J Sports Sci 2012, 30:421-430.

12. Chen LJ, Fox KR, Ku PW, Taun CY: Fitness change and subsequent academic performance in adolescents. J Sch Health 2013, 83:631-638.

13. Hillman CH, Erickson KI, Kramer AF: Be smart, exercise your heart: exercise effects on brain and cognition. Nat Rev Neurosci 2008, 9:58-65.

14. Chaddock L, Erickson KI, Prakash RS, Voss MW, VanPatter M, Pontifex MB, Hillman CH, Kramer AF: A functional MRI investigation of the association between childhood aerobic fitness and neurocognitive control. Biol Psychol 2012, 89:260-268.

15. Hillman CH, Buck SM, Themanson JR, Pontifex MB, Castelli DM: Aerobic fitness and cognitive development: Event-related brain potential and task performance indices of executive control in preadolescent children. Dev Psychol 2009, 45:114-129.

16. Hillman CH, Pontifex MB, Motl RW, O'Leary KC, Johnson CR, Scudder MR, Raine LB, Castelli DM: From ERPs to academics. Dev Cogn Neurosci 2012, 2(Suppl 1):S90-S98.

17. Hillman CH, Castelli DM, Buck SM: Aerobic fitness and neurocognitive function in healthy preadolescent children. Med Sci Sports Exerc 2005, 37:1967-1974.

18. Monti JM, Hillman CH, Cohen NJ: Aerobic fitness enhances relational memory in preadolescent children: the FITKids randomized control trial. Hippocampus 2012, 22:1876-1882.

19. Moore RD, Wu CT, Pontifex MB, O'Leary KC, Scudder MR, Raine LB, Johnson CR, Hillman CH: Aerobic fitness and intra-individual variability of neurocognition in preadolescent children. Brain Cogn 2013, 82:43-57.

20. Bisset S, Foumier M, Pagani L, Janosz M: Predicting academic and cognitive outcomes from weight status trajectories during childhood. Int J Obes 2013, 37:154-159.

21. London RA, Castrechini S: A longitudinal examination of the link between youth physical fitness and academic achievement. J Sch Health 2011, 81:400-408.

22. Rauner RR, Walters RW, Avery M, Wanser TJ: Evidence that aerobic fitness is more salient than weight status in predicting standardized math and reading outcomes in fourth- through eighth-grade students. J Pediatr 2013, 163:344-348.

23. Davis CL, Cooper S: Fitness, fatness, cognition, behavior, and academic achievement among overweight children: do cross-sectional associations correspond to exercise trial outcomes? Prev Med 2011, 52(Suppl 1):S65-S69.

24. Kristjánsson AL, Sigfúsdóttir ID, Allegrante JP: Health behavior and academic achievement among adolescents: the relative contribution of dietary habits, physical activity, body mass index, and self-esteem. Health Educ Behav 2010, 37:51-64.

25. Krukowski RA, West DS, Philyaw Perez A, Bursac Z, Phillips MM, Raczynski JM: Overweight children, weight-based teasing and academic performance. Int J Pediatr Obes 2009, 4:274-280.

26. Torrijos-Nino C, Martinez-Vizcaino V, Pardo-Guijarro MJ, Garcia-Prieto JC, Arias-Palencia NM, Sanchez-Lopez M: Physical Fitness, Obesity, and Academic Achievement in Schoolchildren. J Pediatr 2014. doi:10.1016/j.jpeds.2014.02.041. [Epub ahead of print]

27. Hanushek E, Woessmann L: Education and Economic Growth. In International Encyclopedia of Education, Volume 2. Edited by Peterson P, Baker E, McGaw B. Oxford: Elsevier; 2010:245-252.

28. Ammerman AS, Farrelly MA, Cavallo DN, Ickes SB, Hoerger TJ: Health economics in public health. Am J Prev Med 2009, 36:273-275.

29. Hale J: What contribution can health economics make to health promotion? Health Promot Int 2000, 15:341-348.

30. Harriss DJ, Atkinson G: Update – Ethical standards in sport and exercise science research. Int J Sports Med 2011, 32:819-821.

31. Cooper Institute: Fitnessgram/Activitygram: Test administration manual. Human Kinetics: Champaign; 2007.

32. Cole TJ, Bellizzi MC, Flegal KM, Dietz WH: Establishing a standard definition for child overweight and obesity worldwide: international survey. Br Med J 2000, 320:1240-1243.

33. Donnelly JE, Greene JL, Gibson CA, Sullivan DK, Hansen DM, Hillman CH, Poggio J, Mayo MS, Smith BK, Lambourne K, Herrmann SD, Scudder M, Betts JL, Honas JJ, Washburn RA: Physical activity and academic achievement across the curriculum (A+PAAC): rationale and design of a 3-year, cluster-randomized trial. BMC Public Health 2013, 13:307.

34. Rasberry CN, Lee SM, Robin L, Laris BA, Russell LA, Coyle KK, Nihiser AJ: The association between school-based physical activity, including physical education,

and academic performance: a systematic review of the literature. Prev Med 2011, 52(Suppl 1):S10-S20.

35. Singh A, Uijtdewilligen L, Twisk JW, van Mechelen W, Chinapaw MJ: Physical activity and performance at school: a systematic review of the literature including a methodological quality assessment. Arch Pediatr Adolesc Med 2012, 166:49-55.

36. Chomitz VR, Slining MM, McGowan RJ, Mitchell SE, Dawson GF, Hacker KA: Is there a relationship between physical fitness and academic achievement? Positive results from public school children in the northeastern United States. J Sch Health 2009, 79:30-37.

37. Wittberg RA, Northrup KL, Cottrell LA: Children's aerobic fitness and academic achievement: a longitudinal examination of students during their fifth and seventh grade years. Am J Public Health 2012, 102:2303-2307.

38. Blom L, Alvarez J, Zhang L, Kolbo J: Associations between health-related physical fitness, academic achievement and selected academic behaviors of elementary and middle school students in the state of Mississippi. ICHPER-SD Journal of Research 2011, 6:13-19.

39. Kramer AF, Colcombe S, Erickson K, Belopolsky A, McAuley E, Cohen NJ, Webb A, Jerome GJ, Marquez DX, Wszalek TM: Effects of aerobic fitness training on human cortical function: a proposal. J Mol Neurosci 2002, 19:227-231.

40. Fleshner M: Exercise and neuroendocrine regulation of antibody production: protective effect of physical activity on stress-induced suppression of the specific antibody response. Int J Sports Med 2000, 21(Suppl 1):S14-S19.

41. Etnier JL, Salazar W, Landers DM, Petruzzello SJ, Han M, Nowell P: The influence of physical fitness and exercise upon cognitive functioning: A meta-analysis. J Sport Exerc Psychol 1997, 19:249-277.

42. Ratey JJ, Loehr JE: The positive impact of physical activity on cognition during adulthood: a review of underlying mechanisms, evidence and recommendations. Rev Neurosci 2011, 22:171-185.

43. Cotman CW, Berchtold NC, Christie LA: Exercise builds brain health: key roles of growth factor cascades and inflammation. Trends Neurosci 2007, 30:464-472.

44. Tremblay M, Inman J, Willms J: The relationship between physical activity, self-esteem, and academic achievement in 12-years-old children. Pediatr Exerc Sci 2000, 12:312-323.

45. Griffiths LJ, Parsons TJ, Hill AJ: Self-esteem and quality of life in obese children and adolescents: a systematic review. Int J Pediatr Obes 2010, 5:282-304.

46. Datar A, Sturm R: Childhood overweight and elementary school outcomes. Int J Obes 2006, 30:1449-1460.

47. Morrow JR Jr, Fulton JE, Brener ND, Kohl HW 3rd: Prevalence and correlates of physical fitness testing in U.S. schools-2000. Res Q Exerc Sport 2008, 79:141-148.

48. Baptista F, Santos DA, Silva AM, Mota J, Santos R, Vale S, Ferreira JP, Raimundo AM, Moreira H, Sardinha LB: Prevalence of the Portuguese population attaining sufficient physical activity. Med Sci Sports Exerc 2012, 44:466-473.

49. Centers for Disease Control and Prevention: The Association Between School Based Physical Activity, Including Physical Education, and Academic Performance. Atlanta, GA: U.S. Department of Health and Human Services; 2010.

CHAPTER 11

PHYSICAL FITNESS, OVERWEIGHT, AND THE RISK OF EATING DISORDERS IN ADOLESCENTS: THE AVENA AND AFINOS STUDIES

A. M. VESES, D. MARTHNEZ-GÓMEZ, S. GÓMEZ-MARTHNEZ, G. VICENTE-RODRIGUEZ, R. CASTILLO, F. B. ORTEGA, M. GONZÁLEZ-GROSS, M. E. CALLE, O. L. VEIGA, A. MARCOS, FOR THE AVENA AND AFINOS STUDY GROUPS

11.1 INTRODUCTION

Eating disorders are currently a public health concern in developed countries since their prevalence in young people have remarkably increased in the last decade [1]. For example, European and US surveillance studies have found that between 10% and 25% of adolescents scored above the limit for being at risk for developing an eating disorder [2]. Eating disorders constitute the third cause of illness after obesity and asthma in young population. In addition, they present a chronic course, and have an elevated morbidity and mortality ranging from 6% to 15%, respectively [3].

Reprinted with permission from Veses AM, Martínez-Gómez D, Gómez-Martínez S, Vicente-Rodriguez G, Castillo R, Ortega FB, González-Gross M, Calle ME, Veiga OL, and Marcos A. Physical Fitness, Overweight and the Risk of Eating Disorders in Adolescents. The AVENA and AFINOS Studies. Pediatric Obesity 9,1 (2014), DOI: 10.1111/j.2047-6310.2012.00138.x.

Importantly, a variety of biological and psychological factors may play a key role in the development of eating disorders [3].

Eating disorders and obesity are part of a range of weight-related problems, and they are usually seen as opposite pathologies but in fact they share many similarities. Evidence from cross-sectional studies suggests that these disorders can occur simultaneously in the same individual [4]. An excess of body fat has been associated with a later increased risk of developing eating disorders such as anorexia, bulimia nervosa, self-induced vomiting and binge eating in both children [4-6] and adults [7]. Today's society idealizes thinness and stigmatizes fatness, yet high-calorie foods are widely available and heavily advertised. The mass media, family and peers may be sending children and adolescents mixed messages about food and weight that encourage disordered eating [8].

On the other hand, physical fitness, defined as the capacity to perform physical activity, is a powerful marker of health [9]. Most studies have found inverse associations among obesity, physical activity [10] and fitness [11], and there is strong evidence that high physical fitness attenuates the negative effect of obesity on cardiovascular diseases [12]. However, little is known about the influence of physical fitness on the risk of developing eating disorders. In spite of this, some studies have shown that higher levels of fitness might have a positive influence on depression, anxiety, mood status and self-esteem in young people [9]. This fact is important since adolescents who are at risk of developing eating disorders are also likely to develop other mental health disorders [13, 14]. Therefore, the present study aims to examine the individual and combined association of overweight and physical fitness with the risk of developing eating disorders in Spanish adolescents. This research question was tested in two separate studies conducted in Spanish adolescents.

11.2 PATIENTS AND METHODS

11.2.1 STUDY DESIGN AND PARTICIPANTS

The present study involves data from two different research projects: the AVENA (Food and Assessment of the Nutritional Status of Adolescents)

[15] Study and the AFINOS (Physical Activity as a Preventive Measure of the Development of Overweight, Obesity, Allergies, Infections, and Cardiovascular Risk Factors in Adolescents) [16] Study. The AVENA and AFINOS are cross-sectional studies performed in Spain from November 2000 to June 2002, and from November 2007 to February 2008, respectively. The AVENA Study was designed to assess the health and nutritional status of a national representative sample (n=2859) of Spanish adolescents [15]. Participants in this study were recruited in five Spanish cities (Madrid, Murcia, Granada, Santander and Zaragoza). The AFINOS Study was designed to determine the relationship between physical activity and the incidence of overweight, infections and allergies in a representative sample of adolescents (n=2116) from the Madrid region [16]. The final sample used for the current study comprised 3571 adolescents (1864 girls) aged from 13 to 18.5 years with valid data for the analysed variables. Specifically, a total of 1554 adolescents (828 girls) belonged to the AVENA Study, and 2017 adolescents (1036 girls) to the AFINOS Study.

A comprehensive verbal description of the nature and purpose of these studies was given to the adolescents and their parents, and a written consent to participate was requested from both parents and adolescents. The AVENA Study protocol was approved by the Review Committee for Research Involving Human Subjects of the Hospital Universitario Marqués de Valdecilla (Santander), and the AFINOS Study protocol was approved by the Ethics Committee of Puerta de Hierro Hospital (Madrid) and the Bioethics Committee from Spanish National Research Council [15, 16].

11.2.2 MEASUREMENT OF THE RISK OF EATING DISORDERS

In both studies, the risk of eating disorders was assessed using the SCOFF questionnaire [17]. This questionnaire is a screening instrument originally designed to be routinely used in all individuals considered at risk of such disorders, and it has been validated in Spanish adolescents [18]. The SCOFF questionnaire consists of five eating-related questions asking about intentional vomiting, loss of control over eating, weight loss, body dissatisfaction and food intrusive thoughts. Answering positively two or more items of SCOFF questionnaire has been suggested as the threshold for a suspicion of a probable eating disorder case [17].

11.2.3 ANTHROPOMETRIC MEASURES

In the AVENA Study, two anthropometrists in each city performed all measurements [19]. Body weight and height were measured to 0.05 kg and 0.1 cm using a beam balance including a stadiometer (SECA 861, SECA, Hamburg, Germany). In the AFINOS Study, body weight and height were self-reported by the adolescents. In both studies, body mass index (BMI) was calculated as weight/height squared ($kg\,m^{-2}$). The International Obesity Task Force-proposed gender- and age-adjusted cut-off points were used to classify adolescents according to their weight status in underweight, normal-weight, overweight and obesity [20, 21].

11.2.4 MEASUREMENTS OF PHYSICAL FITNESS

Cardiorespiratory fitness (CRF) in the AVENA Study was assessed by the 20-m shuttle-run test [22]. The 20-m shuttle-run test is one of the most widely used field tests to assess CRF in youth (http://www.fitnessgram. net). Adolescents ran as long as possible, back and forth, across a 20-m space at a specific sound protocol that became $0.5\,km\,h^{-1}$ faster each minute or period from a starting speed of $8.5\,km\,h^{-1}$.

The test finished when the participant failed to reach the end lines concurrent with the audio signals on two consecutive occasions. Adolescents were instructed to abstain from strenuous exercises within the 48 h preceding the test. Last lap completed was the individual score for each participant. Maximal oxygen consumption (VO_2max, $mL\,kg^{-1}\,min^{-1}$) was estimated by the Leger equation [23]. In the AVENA Study, adolescents were classified according to their CRF levels based on sex- and age-specific tertiles [24].

In the AFINOS Study, the participants completed a questionnaire that assessed their health status and lifestyle based on previous questionnaires used in several national and international health surveys [15]. A question about their physical fitness level was incorporated into the questionnaire:

how is your physical fitness? The response options were scored from 1=poor to 5=excellent. The use of self-reported overall physical fitness has been shown to be useful, reliable and valid in adolescents [25]. In the AFINOS Study, participants were classified into low, medium and high fitness levels according to their response to this question as follows: low (categories 1 and 2), medium (category 3) and high (categories 4 and 5).

11.2.5 DATA ANALYSIS

Characteristics of the sample and output results of the study are described as mean±SD or percentage. The Kolmogorov–Smirnov test was used to test the normality of all continuous variables. Statistical differences by sex in the samples were analysed using the chi-squared test for qualitative variables and by one-way analysis of variance for continuous variables. In both studies, underweight and normal-weight adolescents reported a similar (0.5 vs. 0.6, P=1 in the AVENA Study) or slightly lower (0.6 vs. 0.9, P=0.04 in the AFINOS Study) number of positive responses in the SCOFF questionnaire than normal-weight adolescents, whereas obese adolescents reported a higher number of positive responses in such questionnaire than overweight adolescents (1.5 vs. 1.2, P=0.049 in the AVENA Study, and 2.0 vs. 1.2, P<0.001 in the AFINOS Study). Consequently and for more robust analysis, overweight and obese adolescents were combined in the same group (hereafter called overweight adolescents), whereas underweight and normal-weight adolescents (hereafter called non-overweight adolescents) were also merged.

Logistic regression analysis was performed to examine individual and combined association of weight status (non-overweight and overweight) and levels of fitness (low, middle and high) with the risk of eating disorders development in each study. To analyse the combined association of weight status and fitness level subjects in each study, samples were stratified into six groups (two groups according to BMI status × three groups according to fitness levels) and the non-overweight/high fitness adolescents were used as reference group. All logistic regression analyses were sex- and age-adjusted. For all analyses, the error was fixed at 0.05. All analyses were performed using the SPSS statistical software package (v.17.0) (IBM, Armonk, NY, USA) for windows XP.

TABLE 1: Descriptive characteristics of the study samples

	AVENA Study (2000–2002)			P	AFINOS Study (2007,2008)			P
	All	Boys	Girls		All	Boys	Girls	
	n=1554	n=726	n=828		n=2017	n=981	n=1036	
Age (years)	15.4±1.3	15.4±1.3	15.4±1.3	0.845	14.8±1.3	14.8±1.3	14.8±1.3	0.823
Weight (kg)	60.4±12.1	64.5±12.8	56.3±9.8	<0.001	58.3±11.1	62.4±12.0	54.3±8.4	<0.001
Height (cm)	166.5±8.8	171.4±8.2	161.7±6.2	<0.001	166.5±9.2	170.4±9.7	162.7±6.9	0.001
Body mass index (kg m−2)	21.7±3.5	21.9±3.6	21.5±3.4	0.047	20.9±2.9	21.5±3.1	20.5±2.6	<0.001
Overweighta	22.2	25.9	18.5	0.001	17.6	25.0	10.5	<0.001
Fitness levels								
Low	33.3	34.4	32.4		10.3	8.0	12.5	
Medium	33.3	29.5	36.7	0.006	36.1	29.4	42.6	0.001
High	33.3	36.1	30.9		53.6	62.7	44.9	
SCOFF positive responses								
Q1: Deliberate vomiting	34.3	30.0	38.6	<0.001	37.9	31.9	43.6	<0.001
Q2: Loss of control over eating	11.5	9.8	13.2	0.042	15.8	12.6	18.8	<0.001
Q3: Weight loss	4.7	4.9	4.4	0.728	9.1	9.9	8.3	0.215
Q4: Body image distortion	17.6	9.0	26.3	<0.001	20.1	11.7	28.2	<0.001
Q5: Impact of food on life	5.1	4.1	6.1	0.060	11.8	8.9	13.0	0.008
At risk for eating disorderb	17.7	12.5	22.9	<0.001	25.2	17.6	32.3	<0.001
Self-reported physical fitness (score)c	–	–	–		3.5±0.9	3.7±0.9	3.4±0.9	<0.001
Measured physical fitness (VO2max, mL kg−1 min−1)d	45.7±9.5	49.6±9.9	41.8±7.2	<0.001	–	–	–	

[a]Including obesity. [b]A score of ≥2 in the SCOFF questionnaire indicates a likely case of eating disorders. [c]A question about self-report of fitness levels was considered a measure of overall fitness. [d]Cardiorespiratory fitness measured by the 20-m shuttle-run test Values are expressed as mean±SD or percentage (%).

11.3 RESULTS

The descriptive characteristics for the adolescents of the AVENA and AFI-NOS Studies are shown in Table 1. In general, both studies showed that boys had higher levels of body fat and physical fitness than girls, whereas girls reported higher levels of eating disorders than boys. On the other hand, the prevalence of obesity was 4.6% (3.3% in girls, $P=0.001$) in the AVENA Study and 2.1% (1.0% in girls, $P<0.001$) in the AFINOS Study. The prevalence of underweight adolescents was 4.8% (4.7% in girls, $P=0.923$) in the AVENA Study and 5.3% (6.7% in girls, $P=0.005$) in the AFINOS Study.

Tables S1 and S2 (supporting information) show the proportions of positive responses in the SCOFF questionnaire and the risk of developing eating disorders by weight status and fitness levels. Overall, overweight adolescents and those who had low fitness levels had a greater proportion of positive responses in almost all the questions, as well as a higher risk of developing eating disorders. The associations of weight status and physical fitness levels with the risk of developing eating disorders for each study are shown in Table 2. In both studies, the results of the binary logistic regression analysis showed that the adolescents classified as overweight had a higher risk of developing eating disorders (both $P<0.001$) than those classified as non-overweight. Also, adolescents who had low or middle level of physical fitness were more likely to develop eating disorders than those with high physical fitness (all $P<0.001$).

The combined associations of weight status and physical fitness with the risk of eating disorders for each study are shown in Fig. 1. In the AVENA Study, (A) among non-overweight adolescents only those with low fitness were at an increased risk of developing eating disorders compared with the high fitness group (odds ratio [OR]: 1.65, 95% confidence interval [CI]:1.07–2.55). Among overweight adolescents, the ORs (95% CI) of eating disorders for groups with low, medium and high fitness compared with non-overweight adolescents with high fitness were 3.34 (1.77–6.31), 5.78 (3.46–9.66) and 6.23 (4.00–9.70), respectively.

In the AFINOS Study, (B) the ORs (95% CI) in the non-overweight group were 1.85 (1.44–2.37) and 4.50 (3.06–6.63) according to middle and low fitness groups, respectively, compared with the non-overweight group with high fitness levels. In the overweight group, the ORs (95% CIs) for eating disorders for groups with low, medium and high fitness compared with non-overweight adolescents with high fitness were 1.62 (1.03–2.57), 2.64 (1.84–3.80) and 5.12 (3.20–8.19), respectively.

TABLE 2: Odds ratios (OR) and 95% confidence intervals (CI) for risk of developing eating disorders in adolescents with different weight status and physical fitness levels

	AVENA Study[b]			AFINOS Study[c]		
	n	OR	95% CI	n	OR	95% CI
Weight status						
Non-overweight	1211	1	Ref.	1663	1	Ref.
Overweighta	343	4.91	3.63-6.61	354	2.45	1.83-3.22
Fitness levels						
High	518	1	Ref.	1081	1	Ref.
Medium	518	1.51	1.05-2.16	729	1.73	1.37-2.17
Low	518	2.25	1.60-3.19	207	4.11	2.98-5.65

Analyses were sex- and age-adjusted. [a]Including obesity. [b]Weight status and physical fitness variables were measured. [c]Weight status and physical fitness variables were self-reported.

11.4 DISCUSSION

In the present study, we analysed the associations of physical fitness and overweight with the risk of developing eating disorders in two large samples of Spanish adolescents. The main findings of this study indicate that there is an inverse association between physical fitness levels and the risk of eating disorders in adolescents, independently of weight status. We also found that overweight adolescents had a higher risk of developing eating disorders than non-overweight adolescents. However, overweight adolescents with high levels of physical fitness had a lower risk of eating disorders than overweight adolescents with low levels of physical fitness. To the best of our knowledge, this is the first study suggesting that physical fitness might attenuate the negative influence of body fat on risk for eating disorder in adolescents.

Eating disorders are serious, potentially life-threatening conditions that can lead to very serious physical health problems. The origin of eating disorders is very complex. Individual and familial, biological and psychological characteristics contribute. In addition, a large number of previous research projects have concluded that the period with the greatest prevalence of eating disorders is the adolescence and early youth [26]. In Spain, only one previous study involving 841 students, aged 12–19 years, determined the risk of developing eating disorders using the SCOFF questionnaire [27]. The results of that study showed that 21% of the subjects had significant scores in the questionnaire. This rate is similar to and between the rates found in the AVENA (18%) Study and the AFINOS (25%) Study.

The number of investigations examining the association of physical fitness on health outcomes in youth and adults has increased substantially in recent years. High fitness levels have been consistently associated with physical unhealthy outcomes such as obesity, hypertension, type 2 diabetes, metabolic syndrome, cancer and skeletal health problems[12]. However, the scientific literature focused on the relationship between physical fitness and mental disorders is scarce.

Nowadays, the available information suggests that improvements in physical fitness have short-term and long-term positive effects on depression, anxiety, mood status and self-esteem in young people. For example, a school-based controlled trial involving 198 students aged 15 years from Chile showed that improving physical fitness was beneficial for mental well-being. At the end of the program, anxiety score decreased 13.7% in the intervention group versus 2.8% in the control group, and self-esteem score increased 1.3% in the intervention group and decreased 0.1% in the control group [28]. Another study performed in 66 Hispanic children showed that children included in an aerobic intensity program significantly improved their fitness and reported significantly ($P < 0.05$) less depression after 6 weeks [29]. In a sample of 4888 adult participants examined in 1988–1997, weak but significant correlations were found between CRF and positive and negative emotion [30]. Our findings extend these previous results because we have found a novel link between physical fitness and the risk of developing eating disorders.

Indeed, high physical fitness seems to protect against the risk of such disorders in overweight adolescents regardless of the methodology used to assess physical fitness since in the AVENA Study physical fitness was assessed by a field test [15], while in the AFINOS Study it was assessed using a self-reported question [16, 31-33]. The idea of fat but fit was proposed in 1995 by Blair and colleagues, who showed that within a fatness category, aerobic fitness attenuates the risk of disease [34, 35]. Although there is limited evidence, similar fat but fit findings have been observed in youth related to physical health outcomes [36] but, to date, there is no evidence regarding the fat but fit theory on mental health outcomes in youth.

Another finding in the current study was that the association of physical fitness with eating disorders was unclear in the group of non-overweight adolescents. In the AFINOS Study, where the measure of physical fitness was subjective, physical fitness levels were negatively associated with the risk of eating disorders ($P<0.001$). However, in the AVENA Study, where the measure of physical fitness was objective, the association between physical fitness and eating disorders was notably attenuated ($P=0.078$). Likewise, the association between physical fitness and eating disorders was stronger using self-reported fitness than measured fitness. Self-reported physical fitness may be influenced not only by real physical fitness (i.e. physical health) but also by other health dimensions (e.g. mental health, intellectual health, social health and spiritual health) that might be independent of adolescents' weight status [37]. Whether other dimensions of health affects the answer on self-reported physical fitness is unknown. And the other way round, whether self-reported physical fitness could be considered a proximate estimate of overall health is also to be elucidated. This fact might explain the differences observed in our study using different procedures to measure physical fitness [38]. Taken together, these results suggest that improvements on physical fitness should be developed using a multifactorial approach based on multiple dimensions of health to more effectively prevent eating disorders in adolescents.

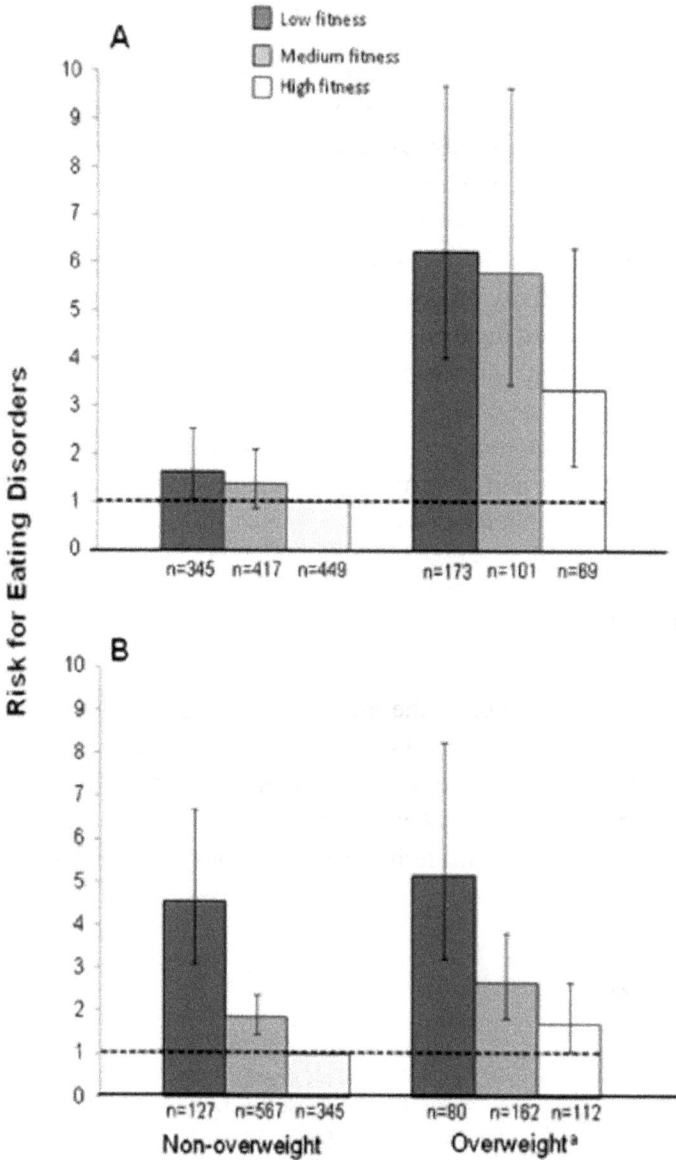

FIGURE 1: Odds ratios and 95% confidence intervals (error bars) to assess the risk of developing eating disorders according to weight status and physical fitness levels. A=AVENA Study (measured variables). B=AFINOS Study (self-reported variables).a Including obesity.

The main limitation of our study is its cross-sectional design, which cannot establish causal relationships. However, the use of two large and heterogeneous samples means that these results can be generalized. Likewise, the results found with the AFINOS Study must be interpreted with caution because we only had self-reported measurements of fatness and fitness. Consequently, our results in the AVENA Study could be more valuable for public health purposes.

Since physical fitness seems to be related to the different health outcomes, physical activity programs should be designed to improve the levels of fitness. Reinforcing the need to include physical fitness testing could also be interesting in health monitoring systems. Longitudinal studies and randomized control trials are still needed in this field to understand the nature and relative importance of alternative determinants of physical fitness during adolescence, and to verify the usefulness of alternative promotion strategies and recommendations.

11.5 CONCLUSION

The present findings support the role of physical fitness in preventing the development of eating disorders in adolescents, especially in overweight or obese adolescents. Hence, it would be important and necessary to develop educational and public health strategies to identify, prevent and treat these health problems considering physical fitness as a relevant measure for prevention.

REFERENCES

1. Herpertz-Dahlmann B. Adolescent eating disorders: definitions, symptomatology, epidemiology and comorbidity. Child Adolesc Psychiatr Clin N Am 2009; 18: 31–47.
2. Austin SB. Prevention research in eating disorders: theory and new directions. Psychol Med 2000; 30: 1249–1262.
3. Lahortiga-Ramos F, De Irala-Estévez J, Cano-Prous A, Gual-García P, Martínez-González MA, Cervera-Enguix S. Incidence of eating disorders in Navarra (Spain). Eur Psychiatry 2005; 20: 179–185.
4. Neumark-Sztainer D. Obesity and eating disorder prevention: an integrated approach. Adolesc Med. 2003; 14: 159–173.

5. Nicholls D, Viner R. Eating disorders and weight problems. BMJ 2005; 30: 950–953.
6. Neumark-Sztainer D, Story M, Hannan PJ. Weight-related concerns and behaviors among overweight and non-overweight adolescents: implications for preventing weight-related disorders. Arch Pediatr Adolesc Med 2002; 156: 171–178.
7. Markey CN, Markey PM. Relations between body image and dieting behaviors: an examination of gender differences. Sex Roles 2005; 53: 519–530.
8. Irving LM, Neumark-Sztainer D. Integrating the prevention of eating disorders and obesity: feasible or futile? Prev Med 2002; 34: 299–309.
9. Ortega FB, Ruiz JR, Castillo MJ, Sjöström M. Physical fitness in childhood and adolescence: a powerful marker of health. Int J Obes (Lond.) 2008; 32: 1–11.
10. Alberga AS, Sigal RJ, Goldfield G, Prud'homme D, Kenny GP. Overweight and obese teenagers: why is adolescence a critical period?. Pediatr Obes 2012; 7: 261–273.
11. Fogelholm M, Stigman S, Huisman T, Metsamuuronen J. Physical fitness in adolescents with normal weight and overweight. Scand J Med Sci Sports 2008; 18: 162–170.
12. LaMonte MJ, Blair SN. Physical activity, cardiorespiratory fitness, and adiposity: contributions to disease risk. Curr Opin Clin Nutr Metab Care 2006; 9: 540–546.
13. Rodgers RF, Paxton SJ, Chabrol H. Depression as a moderator of sociocultural influences on eating disorder symptoms in adolescent females and males. J Youth Adolesc 2010; 39: 393–402.
14. Karpowicz E, Skärsäter I, Nevonen L. Self-esteem in patients treated for anorexia nervosa. Int J Ment Health Nurs 2009; 18: 318–325.
15. González-Gross M, Castillo MJ, Moreno L, et al. Feeding and assessment of nutritional status of Spanish adolescents (AVENA study). Evaluation of risks and interventional proposal. Methodol Nutr Hosp. 2003; 18: 15–28.
16. Veiga OL, Gómez-Martínez S, Martínez-Gómez D, Villagra A, Calle ME, Marcos A. Physical activity as a preventive measure against overweight, obesity, infections, allergies and cardiovascular disease risk factors in adolescents: AFINOS Study protocol. BMC Public Health 2009; 9: 475–486.
17. Morgan JF, Reid F, Lacey JH. The SCOFF questionnaire: assessment of a new screening tool for eating disorder. BMJ 1999; 319: 1467–1468.
18. Rueda GE, Díaz LA, Ortiz DP, Pinzon C, Rodriguez J, Cadena LP. Validation of the SCOFF questionnaire for screening the Eating behaviour disorders of adolescents in school. Aten Primaria 2005; 35: 89–94.
19. Moreno LA, Joyanes M, Mesana MI, et al. Harmonization of anthropometric measurements for a multicenter nutrition survey in Spanish adolescents. Nutrition 2003; 19: 481–486.
20. Cole TJ, Bellizzi MC, Flegal KM, Dietz WH. Establishing a standard definition for child overweight and obesity worldwide. BMJ 2000; 320: 1240–1243.
21. Cole TJ, Flegal KM, Nicholls D, Jackson AA. Body mass index cut offs to define thinness in children and adolescents: international survey. BMJ 2007; 335: 194–202.
22. Léger LA, Mercier D, Gadoury C, Lambert J. The multistage 20 metre shuttle run test for aerobic fitness. J Sports Sci 1988; 6: 93–101.

23. Léger L, Lambert J, Goulet A, Rowan C, Dinelle Y. Aerobic capacity of 6 to 17-year-old Quebecois – 20 meter shuttle run test with 1 minute stages. Can J Appl Sport Sci 1984; 9: 64–69.
24. The Cooper Institute for Aerobics Research. FITNESSGRAM Test Administration. Manual, 3rd edn. Human Kinetics: Champaign, IL, 2004, 38–39.
25. Ortega FB, Ruiz JR, España-Romero V, et al. The International Fitness Scale (IFIS): usefulness of self-reported fitness in youth. Int J Epidemiol 2001; 40: 701–711.
26. Goñi A, Rodríguez A. Variables associated with the risk of eating disorders in adolescents. Salud Mental 2007; 30: 16–23.
27. Jáuregui I, Romero J, Bolaños P, et al. Eating behaviour and body image in a sample of adolescents from Sevilla. Nutr Hosp 2009; 24: 568–573.
28. Bonhauser M, Fernandez G, Püschel K, Yañez F, Thompson B, Coronado G. Improving physical fitness and emotional well-being in adolescents of low socioeconomic status in Chile: results of a school-based controlled trial. Health Promot Int 2005; 20: 113–122.
29. Crews DJ, Lochbaum MR, Landers DM. Aerobic physical activity effects on psychological well-being in low-income Hispanic children. Percept Mot Skills 2004; 98: 319–324.
30. Ortega FB, Lee DC, Sui X, et al. Psychological well-being, cardiorespiratory fitness, and long-term survival. Am J Prev Med 2010; 39: 440–448.
31. Martinez-Gomez D, Veiga OL, Gomez-Martinez S, et al. Gender-specific influence of health behaviors on academic performance in Spanish adolescents; the AFINOS study. Nutr Hosp 2012; 27: 724–730.
32. Martinez-Gomez D, Martín-Matillas M, Veiga OL, Marcos A. Trends in six years participation in extracurricular physical activity in adolescents. The AVENA and AFINOS Studies. Rev Esp Cardiol 2011; 64: 437–438.
33. Martinez-Gomez D, Eisenmann JC, Gomez-Martinez S, et al. Relationships of self-reported physical activity, fitness and body mass index with inflammatory proteins in adolescents. The AFINOS study. Proc Nutr Soc 2012; 69: E273.
34. Lee SL, Kuk JL, Katzmarzyk PT, Blair SN, Church TS, Ross R. Cardiorespiratory fitness attenuates metabolic risk independent of abdominal subcutaneous and visceral fat in men. Diabetes Care 2005; 28: 895–901.
35. Barlow CE, Kohl HW 3rd, Gibbons LW, Blair SN. Physical fitness, mortality and obesity. Int J Obes Relat Metab Disord 1995; 19: 41–44.
36. Eisenmann JC. Aerobic fitness, fatness and the metabolic syndrome in children and adolescents. Acta Paediatr 2007; 96: 1723–1729.
37. Corbin CB, Welk GJ, Corbin WR, Welk KA. Concepts of Physical Fitness: Active Lifestyles for Wellness, 14th edn. McGraw-Hill: London, 2008.
38. Fonseca H, Matos MG, Guerra A, Pedro JG. Are overweight and obese adolescents different from their peers? Int J Pediatr Obes 2009; 4: 166–174.

There are several supplemental files that are not available in this version of the article. To view this additional information, please use the citation on the first page of this chapter.

CHAPTER 12

ADOLESCENT OBESITY, JOINT PAIN, AND HYPERMOBILITY

SHARON BOUT-TABAKU, SARAH B. KLIEGER,
BRIAN H. WROTNIAK, DAVID D. SHERRY, BABETTE S. ZEMEL,
AND NICOLAS STETTLER

12.1 INTRODUCTION

Non- inflammatory joint pain referrals to pediatric rheumatologists are common. The underlying etiologies include trauma, overuse and hypermobility [1-3] With the current obesity epidemic, 16.9 percent of United States (U.S.) children and adolescents are obese and joint pain is more prevalent in obese than healthy weight children [4-6]. One mechanism of obesity related joint pain is that greater load bearing causes micro injury. However little is known about other factors that alter joint loads and possibly cause micro injury among obese children, such as hypermobility.

Hypermobility and obesity together, during rapid growth in puberty, may cause more children to have joint pain and damage, as greater loading stresses are applied to the joint. A single study to date, in British adolescents, found that hypermobility and obesity was a risk factor for musculoskeletal pain [7]. Specifically, the odds ratio of knee pain was 11 in obese, hypermobile subjects compared to 1.57 in non-obese, hypermobile

Adolescent Obesity, Joint Pain, and Hypermobility. © *Bout-Tabaku S, Klieger SB, Wrotniak BH, Sherry DD, Zemel BS and Stettler N.* Pediatric Rheumatology *12,11 (2014);* doi:10.1186/1546-0096-12-11. *Licensed under Creative Commons Attribution 2.0 Generic License, http://creativecommons. org/licenses/by/2.0/.*

subjects, suggesting that two factors affecting load on the lower extremity joints may be markers for joint stress [7].

We characterized the association of obesity and non-traumatic lower extremity (LE) joint pain in US adolescents and evaluated the modifying effect of hypermobility on this association. We hypothesized that obese adolescents would have a greater prevalence of LE pain compared to healthy weight peers, and that hypermobile, obese adolescents would have a greater prevalence of LE pain than non-hypermobile, obese adolescents.

12.2 FINDINGS

12.2.1 SUBJECTS

Analysis for this sub study was based on baseline data from obese subjects and a healthy weight control (HW) group enrolled in a randomized clinical control trial examining the impact of weight loss, on bone health in adolescents between January 2008 and August 2011. The study was a nested case–control powered on detecting differences in bone strength between obese and HW subjects required 51 HW subjects. The number of obese subjects was determined based on power analysis to detect change in bone strength between obese subjects in the RCT phase who received standard care or comprehensive weight control.

Subjects were recruited using flyers and radio announcements from the community. They were invited to participate based on inclusion and exclusion criteria. Subjects were excluded for syndromic or secondary obesity, developmental delay, significant psychological or psychiatric disorder, diabetes, any chronic disease or medication interfering with bone health or weight loss, inability of parents to participate in the study visits, cigarette smoking, or recent significant weight loss. All the participants who participated in the RCT had data collected for this sub study at baseline. Baseline visits included the collection of self-reported pain and hypermobility data in addition to the multiple measures related to the primary outcomes of the study of bone health and weight loss. The RCT and the sub study received approval from the Children's Hospital of Philadelphia institutional review board and all subjects signed informed consents.

12.2.2 ANTHROPOMETRIC MEASURES

Anthropometric data were collected at the study visit per study protocol. Height was measured using a stadiometer (Holtain, Crymych, UK) to the nearest 0.1 centimeter. Weight was measured on a digital electronic scale (Seca, Munich, Germany) to the nearest 0.1 kilogram. Body mass index (BMI=kg/m^2) was calculated and obesity status determined using US CDC 2000 growth charts. Obesity was defined as having a BMI≥95th percentile for sex and age. BMI Z-scores were generated similarly [8]. Younger obese adolescents and slightly older adolescent HW subjects were recruited to account for the advanced maturation expected in the obese subjects [9].

12.2.3 MEASUREMENT OF PAIN

The PEDS™ Pediatric Pain Questionnaire™ assessed present pain and worst pain over the past week [10]. A body map localized areas of musculoskeletal pain across 14 areas including joints. We analyzed pain data that was reported by the adolescent [11]. Anyone answering "yes" to pain at a specific body part was considered to have pain. Adolescents with trauma related pain, headaches and stomach pain were categorized as no pain. Then two pain variables were generated to characterize pain 1) any musculoskeletal pain (including all extremities, neck and back) and 2) pain only in the LE (including the hips, legs, thighs, knees or ankles). This allowed us to separate the effects of weight bearing associated pain vs. pain unrelated to weight bearing.

12.2.3.1 HYPERMOBILITY MEASURES

Hypermobility measurements were performed by a trained pediatric rheumatologist (SBT) and trained examiners (SK, SN) using the modified Beighton nine-point scoring system [12]. We defined hypermobility two ways: ≥4 hypermobile joints and a more stringent definition, ≥ 6 hypermobile joints [13]. We assessed the popliteal angle to measure hamstring flexibility with a goniometer according to standard technique [14,15]. The inter-observer correlation coefficient of two measurers on a total of 129 subjects was 0.92 and 0.90 for the right and left popliteal angles, respectively.

12.2.3.2 OTHER MEASUREMENTS

Sex, age, race, Tanner stage and physical activity were covariates. Tanner stage was self-reported using a validated questionnaire [16]. Physical activity was assessed using the Actitrac activity monitor (IM Systems, Baltimore, MD), a two-dimensional accelerometer worn on the belt for seven days. The average number of activity counts per minute (cpm) was used as a measure of activity and as a continuous variable in the analysis.

12.2.4 STATISTICAL ANALYSIS

Categorical variables were reported as percentages, and continuous variables as means and standard deviations. Between group differences in pain and hypermobility were tested with chi-square or Fisher's exact test, and t-tests for normally distributed variables, or Kruskal-Wallis tests for non-normal distributions. The relationship between obesity and LE pain and obesity and hypermobility, were examined using multivariate logistic regression models. A separate model assessed whether the association between obesity and joint pain is modified by hypermobility. A two-tailed p-value <0.05 was considered statistically significant. Stata12.0. (StataCorp) was used for the analyses.

12.2.5 CHARACTERISTICS OF THE COHORT

Data were obtained on 142 subjects (91 were obese and 51 were healthy weight). The demographic characteristics of the subjects are shown in Table 1. The HW subjects were older than their obese counterparts by design

(14.5 vs. 12.2 years, p<0.001). As expected, the BMI and BMI-Z-score differed between groups.

TABLE 1: Characteristics of obese subjects and healthy controls

Variable	Obese (n=91)	Controls (n=51)	p value
Age, years (median)	12.2	14.5	<0.001
Range	10.2 to 17.6	10.2 to 17.9	
Sex, % male	35.2	37.3	0.80
Race, % black	64.8	64.7	0.99
% Tanner 4 or 5	47.7	70.6	0.055
Physical activity (mean cpm, sd)*	272.8±108.2	255.6±92.3	0.38
BMI (mean)	33.9±4.90	19.70±2.00	<0.001
Range	26.3 to 49.6	15.1 to 23.2	
BMI-Z- score (mean)	2.38±0.23	- 0.02±0.62	<0.001
Range	1.93 to 2.88	-1.54 to 0.99	

*Statistical analysis for continuous variables was performed using t-tests for normally distributed variables. For categorical variables, the Chi 2 test was used. SD = standard deviation. Physical activity is in counts per minute (cpm) of physical activity. *Physical activity data were available on 125 subject (obese = 82, non obese = 43). Body Mass index (BMI). BMI-Z-score adjusted for age and gender based on US 2000 CDC growth charts.*

12.2.6 OBESITY, HYPERMOBILITY AND JOINT PAIN

LE pain prevalence was 14% among obese and 10% among HW subjects; but obesity was not associated with any musculoskeletal pain (OR 0.96, CI 0.64-1.44, p=0.8) or LE pain (OR 1.29, CI 0.75-2.23, p=0.3) in unadjusted and adjusted models (Table 2). Hypermobility (defined as≥to 4 joints) prevalence was 14% among obese, and 9% among HW subjects. With the stringent definition, (hypermobility≥6 joints), the prevalence was 2% for both groups. (Table 3) Obesity was not associated with hypermobility (OR 1.23, CI 0.72-2.14, p=0.3 in unadjusted and adjusted models. (Table 4) Hypermobility did not differ by sex or race.

TABLE 2: Association of pain with BMI Z-score and obesity

		1. Unadjusted		2. Adjusted	
Pain	Covariate	OR	95% CI	OR	95% CI
Musculoskeletal	BMI-Z-score	0.99	0.72 - 1.36	1.01	0.64 - 1.58
Lower Extremity	BMI-Z-score	1.10	0.73 - 1.66	0.98	0.56 - 1.72
Musculoskeletal	Obesity	0.96	0.64 - 1.44	0.86	0.49 - 1.50
Lower Extremity	Obesity	1.29	0.75 - 2.33	1.02	0.49 - 2.15

Adjusted for sex, age, race, Tanner stage, hypermobility and physical activity.
Odds ratios (OR's) > 1 indicate increased odds of having any musculoskeletal pain or lower extremity pain. OR's <1 indicate a decreased odds of having any musculoskeletal pain or lower extremity pain. Results are considered statistically significant if the 95% Confidence interval (CI) does not include 1.

TABLE 3: Pain and hypermobility

	Obese (n=91)	Non-obese (n=51)	p value
Musculoskeletal pain			
Any musculoskeletal pain (%)	22	24	0.83
Lower extremity pain (%)	14	10	0.31
Hypermobility			
Hypermobile 6 (%)	2	2	0.71
(≥6 Beighton score)			
Hypermobile 4 (%)	14	10	0.31
(≥4 on Beighton score)			
Thumbs (%)	24	25	0.86
Elbows (%)	8	22	0.02
Knees (%)	13	12	0.81
Fingers (%)	9	2	0.10
Trunk (%)	4	2	0.41

All values are percentages. For categorical variables, the Chi 2 or the Fisher's exact test was used where appropriate.

TABLE 4: Association of hypermobility with BMI Z-score and obesity

		1. Unadjusted		2. Adjusted	
	Covariate	OR	95% CI	OR	95% CI
Hypermobility4*	BMI-Z-score	1.12	0.74 -1.72	0.72	0.42- 1.22
Hypermobility4	Obesity	1.23	0.72 – 2.14	0.79	0.39- 1.60

Adjusted for sex, age. Race, Tanner stage, and physical activity. *Hypermobility4 is the less stringent level of the Beighton score (4/9). Odds ratios (OR's) > 1 indicate increased odds of having hypermobility. OR's <1 indicate a decreased odds of having hypermobility. Results are considered statistically significant if the 95% Confidence interval (CI) does not include 1.

TABLE 5: Association of hypermobility and pain

		1. Unadjusted		2. Adjusted	
	Covariate	OR	95% CI	OR	95% CI
MSK pain	Hypermobility4	1.88	0.65 - 5.50	2.61	0.76 - 8.89
LE pain	Hypermobility4	1.35	0.35 – 5.19	1.46	0.32 - 6.55
MSK pain	Hypermobility4x Obesity§			0.80	0.45 - 1.42
LE pain	Hypermobility4x Obesity§			0.98	0.46 – 2.08

Adjusted for sex, age, race, Tanner stage, obesity and physical activity. Odds ratios (OR's) > 1 indicate increased odds of having MSK pain or Le pain. OR's <1 indicate a decreased odds of having MSK pain or LE pain. Results are considered statistically significant if the 95% Confidence interval (CI) does not include 1. §Hypermobility4xObesity is the interaction term in the model looking at the association of obesity and joint pain.

The mean right popliteal angles were 136° and 119°, for the obese and HW subjects, respectively. The mean left popliteal angles were 136° and 120° for the obese and HW subjects, respectively. The standard deviation was 15°. These angles differed by obesity status with a $p < 0.001$.

There was no effect modification by hypermobility status, on the association between obesity and LE pain 0.98 (95% CI = 0.46 - 2.08) or musculoskeletal pain 0.80 (95% CI = 0.45 -1.42) (Table 5).

12.3 DISCUSSION

We are the first to examine the associations between obesity, hypermobility and non-traumatic LE pain in US adolescents. Obese adolescents compared to healthy weight subjects did not have a greater prevalence of LE pain or hypermobility. We found that the combination of obesity and hypermobility did not confer greater odds of reporting LE joint pain.

Consistent with our findings of 14%, the prevalence of LE joint pain in obese adolescents ranges from 12- 44% [5,17-19]. A recent study in 5000 British 17 year olds showed an association between obesity and knee pain (OR 1.81 CI 1.27–2.74) [6]. Although this was a large study the population was racially homogenous and limited to only 17 year olds. Our data, with fewer subjects and greater racial heterogeneity, showed a greater percent of adolescents with LE pain were obese but there was no statistical difference from the HW subjects. In a post hoc analysis assuming the prevalence of LE between the two groups (14% vs. 10%), at a significance level of 0.05 and power of 80%, we would have needed a total sample size of 2210 subjects.

The combination of hypermobility and obesity, two pathways associated with joint instability and micro trauma, is a plausible mechanistic hypothesis for why more obese subjects have lower extremity joint pain than non-obese ones [20]. Tobias et al. found that knee pain was prevalent among 17 year olds if at 14 years, they were hypermobile and obese compared to those at 14 years who were hypermobile and non-obese [7]. However, they did not exclude children with injuries, thus the positive association and interaction between obesity and hypermobility on pain could be due to injury instead. Our data excluded children with injuries and we found no evidence to suggest that hypermobility, together with obesity, was associated with LE non-traumatic joint pain. Our findings may differ due to the racial heterogeneity and younger age of our subjects. Our study had more black subjects, who have a lower prevalence of hypermobility than whites, which may account for the lack of association in our group [21]. It is possible that obesity and hypermobility manifests with pain in older adolescents rather than younger ones, as adolescents have completed their bone and peri-articular tissue growth, while younger adolescents may be more resilient and heal from micro injuries.

Popliteal angles were measured to assess hamstring tightness, which has been associated with knee and back pain. Typically as children get older the popliteal angle decreases indicating less hamstring flexibility. Interestingly among our subjects the obese children had larger popliteal angles than the HW ones, indicating more hamstring flexibility which differs from de Sa Pinto et al., who found no difference between obese and HW subjects [19]. As the prevalence of both knee and back pain were low in our study we could not determine how hamstring flexibility among obese children relates to knee or back pain.

Our major limitation is our small sample size, since we were not powered to study obesity and joint pain. In particular the prevalence of hypermobility was low in our subjects, and larger numbers would be necessary to test associations as has been the case in the larger cross-sectional studies [13]. Another limitation was that we did not assess pain intensity since our focus was pain prevalence. Finally, our subjects may not be representative of the general population as they agreed to join an RCT and are possibly more motivated due to greater obesity and more obesity related problems, such as pain.

Our findings add to the sparse evidence about obesity, hypermobility and LE pain in U.S. adolescents. Furthermore, the clinical significance of a difference of 4% greater prevalence of LE pain in obese children may be important, as pain likely limits their interest, function and ability to participate in weight loss programs involving physical activities [22]. Prospective studies with sufficient power and sampling children at different developmental stages are needed to understand how obesity mediated altered mechanics affects the function and structure of the LE joints.

REFERENCES

1. Berard R: Approach to the child with joint inflammation. Pediatr Clin North Am 2012, 59:245-262.
2. Weiser P: Approach to the patient with noninflammatory musculoskeletal pain. Pediatr Clin North Am 2012, 59:471-492.
3. Bird HA: Joint hypermobility. Musculoskeletal Care 2007, 5:4-19.
4. Ogden CL, Carroll MD, Kit BK, Flegal KM: Prevalence of obesity and trends in body mass index among US children and adolescents, 1999–2010. JAMA 2012, 307:483-490.

5. Krul M, van der Wouden JC, Schellevis FG, van Suijlekom-Smit LW, Koes BW: Musculoskeletal problems in overweight and obese children. Ann Fam Med 2009, 7:352-356.

6. Deere KC, Clinch J, Holliday K, McBeth J, Crawley EM, Sayers A, Palmer S, Doerner R, Clark EM, Tobias JH: Obesity is a risk factor for musculoskeletal pain in adolescents: findings from a population-based cohort. Pain 2012, 153:1932-1938.

7. Tobias JH, Deere K, Palmer S, Clark EM, Clinch J: Joint hypermobility is a risk factor for musculoskeletal pain during adolescence: findings of a prospective cohort study. Arthritis Rheum 2013, 65:1107-1115.

8. Kuczmarski RJ, Ogden CL, Grummer-Strawn LM, Flegal KM, Guo SS, Wei R, Mei Z, Curtin LR, Roche AF, Johnson CL: CDC growth charts: United States. Adv Data 2000, 314:1-27.

9. Johnson W, Stovitz SD, Choh AC, Czerwinski SA, Towne B, Demerath EW: Patterns of linear growth and skeletal maturation from birth to 18 years of age in overweight young adults. Int J Obes (Lond) 2012, 36:535-541.

10. Varni JW, Thompson KL, Hanson V: The Varni/Thompson Pediatric Pain Questionnaire. I. Chronic musculoskeletal pain in juvenile rheumatoid arthritis. Pain 1987, 28:27-38.

11. Vetter TR, Bridgewater CL, McGwin G Jr: An observational study of patient versus parental perceptions of health-related quality of life in children and adolescents with a chronic pain condition: who should the clinician believe? Health Qual Life Outcomes 2012, 10:85.

12. Beighton P, Solomon L, Soskolne CL: Articular mobility in an African population. Ann Rheum Dis 1973, 32:413-418.

13. Clinch J, Deere K, Sayers A, Palmer S, Riddoch C, Tobias JH, Clark EM: Epidemiology of generalized joint laxity (hypermobility) in fourteen-year-old children from the UK: a population-based evaluation. Arthritis Rheum 2011, 63:2819-2827.

14. Katz K, Rosenthal A, Yosipovitch Z: Normal ranges of popliteal angle in children. J Pediatr Orthop 1992, 12:229-231.

15. Woolston SL, Beukelman T, Sherry DD: Back mobility and interincisor distance ranges in racially diverse North American healthy children and relationship to generalized hypermobility. Pediatr Rheumatol Online J 2012, 10:17.

16. Duke PM, Litt IF, Gross RT: Adolescents' self-assessment of sexual maturation. Pediatrics 1980, 66:918-920.

17. Taylor ED, Theim KR, Mirch MC, Ghorbani S, Tanofsky-Kraff M, Adler-Wailes DC, Brady S, Reynolds JC, Calis KA, Yanovksi JA: Orthopedic complications of overweight in children and adolescents. Pediatrics 2006, 117:2167-2174.

18. El-Metwally A, Salminen JJ, Auvinen A, Kautiainen H, Mikkelsson M: Risk factors for traumatic and non-traumatic lower limb pain among preadolescents: a population-based study of Finnish schoolchildren. BMC Musculoskelet Disord 2006, 7:3.

19. de Sa Pinto AL, de Barros Holanda PM, Radu AS, Villares SM, Lima FR: Musculoskeletal findings in obese children. J Paediatr Child Health 2006, 42:341-344.

20. Pacey V, Nicholson LL, Adams RD, Munn J, Munns CF: Generalized joint hypermobility and risk of lower limb joint injury during sport: a systematic review with meta-analysis. Am J Sports Med 2010, 38:1487-1497.

21. Scher DL, Owens BD, Sturdivant RX, Wolf JM: Incidence of joint hypermobility syndrome in a military population: impact of gender and race. Clin Orthop Relat Res 2010, 468:1790-1795.
22. Bout-Tabaku S, Briggs MS, Schmitt LC: Lower extremity pain is associated with reduced function and psychosocial health in obese children. Clin Orthop Relat Res 2012, 471:1236-1244.

CHAPTER 13

FTO, OBESITY, AND THE ADOLESCENT BRAIN

MELKAYE G. MELKA, JESSE GILLIS, MANON BERNARD, MICHAL ABRAHAMOWICZ, M. MALLAR CHAKRAVARTY, GABRIEL T. LEONARD, MICHEL PERRON, LOUIS RICHER, SUZANNE VEILLETTE, TOBIAS BANASCHEWSKI, GARETH J. BARKER, CHRISTIAN BÜCHEL, PATRICIA CONROD, HERTA FLOR, ANDREAS HEINZ, HUGH GARAVAN, RÜDIGER BRÜHL, KARL MANN, ERIC ARTIGES, ANBARASU LOURDUSAMY, MARK LATHROP, EVA LOTH, YANNICK SCHWARTZ, VINCENT FROUIN, MARCELLA RIETSCHEL, MICHAEL N. SMOLKA, ANDREAS STRÖHLE, JÜRGEN GALLINAT, MAREN STRUVE, EVA LATTKA, MELANIE WALDENBERGER, GUNTER SCHUMANN, PAUL PAVLIDIS, DANIEL GAUDET, TOMÁŠ PAUS, AND ZDENKA PAUSOVA

13.1 INTRODUCTION

The fat mass and obesity-associated gene (*FTO*) is a well-replicated gene locus of obesity (1–4). It was originally identified as a gene locus of type-2 diabetes, and only later it was discovered that it increases risk of this disease through its primary effect on adiposity (1). However, the mechanisms

Reprinted with permission from Melka MG et al. FTO, Obesity and the Adolescent Brain. Human Molecular Genetics **22**,5 (2012), doi: 10.1093/hmg/dds504.

through which *FTO* may increase adiposity are still not clear. In vitro studies suggest that *FTO* encodes 2-oxoglutarate-dependent nucleic-acid demethylase that may regulate gene expression (5–7). Beginning from early embryogenesis, the gene is expressed throughout the body and the brain (5,8,9). The relatively high expression of *FTO* in the adult hypothalamus, a brain structure regulating energy balance, suggested that *FTO* might influence adiposity through its impact on energy homeostasis. Conflicting results of both human and animal studies exist, however, as to whether the gene influences either food intake or energy expenditure in a way that would increase risk for obesity [reviewed in (3,4)].

Obesity is a major risk factor for cognitive decline (10). In part, this association may be mediated through the cardiometabolic sequelae of obesity that promote cerebrovascular disease and subsequent neuronal degeneration (11,12). Recently, the *FTO*-risk allele for obesity has been associated with lower regional volumes of (cortical) brain tissue in elderly (13). These differences were not, however, associated with differences in cholesterol levels, hypertension or white-matter hyperintensities (13), suggesting that other factors may be at play.

The aim of the present study was to investigate an association between *FTO*, brain and adiposity in a developmental context. For this reason, we have focused on adolescence and used total brain volume as the main dependent variable. Total brain volume reaches 83% of adult values by the end of the second year of postnatal life (14) and 95% by 6 years of age (15). Thus, values of the total brain volume obtained in adolescence are likely to reflect mainly biological processes at play in utero and during early postnatal years. We performed these studies in a sample of 598 adolescents recruited from the French Canadian founder population as part of the Saguenay Youth Study (SYS-Discovery) and replicated our findings in 413 adolescents who were recruited and phenotyped later in the same study (SYS-Replication) and in 718 adolescents of mixed European background who were recruited as part of the IMAGEN study. In all three samples, brain volumes were assessed with magnetic resonance imaging (MRI), and a variant of *FTO* (i.e. rs9930333) previously reported as associated with body mass index (BMI) (16) was studied.

TABLE 1: Basic characteristics of studied participants

Outcome	SYS-Discovery		SYS-Replication		IMAGEN	
	Number	Mean ± SD	Number	Mean ± SD	Number	Mean ± SD
Age (years)	592	15.1 ± 1.9	416	14.4 ± 1.8	710	14.5 ± 0.4
Sex (males/females)	592	282/310	416	210/206	718	348/370
Height (cm)	590	163.3 ± 9.5	415	163.1 ± 9.5	663	168.4 ± 8.0
Body weight (log kg)	581	1.7 ± 0.1	412	1.8 ± 0.1	669	1.8 ± 0.1
BMI (log kg/m^2)	582	1.3 ± 0.1	413	1.3 ± 0.1	658	1.3 ± 0.01
Overweight/obesity (y/n)	582	139/443	413	135/278	654	124/530
TBF (log kg)	559	1.0 ± 0.3	397	1.0 ± 0.3	N/A	N/A
LBM (log kg)	566	1.7 ± 0.1	389	1.7 ± 0.1	N/A	N/A
Brain volume (cm^3)	562	1301 ± 119	395	1235 ± 112	712	1195 ± 113
IC volume (cm^3)	529	1813.5 ± 156	355	1811.5 ± 151	653	1818.1 ± 156
Ventricular volume (log cm^3)	558	1.0 ± 0.2	401	1.0 ± 0.2	708	1.1 ± 0.2
MAF (rs99930333)	594	0.31	422	0.36	717	0.34

Ventricular volume is defined as the sum of volumes of the left lateral, right lateral, third and fourth ventricles. MAF, minor allele frequency.

13.2 RESULTS

13.2.1 FTO ASSOCIATIONS WITH BMI AND BRAIN VOLUME

Basic characteristics of the SYS-Discovery, SYS-Replication and IMA-GEN samples are provided in Table 1. The prevalence of overweight or obesity was 23.9, 32.7 and 19.0% in the SYS-Discovery, SYS-Replication and IMAGEN samples, respectively, which is similar to that of current adolescent populations (17,18). In the SYS, the G allele of rs9930333 was associated with higher BMI ($P = 1.1 \times 10^{-4}$) and lower brain volume ($P = 0.005$, Fig. 1 and Table 2). Similar associations were observed in the replication (SYS-Replication and IMAGEN) samples, and the G allele was associated with higher BMI ($P = 0.005$ and $P = 1.4 \times 10^{-5}$, respectively) and trends towards lower brain volume ($P = 0.05$ and $P = 0.06$, respectively; Fig. 1 and Table 2). In a meta-analysis involving 1729 SYS-Discovery,

SYS-Replication and IMAGEN adolescents, the G allele was associated with higher BMI (P = 8.9×10^{-11}) and lower brain volume (P = 1.5×10^{-4}, Table 3). These results suggest that *FTO* may impact inversely on BMI and brain volume.

TABLE 2: Associations between *FTO* (rs9930333) and body and brain outcomes

Outcome	Effect size ± SE (G allele)			P-value		
	SYS-Discovery	SYS-Replication	IMAGEN	SYS-Discovery	SYS-Replication	IMAGEN
BMI (log kg/m²)	0.017 ± 0.004	0.017 ± 0.006	0.016 ± 0.004	1.1×10^{-4}	0.005	1.4×10^{-5}
Body weight (log kg)	0.016 ± 0.005	0.021 ± 0.007	0.013 ± 0.004	0.003	0.004	0.003
TBF (log kg)	0.052 ± 0.016	0.063 ± 0.022	–	0.002	0.004	–
LBM (log kg)	0.008 ± 0.004	0.008 ± 0.005	–	0.05	0.11	–
Height (cm)	0.001 ± 0.488	0.60 ± 0.53	−0.001 ± 0.004	1.00	0.26	0.72
Brain volume (cm³)	−16.8 ± 6.0	−12.8 ± 6.6	−9.8 ± 5.2	0.005	0.05	0.06
IC volume (cm³)	−17.4 ± 8.0	−3.8 ± 10.0	−8.5 ± 7.4	0.03	0.70	0.25
Ventricular volume (log cm³)	0.002 ± 0.010	0.003 ± 0.01	0.006 ± 0.009	0.84	0.81	0.50
Component 1	0.16 ± 0.09	0.15 ± 0.12	0.05 ± 0.07	0.10	0.21	0.51
Component 2	−0.29 ± 0.06	−0.25 ± 0.07	−0.15 ± 0.06	5.5×10^{-6}	5.9×10^{-4}	0.007

Associations were tested with Merlin-1.1.2. Ventricular volume is defined as the sum of volumes of the left lateral, right lateral, third and fourth ventricles. Components 1 and 2: principal components 1 and 2 from PCA of brain volume and BMI determinants (i.e. TBF, LBM and height). SE, standard error.

TABLE 3: Meta-analysis of *FTO* associations in the SYS (discovery and replication) and IMAGEN samples

Outcome	Effect size ± SE (G allele)	P-value	HetISq	Heterogeneity P-value
BMI (log kg/m²)	−0.020 ± 0.003	8.9×10^{-11}	0.0	0.98
Body weight (log kg)	−0.015 ± 0.003	8.1×10^{-8}	0.0	0.60
Brain volume (cm³)	12.8 ± 3.4	1.5×10^{-4}	0.0	0.68
IC volume (cm³)	10.6 ± 4.8	0.03	0.0	0.53
Component 2	0.22 ± 0.04	1.3×10^{-9}	32.1	0.23

Meta-analysis was performed with METAL. Component 2: principal component 2 from PCA of brain volume and BMI determinants (i.e. TBF, LBM and height). HetISq: I2 statistic that measures heterogeneity on scale of 0–100%. SE, standard error.

13.2.2 FTO ASSOCIATIONS WITH BMI DETERMINANTS AND INTRACRANIAL (IC) AND CEREBROSPINAL VOLUMES

Next, we tested whether the *FTO* association with BMI is mediated mainly through its association with body adiposity. In the SYS, the G allele was associated with higher total body fat (TBF, P = 0.002) and lean body mass (LBM, P = 0.03) and no difference in height (P = 0.99, Table 2). Similar results were observed in the replication samples. In SYS-Replication, the G allele was associated with higher TBF (P = 0.004), a trend towards higher LBM (P = 0.11) and no difference in height (P = 0.26, Table 2). In the IMAGEN sample, the G allele was associated with higher body weight (P = 0.003) and no difference in height (P = 0.72, Table 2). These results suggest that the *FTO* association with BMI is mediated mainly through its association with body adiposity (both SYS samples) and not with longitudinal growth (all three samples).

Furthermore, we tested whether the *FTO* association with brain volume is similar to that with intracranial (IC) volume (an index of cranium/head size) and ventricular volume. The G allele (associated with lower brain volume) was associated with lower IC volume in the SYS-Discovery (P = 0.03). Similar, but non-significant trends were observed in both replication samples (Table 2). In a meta-analysis involving all three samples, the G allele was associated with lower IC volume at P = 0.03 (Table 3). *FTO* was not associated with ventricular volume in any of the three samples (Table 2). These results suggest that *FTO* association with brain volume is likely mediated through processes influencing the growth of the brain and, to some degree, that of the cranium.

13.2.3 FTO ASSOCIATION WITH SHARED VARIANCE BETWEEN BMI DETERMINANTS AND BRAIN VOLUME

Because our results suggest that *FTO* may influence both body adiposity and brain size, we performed principal component analysis (PCA) to examine whether shared variance exists between body adiposity and brain volume that is independent of LBM and height. In the SYS sample, this analysis identified two significant components capturing a total of 75.6% of variance shared among brain volume, TBF, LBM and height. Component 1, which captured 50.6% of variance, was loaded positively by TBF, LBM and height, whereas Component 2, which captured 25.0% of variance, was loaded positively by brain volume and negatively by TBF (Fig. 2). Consistent with the opposite effects of the G allele on TBF and brain volume, this allele was strongly associated with Component 2 that captures the shared inverse variance between TBF and brain volume (P = 5.5×10^{-6}), but not with Component 1 (P = 0.10; see Fig. 2). We obtained similar results in both replication samples (SYS-Replication: Component 1: P = 0.21, Component 2: P = 5.9×10^{-4}; IMAGEN: Component 1: P = 0.51, Component 2: P = 0.007; Fig. 2). In a meta-analysis involving all three samples, *FTO* was associated with Component 2 at P = 1.3×10^{-9} (Table 3).

In addition, we performed a conditional analysis in the discovery sample in which we tested for association between *FTO* and Component 2, now including TBF as a covariate. This analysis continued to show a significant association between *FTO* and Component 2 (effect size = −0.20, P = 5×10^{-4}), confirming that this association is not driven entirely by TBF alone.

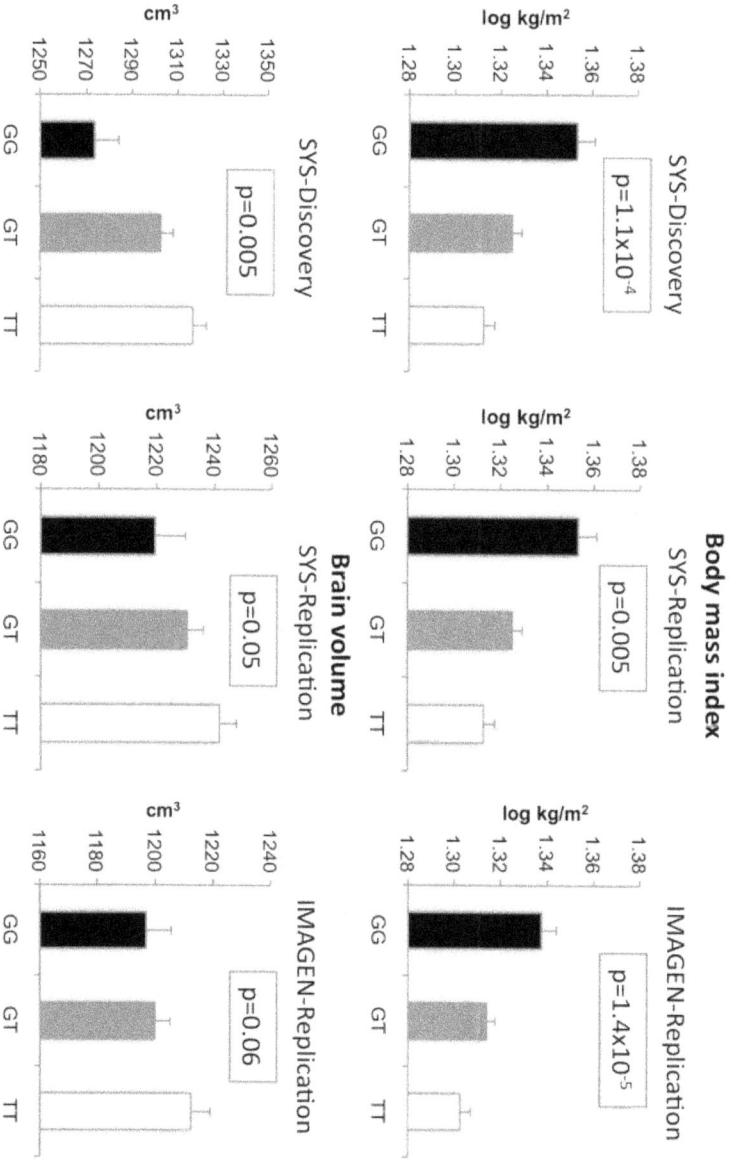

FIGURE 1: FTO associations with BMI and brain volume in the SYS-Discovery, SYS-Replication and IMAGEN samples. Associations between *FTO* (rs99930333) and the body and brain variables were tested with Merlin-1.1.2 under an additive model.

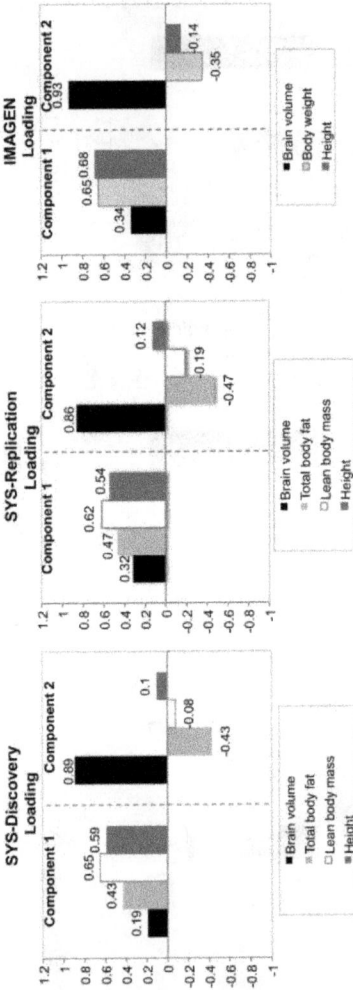

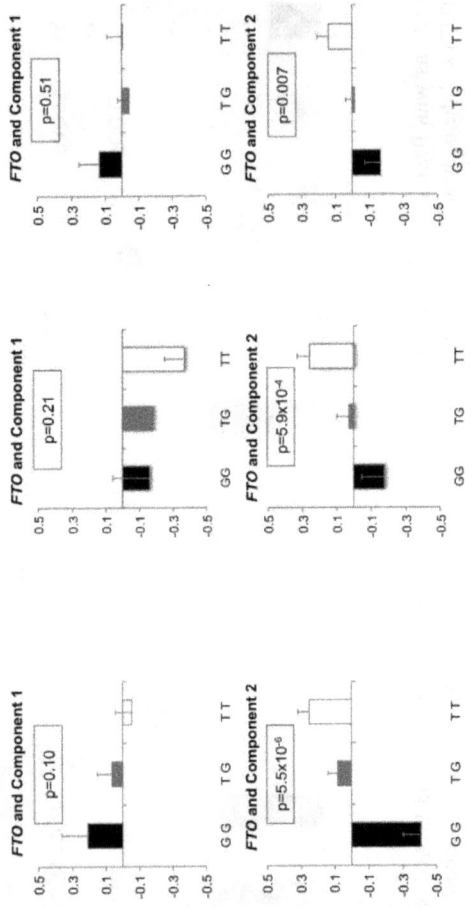

FIGURE 2: FTO and shared variance between brain volume and BMI determinants in the SYS-Discovery, SYS-Replication and IMAGEN samples. (A) Two significant components (and their respective loadings) identified with PCA involving four variables (i.e. brain volume, TBF, LBM and height) in the SYS-Discovery and SYS-Replication samples and three variables (i.e. brain volume, body weight and height) in the IMAGEN sample are presented. Component 1 explained 50.6, 54.9 and 54.5% of variance in the SYS-Discovery, SYS-Replication and IMAGEN samples, respectively. Component 2 explained 25.0, 22.6 and 31.0% of variance in the SYS-Discovery, SYS-Replication and IMAGEN samples, respectively. (B) Association between FTO (rs9930333) and each of the two significant components were tested with Merlin-1.1.2.

13.2.4 META-ANALYSIS OF *FTO* CO-EXPRESSION NETWORKS DURING DEVELOPMENT

In the present study, *FTO* is associated with a shared (inverse) variance between body adiposity and total brain volume, suggesting that this gene may exert opposing effects on the growth of adipose and brain tissues. As pointed out in the Discussion section, we speculate that such effects may occur during early embryogenesis when a single factor may influence developmentally distant tissues. *FTO* being expressed during early embryogenesis (5,8,9) and encoding a nucleic acid demethylase (5–7) may modulate expression of such a factor. Based on the existing literature, we identified bone morphogenetic protein 4 (*BMP4*) as a possible candidate for this role. *BMP4* is critical for embryonic development (19) and shows opposing effects on adipose and brain tissues (20,21) (Supplementary Material, Fig. S1). To explore the possibility that *FTO* may exert at least some opposing effects on body adiposity and brain volume via its interaction with *BMP4* during embryogenesis, we performed a meta-analysis of *FTO* co-expression networks during development. We found that *FTO* and *BMP4* exhibited the most significant positive or negative co-expressions (P < 0.01) in datasets annotated as 'embryonic', suggesting that the two genes may interact in embryonic tissues. Next, we searched for genes whose correlation strength with *FTO* was similar to that of *FTO* with *BMP4*. Ranking such 'FTO co-expressed' genes in this way produced a list that was enriched for functions related to the nervous system (e.g. synaptic transmission; corrected P < 0.01). The 165 top-ranking genes (r

> 0.25, P < 0.01) showed significant modularity (P < 0.01) in a network constructed from the brain-derived expression data, but not in a network constructed from the non-brain-derived expression data (size and platform matched). We noted that *FTO* exhibited particularly strong interaction with the protocadherin α-gene cluster (Supplementary Material, Fig. S2) that is involved in the regulation of neural circuit assembly and neuronal survival (22,23).

13.2.5 FTO ASSOCIATION WITH BODY FAT, BRAIN VOLUME AND SHARED VARIANCE BETWEEN BODY FAT AND BRAIN VOLUME: POTENTIALLY CONFOUNDING FACTORS

All statistical analyses presented above were carried out while adjusting for age and sex. But, several other potentially confounding factors might influence adiposity and brain development. In all discovery and replication samples, the participants were high-school students—therefore, the level of education did not vary among them. Data on nutrition, exercise, maternal education and family income were collected only in the SYS. Additional adjusting for these potentially confounding factors did not change the *FTO* associations with TBF, brain volume and the shared variance between the two variables captured by Component 2 (Supplementary Material, Table S2).

13.3 DISCUSSION

The results of the present study show that *FTO* is associated with shared inverse variance between body adiposity and total brain volume, suggesting that this gene may exert inverse effects on adipose and brain tissues. Given the completion of the overall brain growth in early childhood, it is plausible that these effects occur during development.

Early embryogenesis is a period of human development when such opposing effects of *FTO* on adipose and brain tissues may take place. As described below, a single factor may influence developmentally distant tissues, such as adipose tissue (derived from mesoderm) and brain tissue (derived from ectoderm), and this influence may be of the opposite direction. *FTO*, as a gene encoding nucleic acid demethylase (5–7) and expressed during early embryogenesis (5,8,9), may act as a modulator of such a factor. For example, *BMP4* is a protein involved in the regulation of cell proliferation and differentiation during embryonic development [reviewed in (19)], and its inhibition in ectoderm is critical for neural induction and the development of the brain (20), whereas its inhibition in mesoderm may attenuate the development of adipose tissue (21). We speculate that a moderate increase in *BMP4* expression, because of greater demethylating activity of *FTO*, would lead to a decrease in allocating stem cells towards brain cell lineages and an increase in allocating stem cells towards adipose tissue lineages (Supplementary Material, Fig. S1). Such relative differences in stem cell allocation, and thus life-long potential for growth of the respective tissues, would then result in a lower brain volume and a higher body fat mass postnatally. The former would be realized during major periods of brain development (prenatal and early postnatal period), whereas the latter would become apparent gradually during postnatal life as a result of a chronic positive energy balance (life-long risk for obesity) (24,25). Our meta-analysis of co-expression networks provided some support for (i) the possible existence of such *FTO–BMP4* interactions during embryogenesis and (ii) the possibility that these interactions are involved in the processes of brain development. It also suggested that the latter might include the protocadherin α-gene cluster that is critical for the regulation of neural circuit assembly and neuronal survival (22,23). Further experimental studies are required to confirm these findings.

Consistent with the above hypothesis, previous research in experimental animals and humans suggests that *FTO* effects observed in childhood and adulthood may stem from its effects during early development. *FTO* deletion in mice results in growth retardation present already at birth and a significant reduction in fat mass and, less so, in LBM (26,27). Similarly, a loss-of-function mutation in the human *FTO* results in severe growth retardation and development of multiple malformations, including those affecting the brain (8). In addition, duplication of a chromosomal region, including *FTO* in humans leads to obesity and mental retardation (28).

In the present study, *FTO* was associated with brain and cranium volumes, but not with height (an index of axial growth). These results are consistent with the fact that (i) the brain and cranium versus axial skeleton exhibit different developmental growth patterns: while most of the brain and cranium growth is completed during the first few years of life, the axial skeleton shows major growth during adolescence; and (ii) most of the cranium, but not the axial skeleton is of the same ectodermal origin as the brain (29). In agreement with this closer developmental relationship of the cranium with the brain than of the cranium with the axial skeleton, we show here that IC volume correlates much closer with brain volume ($r^2 = 0.75$) than it does with height ($r^2 = 0.12$), and note also that height is only weakly associated with brain volume ($r^2 = 0.04$; Supplementary Material, Fig. S3). Taken together, there are likely a number of factors that influence the growth and development of the brain and cranium, but not that of the axial skeleton (e.g. *FTO*), and vice versa. Also supporting our results, it has been shown previously that *FTO* is not associated with height, despite being strongly associated with BMI (24). Whether *FTO* impacts primarily growth of the skull and only secondarily growth of the brain is also a possibility that requires further developmental studies.

In summary, our results suggest that *FTO* may exert inverse effects on adipose and brain tissues. Given the fact that these effects are detected already in adolescence, they may occur during early development.

13.4 MATERIALS AND METHODS

13.4.1 ADOLESCENT SAMPLES

13.4.1.1 DISCOVERY SAMPLE (SYS DISCOVERY) AND REPLICATION SAMPLE 1 (SYS REPLICATION)

Discovery sample (SYS-Discovery) included 598 SYS adolescents recruited between November 2003 and June 2009, and Replication sample 1 (SYS-Replication) included 413 SYS adolescents recruited between September 2009 and February 2012. Both SYS samples were white Caucasian adolescents (aged 12–18 years) drawn from the French Canadian genetic founder population living in the Saguenay-Lac St. Jean region of Quebec,

Canada (30). The SYS is a population-based, cross-sectional study of cardiovascular, metabolic and mental health in adolescence, and recruitment and selection criteria have been described previously (30). Written consent of the parents and assent of the adolescents were obtained before the commencement of data collection. The Research Ethics Committee of the Chicoutimi Hospital approved the study protocol.

13.4.1.2 REPLICATION SAMPLE 2 (IMAGEN)

Replication sample 2 was the IMAGEN Study involving white Caucasian adolescents (n = 718; aged 13–15 years) of mixed European background (German, English, Irish and French). The IMAGEN Study is a European multicentre study on impulsivity, reinforcement sensitivity and emotional reactivity in adolescents. The IMAGEN sample comprises 718 healthy adolescents recruited between 2008 and 2010 in local schools from 8 participating sites in Germany (Berlin, Dresden, Hamburg and Manheim), UK (London and Nottingham), France (Paris) and Ireland (Dublin). All participants and their parents provided informed written assent and consent, respectively. The local ethics committees approved the study protocol (31).

Basic characteristics of all three samples are provided in Table 1. Adolescents were defined as obese or overweight, if their BMI was ≥85th age- and sex-specific percentile of the Centers for Disease Control and Prevention BMI curves (http://www.cdc.gov/growthcharts). The prevalence of overweight or obesity was 23.9, 32.7 and 19.0% in the SYS-Discovery, SYS-Replication and IMAGEN sample (Table 1), which is similar to that in the Canadian (2004 Canadian Community Health Survey) and European adolescent populations (17,18).

13.4.2 PHENOTYPING

13.4.2.1 ANTHROPOMETRY AND BIOIMPEDANCE

In the SYS-Discovery, SYS-Replication and IMAGEN samples, weight (0.1 kg precision) and height (1 mm precision) were measured, and the

BMI was calculated as weight in kilograms divided by squared height in metres. In both SYS samples, but not in the IMAGEN sample, TBF and LBM were assessed using multi-frequency bioimpedance analysis (Xitron Technologies, Inc., San Diego, CA, USA).

13.4.2.2 MRI OF THE BRAIN

In the SYS-Discovery and SYS-Replication samples, structural magnetic resonance (MR) images of the brain were collected on a Phillips 1.0-T superconducting magnet. High-resolution anatomical T1-weighted images were acquired using the following parameters: 3D radiofrequency-spoiled gradient echo scan with 140–160 sagittal slices, 1-mm isotropic voxel size, time repetition (TR) = 25 ms, echo time (TE) = 5 ms and flip angle = 30°. In the IMAGEN study, structural MR images were obtained using 3.0-T scanners (Siemens, Phillips and General Electric). The details of the entire MR protocol are described elsewhere (31). High-resolution T1-weighted anatomical images were acquired using a 3D Magnetization Prepared Rapid Acquisition Gradient Echo sequence with 160 or 170 sagittal slices (depending on the manufacturer), 1-mm isotropic voxel size, TR = 2300 ms, TE = 2.8 ms, inversion time (TI) = 900 ms and flip angle = 9°. In all three samples, total brain and ventricular volumes were derived using FreeSurfer (32), and IC volumes were estimated using the whole cranium/face model as described previously (33). For the latter, brains were removed from all MR images using the brain extraction tool algorithm, and all individual images were normalized in the same space to the average linear dimensions of the entire group. The first population average was then created via voxel-by-voxel averaging. A hierarchical iterative model-building step was then initiated, where each image was non-linearly registered to the populating average and subsequently to the model created in the previous non-linear registration step. At each iteration, finer resolution non-linear transformations were estimated. One of the outputs at the end of the model-building process is a non-linear transformation that maps each individual to the average of the group. All transformations were estimated using the minc suite of software tools (http://www.bic.mni.mc-gill.ca/ServicesSoftware/HomePage) (34,35). The IC space was manually defined on the resulting population model by one of the authors (M.M.C.) and then transformed to fit each individual using the inverse transformation previously described (34,35). An example of IC mask is shown in the Supplementary Material, Fig. S4.

13.4.3 FTO GENOTYPING

Both the SYS-Discovery and IMAGEN samples were genotyped with the Illumina Human610-Quad BeadChip (Illumina, San Diego, CA, USA). The genotyping was conducted at the Centre National de Génotypage (Paris, France). The SYS-Replication sample was genotyped with the HumanOmniExpress BeadChip (Illumina). The genotyping was conducted at the Genome Analysis Centre of Helmholtz Zentrum München (Munich, Germany). In all three samples, single nucleotide polymorphisms (SNPs) with call rate <95% and minor allele frequency <0.01 and SNPs that were not in Hardy–Weinberg equilibrium ($P < 1 \times 10^{-4}$) were excluded. A variant of *FTO* that showed the most significant association with BMI in our previously reported genome-wide association study (i.e. rs9930333) (16) was then tested for association with other outcomes in the SYS-Discovery sample and with all outcomes in the replication samples (SYS-Replication and IMAGEN). This variant was in linkage disequilibrium and showed the same direction of effect on BMI, as the previously reported *FTO* SNPs (1,2,36).

13.4.4 STATISTICAL METHODS

13.4.4.1 GENOTYPE–PHENOTYPE ASSOCIATION TESTS

Genotype–phenotype association tests were conducted with Merlin (version 1.1.2) under an additive model (37,38). With Merlin, a simple regression model is fitted to each studied outcome, and a variance component approach is used to account for correlation between different observed phenotypes within each family (if required). For all primary and derived traits, values outside mean ± 3 SDs were excluded. Variables were log transformed, if they did not follow normal distribution. Age and sex were included as potential confounders for all variables, except for principal components that were already adjusted for age and sex prior to PCA. To combine the evidence for association from the SYS-Discovery, SYS-Replication and IMAGEN samples, we used METAL (39), which converts the direction of effect and P-value observed in each study into a signed Z-score combined across samples in a weighted sum, with weights proportional to the square root of the sample size for each study (39).

13.4.4.2 PRINCIPAL COMPONENT ANALYSIS

PCA was used to identify components of shared variance between individual BMI determinants and brain volume. In the SYS-Discovery and SYS-Replication samples, the BMI determinants were TBF, LBM and height. In the IMAGEN sample, only body weight and height were available. PCA is a multivariate statistical technique used to extract shared variance from correlated data (40). It transforms a number of possibly correlated variables into a number of uncorrelated variables, the so-called principal components. Each principal component represents a different linear combination of the original correlated variables. The original variables are first normalized to their respective means and then used to generate a correlation matrix. PCA is then performed by eigenvalue decomposition of the correlation matrix. Loadings of significant principal components are described in terms of eigenvectors. The significant principal components were tested for association with the studied *FTO* SNP (rs9930333) as described above.

13.4.4.3 META-ANALYSIS OF FTO CO-EXPRESSION NETWORKS

To identify genes frequently co-expressed with *FTO*, we assembled 721 diverse, publicly available expression datasets containing a total of 34 019 microarrays (http://www.chibi.ubc.ca/Gemma). Using these data, we conducted co-expression analysis as previously described (41). In brief, correlations between *FTO*-expression profile and expression profiles of 14

184 genes (identified as all genes present in at least 500 datasets) were determined for each dataset. These correlations were then ranked to give a score of similarity between *FTO*-expression profile and expression profiles of all other genes in each dataset. Next, each dataset was annotated from a set of 128 terms (describing factors such as the tissue, treatment, developmental stage and/or disease); an annotation was given, if the term was present in at least 5 (and up to 25) datasets. Finally, analysis of gene function enrichment was applied to test for enrichment across dataset annotations (42). Further details on co-expression methods and results are available in Supplementary Information and at http://www.chibi.ubc.ca/FTO.

REFERENCES

1. Frayling T.M., Timpson N.J., Weedon M.N., Zeggini E., Freathy R.M., Lindgren C.M., Perry J.R., Elliott K.S., Lango H., Rayner N.W., et al. A common variant in the *FTO* gene is associated with body mass index and predisposes to childhood and adult obesity. Science 2007;316:889-894.

2. Speliotes E.K., Willer C.J., Berndt S.I., Monda K.L., Thorleifsson G., Jackson A.U., Allen H.L., Lindgren C.M., Luan J., Magi R., et al. Association analyses of 249 796 individuals reveal 18 new loci associated with body mass index. Nat. Genet. 2010;42:937-948.

3. Fawcett K.A., Barroso I. The genetics of obesity: *FTO* leads the way. Trends Genet. 2010;26:266-274.

4. Larder R., Cheung M.K., Tung Y.C., Yeo G.S., Coll A.P. Where to go with *FTO*? Trends Endocrinol. Metab. 2011;22:53-59.

5. Gerken T., Girard C.A., Tung Y.C., Webby C.J., Saudek V., Hewitson K.S., Yeo G.S., McDonough M.A., Cunliffe S., McNeill L.A., et al. The obesity-associated *FTO* gene encodes a 2-oxoglutarate-dependent nucleic acid demethylase. Science 2007;318:1469-1472.

6. Jia G., Yang C.G., Yang S., Jian X., Yi C., Zhou Z., He C. Oxidative demethylation of 3-methylthymine and 3-methyluracil in single-stranded DNA and RNA by mouse and human *FTO*. FEBS Lett. 2008;582:3313-3319.

7. Han Z., Niu T., Chang J., Lei X., Zhao M., Wang Q., Cheng W., Wang J., Feng Y., Chai J. Crystal structure of the *FTO* protein reveals basis for its substrate specificity. Nature 2010;464:1205-1209.

8. Boissel S., Reish O., Proulx K., Kawagoe-Takaki H., Sedgwick B., Yeo G.S., Meyre D., Golzio C., Molinari F., Kadhom N., et al. Loss-of-function mutation in the dioxygenase-encoding *FTO* gene causes severe growth retardation and multiple malformations. Am. J. Hum. Genet. 2009;85:106-111.

9. Stratigopoulos G., Padilla S.L., LeDuc C.A., Watson E., Hattersley A.T., McCarthy M.I., Zeltser L.M., Chung W.K., Leibel R.L. Regulation of *FTO*/Ftm gene

expression in mice and humans. Am. J. Physiol. Regul. Integr. Comp. Physiol. 2008;294:R1185-R1196.

10. Gustafson D., Rothenberg E., Blennow K., Steen B., Skoog I. An 18-year follow-up of overweight and risk of Alzheimer disease. Arch. Intern. Med. 2003;163:1524-1528.

11. Gustafson D., Lissner L., Bengtsson C., Bjorkelund C., Skoog I. A 24-year follow-up of body mass index and cerebral atrophy. Neurology 2004;63:1876-1881.

12. Debette S., Beiser A., Hoffmann U., Decarli C., O'Donnell C.J., Massaro J.M., Au R., Himali J.J., Wolf P.A., Fox C.S., et al. Visceral fat is associated with lower brain volume in healthy middle-aged adults. Ann. Neurol. 2010;68:136-144.

13. Ho A.J., Stein J.L., Hua X., Lee S., Hibar D.P., Leow A.D., Dinov I.D., Toga A.W., Saykin A.J., Shen L., et al. A commonly carried allele of the obesity-related *FTO* gene is associated with reduced brain volume in the healthy elderly. Proc. Natl. Acad. Sci. USA 2010;107:8404-8409.

14. Knickmeyer R.C., Gouttard S., Kang C., Evans D., Wilber K., Smith J.K., Hamer R.M., Lin W., Gerig G., Gilmore J.H. A structural MRI study of human brain development from birth to 2 years. J. Neurosci. 2008;28:12176-12182.

15. Lenroot R.K., Giedd J.N. Brain development in children and adolescents: insights from anatomical magnetic resonance imaging. Neurosci. Biobehav. Rev. 2006;30:718-729.

16. Melka M.G., Bernard M., Mahboubi A., Abrahamowicz M., Paterson A.D., Syme C., Lourdusamy A., Schumann G., Leonard G.T., Perron M., et al. Genome-wide scan for loci of adolescent obesity and their relationship with blood pressure. J. Clin. Endocrinol. Metab. 2012;97:E145-E150.

17. Shields M. Overweight and obesity among children and youth. Health Rep. 2006;17:27-42.

18. Lobstein T., Frelut M.L. Prevalence of overweight among children in Europe. Obes. Rev. 2003;4:195-200.

19. Chen D., Zhao M., Mundy G.R. Bone morphogenetic proteins. Growth Factors 2004;22:233-241.

20. Finley M.F., Devata S., Huettner J.E. BMP-4 inhibits neural differentiation of murine embryonic stem cells. J. Neurobiol. 1999;40:271-287.

21. Bowers R.R., Kim J.W., Otto T.C., Lane M.D. Stable stem cell commitment to the adipocyte lineage by inhibition of DNA methylation: role of the BMP-4 gene. Proc. Natl. Acad. Sci. USA 2006;103:13022-13027.

22. Zipursky S.L., Sanes J.R. Chemoaffinity revisited: dscams, protocadherins, and neural circuit assembly. Cell 2010;143:343-353.

23. Kehayova P., Monahan K., Chen W., Maniatis T. Regulatory elements required for the activation and repression of the protocadherin-alpha gene cluster. Proc. Natl. Acad. Sci. USA 2011;108:17195-17200.

24. Hardy R., Wills A.K., Wong A., Elks C.E., Wareham N.J., Loos R.J., Kuh D., Ong K.K. Life course variations in the associations between *FTO* and MC4R gene variants and body size. Hum. Mol. Genet. 2010;19:545-552.

25. Sovio U., Mook-Kanamori D.O., Warrington N.M., Lawrence R., Briollais L., Palmer C.N., Cecil J., Sandling J.K., Syvanen A.C., Kaakinen M., et al. Association between common variation at the *FTO* locus and changes in body mass index from

infancy to late childhood: the complex nature of genetic association through growth and development. PLoS Genet. 2011;7:e1001307.

26. Fischer J., Koch L., Emmerling C., Vierkotten J., Peters T., Bruning J.C., Ruther U. Inactivation of the *FTO* gene protects from obesity. Nature 2009;458:894-898.

27. Gao X., Shin Y.H., Li M., Wang F., Tong Q., Zhang P. The fat mass and obesity associated gene *FTO* functions in the brain to regulate postnatal growth in mice. PLoS One 2010;5:e14005.

28. Stratakis C.A., Lafferty A., Taymans S.E., Gafni R.I., Meck J.M., Blancato J. Anisomastia associated with interstitial duplication of chromosome 16, mental retardation, obesity, dysmorphic facies, and digital anomalies: molecular mapping of a new syndrome by fluorescent in situ hybridization and microsatellites to 16q13 (D16S419-D16S503). J. Clin. Endocrinol. Metab. 2000;85:3396-3401.

29. Lieberman D.E. The Evolution of the Human Head. Cambridge, MA: Harvard University Press; 2011. p. 56-95.

30. Pausova Z., Paus T., Abrahamowicz M., Almerigi J., Arbour N., Bernard M., Gaudet D., Hanzalek P., Hamet P., Evans A.C., et al. Genes, maternal smoking, and the offspring brain and body during adolescence: design of the Saguenay Youth Study. Hum. Brain Mapp. 2007;28:502-518.

31. Schumann G., Loth E., Banaschewski T., Barbot A., Barker G., Buchel C., Conrod P.J., Dalley J.W., Flor H., Gallinat J., et al. The IMAGEN study: reinforcement-related behaviour in normal brain function and psychopathology. Mol. Psychiatry 2010;15:1128-1139.

32. Dale A.M., Fischl B., Sereno M.I. Cortical surface-based analysis. I. Segmentation and surface reconstruction. Neuroimage 1999;9:179-194.

33. Chakravarty M.M., Aleong R., Leonard G., Perron M., Pike G.B., Richer L., Veillette S., Pausova Z., Paus T. Automated analysis of craniofacial morphology using magnetic resonance images. PLoS One 2011;6:e20241.

34. Collins D.L., Holmes C.J., Peters T.M., Evans A.C. Automatic 3-D model-based neuroanatomical segmentation. Hum. Brain Mapp 1995;3:190-208.

35. Collins D.L., Evans A.C. ANIMAL: validation and applications of non-linear registration-based segmentation. Int. J. Pattern Recogn. 1997;11:1271-1294.

36. Chanock S.J., Manolio T., Boehnke M., Boerwinkle E., Hunter D.J., Thomas G., Hirschhorn J.N., Abecasis G., Altshuler D., Bailey-Wilson J.E., et al. Replicating genotype-phenotype associations. Nature 2007;447:655-660.

37. Abecasis G.R., Cherny S.S., Cookson W.O., Cardon L.R. Merlin–rapid analysis of dense genetic maps using sparse gene flow trees. Nat. Genet. 2002;30:97-101.

38. Abecasis G.R., Wigginton J.E. Handling marker-marker linkage disequilibrium: pedigree analysis with clustered markers. Am. J. Hum. Genet. 2005;77:754-767.

39. Willer C.J., Li Y., Abecasis G.R. METAL: fast and efficient meta-analysis of genomewide association scans. Bioinformatics 2010;26:2190-2191.

40. Jolliffe I.T. Principal Component Analysis. New York: Springer; 2002.

41. Gillis J., Pavlidis P. The role of indirect connections in gene networks in predicting function. Bioinformatics 2011;27:1860-1866.

42. Gillis J., Mistry M., Pavlidis P. Gene function analysis in complex data sets using ErmineJ. Nat. Protoc. 2010;5:1148-1159.

There are several supplemental files that are not available in this version of the article. To view this additional information, please use the citation on the first page of this chapter.

PART IV

CONSIDERATIONS FOR FUTURE ACTION

CHAPTER 14

CHANGES IN ADOLESCENTS' INTAKE OF SUGAR-SWEETENED BEVERAGES AND SEDENTARY BEHAVIOR: RESULTS AT 8 MONTH MID-WAY ASSESSMENT OF THE HEIA STUDY—A COMPREHENSIVE, MULTI-COMPONENT SCHOOL-BASED RANDOMIZED TRIAL

MONA BJELLAND, INGUNN H. BERGH, MAY GRYDELAND, KNUT-INGE KLEPP, LENE F. ANDERSEN, SIGMUND A. ANDERSSEN, YNGVAR OMMUNDSEN, AND NANNA LIEN

14.1 BACKGROUND

Interventions to prevent unhealthy weight gain should aim at making a change in energy balance related behaviours (EBRB) [1]. The consumption of sugar-sweetened beverages (SSB), television viewing and computer use are behaviours that have been associated with increased risk for obesity [2]. Lack of effective school-based obesity prevention interventions [3,4] has initiated a debate about the best intervention strategies and evaluation designs [4,5]. Intervention strategies tailored to specific subgroups (like gender) [3,6], including family components [7,8], and evaluated by the target groups [9] seem needed in order to examine for whom and why obesity prevention programmes works.

Schools are often used as a setting for implementing interventions developed to reduce the prevalence of obesity in children and adolescents, because it offers continued and intensive contact with a large population across ethnic and socio-economic groups [3,7]. However, including the home- and family environment could increase the effectiveness of school-based prevention of obesity [10,11], and such interventions have been requested [7,8]. Process evaluation of environment-focused interventions is also requested, including the social environment [4]. Both dietary habits and sedentary behaviours are mainly performed in the home and family environment [12,13], with parents being key persons in children and adolescents' social environment. Nevertheless, the effects of parental involvement in obesity prevention programs are still unclear [8].

Obesity risk may differ across subgroups, and intervention strategies may not be equally effective across these groups [14]. Gender is the most convincing and most frequently examined moderator of school-based interventions aimed at EBRB, and the interventions seem to work better for girls than for boys [15,16]. It may be that in early adolescence, boys and girls respond differently to various intervention strategies [3]. Weight status (WS) and socio-economic status (SES) have not been shown to be consistently moderators of EBRB [15,16]. The WS of children and adolescents may affect their dietary habits and sedentary behaviours of which TV-viewing is an example [12]. Watching TV may be a risk factor for obesity, but the causal arrow may be backward; that obesity itself increases TV-viewing [17,18]. Lower SES children have a higher risk of obesity, and parental education has been found to be inversely associated with sedentary behaviours and consumption of SSB in adolescents [19,20]. More research is needed exploring further the moderating effect of WS and SES in obesity prevention studies [15,16].

Process evaluation data might serve to better interpret the intervention effects, but a limited number of published intervention studies report on process evaluation, including data on implementation quality and quantity of exposure [8,9]. In health promoting interventions parental involvement could be assessed by the awareness of the intervention components, the dose received and the satisfaction with the components [21-23]. Conducting process evaluation is important in order to identify the reach and dose received by the participants [24,25], and indices of dose received can be assessed in terms of both intervention exposure and satisfaction [26].

The overall goal of the HEalth In Adolescents (HEIA) study was to design, implement and evaluate a comprehensive, intervention program to promote healthy weight development among young adolescent schoolchildren (11-13 year olds). The targeted changes in the behaviours were to decrease consumption of SSB and sedentary behaviour, and to increase the physical activity and the consumption of fruit and vegetables [27]. In this study, the two behaviours to be reduced were explored in relation to the important issues raised in the literature and summarised above.

The aim of this paper was three-fold. Firstly, to determine if a multi-component health promotion intervention targeting 11-12 year olds influenced their consumption of SSB, television viewing and/or computer/game-use. Secondly, the aim was to explore whether the results varied by gender, adolescent WS or by parental educational level. Finally, the aim was to assess whether parental involvement differed by parental educational level or by the adolescents' gender or WS.

14.2 METHODS

14.2.1 STUDY DESIGN AND SUBJECTS

Eligible schools were located in the Eastern part of Norway and had more than 40 pupils in 6th grade. Such schools are mainly located in larger towns/municipalities, and 37 schools were recruited from the largest towns/municipalities in seven counties surrounding Oslo (Figure 1) [27]. All 6th graders in these 37 schools (n = 2165) and their parents/legal guardians were invited to participate. Of these, 1580 returned a parent signed informed consent form for the adolescent. A cluster randomized controlled pre-post study design was used to evaluate the effectiveness of the intervention; 12 schools were randomly assigned by simple drawing to the intervention group and 25 to the control group. The pre-test data collection took place during four weeks in September 2007, while the 8 month mid-way assessment took place in May 2008.

The adolescents who participated in both data collections were included in this paper, as were the parents in the intervention schools who answered the process evaluation questions at the mid-way assessment (one question-naire per pupil). A total of 1465 adolescents (92.7% of those 1580 returning consent) and 349 parents (82.5% mothers and 17.5% fathers, in total 65.7% of the parents in the intervention group) were included in the analyses. There were no significant differences in demographic and behavioural variables between those participating both at the pre-test and at the mid-way assess-ment compared to those lost to the mid-way assessment (n = 63).

The intervention program in the HEIA study consisted of a mixture of individual-, group-, and environmental level strategies and activities. Strat-egies and activities in the 6th grade were: Lessons with student booklet, posters, weekly fruit and vegetable breaks and activity breaks in classroom, sports equipment for recess activities, active commuting, fact sheets for par-ents and an inspirational course for physical education teachers [27].

Ethical approval and research clearance was obtained from the Region-al Committees for Medical Research Ethics and the Norwegian Social Sci-ence Data Service.

14.2.2 QUESTIONNAIRE DATA

The Internet based child questionnaire comprised mostly questions with pre-coded answer categories and could be completed in about 45 minutes. The parental process evaluation questionnaire (paper-pencil format) were sent home with the adolescent at the mid-way assessment, completed by one of the parents, returned to the teachers in a sealed envelope and col-lected from the schools by project staff. Process evaluation questions that tapped into the parents' perceived exposure and satisfaction are included in this paper.

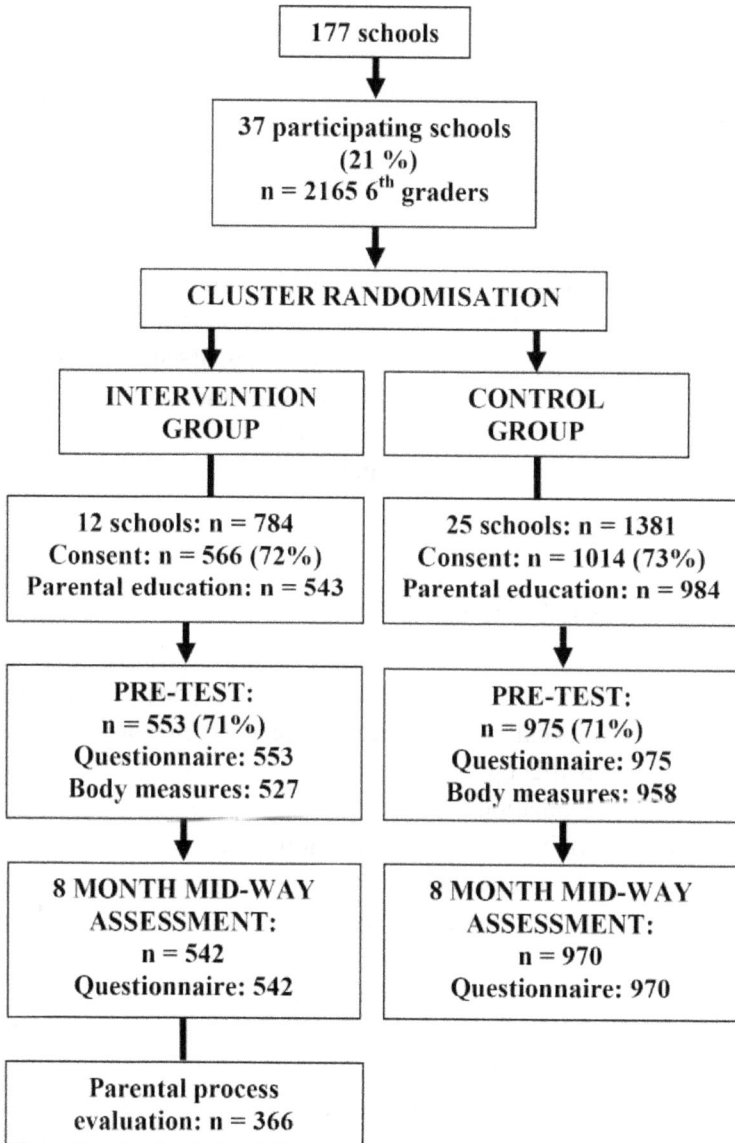

FIGURE 1: Flow diagram of recruitment, randomization and participation of adolescents and parents in the HEIA study.

14.2.3 BEHAVIOURAL OUTCOMES

The intake of beverages was assessed by frequency (six categories, from never/seldom to every weekday) and amount (in glasses, four categories: from 1 glass to 4 glasses or more) for weekdays and by amount for weekends (in glasses, eight categories: from never/seldom to 7 glasses or more). Soft drinks with sugar and sugar-sweetened fruit drinks were the targeted beverages (summed and presented as SSB). Two questions assessed the number of hours spent on watching TV and/or DVD during a regular weekday and weekend day (six categories, 0.5 - 5 hours). Similarly, two questions assessed the number of hours spent on the computer, playing TV-games or other electronic games on a regular weekday and a weekend day, respectively (six categories, 0 to 4 hours). The test-retest correlation coefficients for the outcome measures were moderate to high ($r = 0.46$-0.78) [27].

14.2.4 PROCESS EVALUATION

Process evaluation is used to explore what happened in the intervention program, to what extent the intervention reached intended participants, and how that could affect program impacts or outcomes. Some of the elements in a process evaluation are reach and dose received [26]. Reach can be defined as participation rate and a quantification of how many within the intended target audience who participated in the intervention [26]. Dose received in the meaning of exposure are used to describe and quantify how much of the intervention that was received, whereas dose received related to satisfaction is used to describe and rate the participants' liking [26].

The process evaluation questions for parents comprised parental awareness of the intervention components/program activities for the adolescents at school (Have you heard of these components? Seven components, yes = 1/no = 0) as an indication of to which extend the adolescents talked about the project at home. The answers were summed and recoded into tertiles; low to moderate awareness (0-3 components), moderate to high (4-5) and high (6-7). Dose received was assessed with regards to the fact sheets handed out at school and sent home with the adolescent (Have you received or read the following fact sheets? Seven sheets and topics, three categories for each sheet: received = 1/read = 2/not aware of it = 0). The answers were summed and recoded into tertiles; low to moderate dose (0-7), moderate to high (8-13) and high (14). Parents also reported what they thought about the intervention (Overall, what do you think about the HEIA project in grade 6? Four response categories: did not like it at all = 0 to liked it very much = 3, those answering "I do not know the HEIA project" were excluded). The answers were combined into tertiles; low to moderate liking (0-1), moderate to high (2), and high (3). Finally, they were asked to give their opinion on the fact sheets (Overall, what do you think about the fact sheets? Three statements related to (1) appreciation of receiving the sheets, (2) interesting content and (3) useful tips, four response categories for each statement: not at all = 0 to a high degree = 3). The answers were summed and recoded into tertiles; low to moderate liking (0-6), moderate to high (7-8) and high (9).

TABLE 1: Pre-test characteristics (demographic) for the control and the intervention group in the HEIA study

	Pre-test		
	Control	Intervention	
	n† = 910	n† = 510	p
Age (mean (SD))	11.2 (0.27)	11.2 (0.26)	0.30
Gender			
Boys (%)	52.0	50.7	0.61
Girls (%)	48.0	49.3	
Weight status			
Normal weight (%)	84.9	88.5	0.06
Overweight (%)	15.1	11.5	
Parental educational level			
< 12 years (%)	32.0	26.3	0.07
13-16 years (%)	35.7	37.8	
> 16 years (%)	32.3	35.9	

p = Pearson Chi-Square/T-test (age) †n vary slightly

14.2.5 WEIGHT STATUS AND PARENTAL EDUCATION

The age- and gender specific body mass index (BMI) cut-off values proposed by the International Obesity Task Force [28] were used to categorize the adolescents as normal weight and overweight. Due to few obese adolescents (1.6%) these were included in the same group as the overweight adolescents in the analyses. Details of the anthropometrics of the participants and test-retest values of the measures have been reported elsewhere [27,29]. Parental education was collected as part of the informed consent form filled in by parents for the adolescent. Education was categorized into three levels: 12 years or less, between 13 and 16 years and more than 16 years. The parent with the longest education was used in the analyses, or else the one available.

14.2.6 DATA ANALYSIS

Clustering effects due to schools being the unit of recruitment was checked by the Linear Mixed Model procedure. Only 1-3% of the unexplained variance in the behaviours was on group level, and it was therefore decided to not conduct multilevel analysis.

The characteristics at the pre-test are presented as proportions (demographic variables), means and standard deviations (SD) (behavioural variables). Continuous variables were tested for differences between the intervention group and the control group with independent sample t-tests, and Chi-square test of proportions was used for categorical variables.

The effect of the intervention was determined using one-way ANCOVA with the mid-way value for the outcomes as the dependent variables, the experimental group as the independent variable and the pre-test values of the outcomes as covariates. The data were checked to ensure that there were no violations of the assumptions. Interaction effects by WS and parental educational level were tested in separate analyses as a second step, using two-way ANCOVA. To further explore gender differences by WS for the behavioural variables one-way ANCOVA were used. For secondary analyses a magnitude-based inference were made using a spreadsheet [30].

Chi-square test of proportions were used to assess whether the parental involvement in the intervention differed by gender, WS or parental educational level. The significance level was set at p <.05.

Data were analysed using SPSS Statistics, version 16 (IBM Corporation, New York, USA).

TABLE 2. Pre-test characteristics (behaviours) for the control and the intervention group in the HEIA study

| | Pre-test | | | | |
| | Control n† = 881 | | Intervention n† = 490 | | |
	Mean	SD	Mean	SD	p
SSB, dl/d					
- week	1.2	(1.7)	1.1	(1.6)	0.28
- weekend	2.3	(2.0)	2.3	(2.0)	0.76
TV/DVD, hours/d					
- week	1.5	(1.0)	1.5	(1.1)	0.65
- weekend	2.1	(1.2)	2.2	(1.3)	0.13
Computer/games, hours/d					
- week	1.1	(0.9)	1.1	(0.9)	0.16
- weekend	1.5	(1.1)	1.5	(1.1)	0.69

SSB = Sugar-sweetened beverages p = T-test †n vary slightly

14.3 RESULTS

The pre-test characteristics of the control and intervention group are presented in Table 1 and Table 2. No significant differences were found between the groups with respect to demographic and behavioural variables.

The changes in outcome variables in the control and intervention groups from the pre-test to the mid-way assessment are summarized in Table 3. In the total sample, significant differences were found between the intervention group and control group in the number of hours watching TV/DVD during week days (p = 0.002) and weekend days (p = 0.04), and time spent on computer/games during weekend days (p = 0.003). Stratified by gender, the results showed effects for girls only. The girls in the intervention group spent significantly less time on watching TV/DVD and computer/game-use compared to the girls in the control group, and the intake of SSB during weekend days was significantly lower among the girls in the intervention group.

Analyses of moderating effects by the adolescents' WS and parental education on pre-test to mid-way changes in the control and intervention groups, revealed an interaction of WS; number of hours spent on watching TV/DVD (borderline, p = 0.05) and computer/game-use during week days (p = 0.01) for the total sample. For boys, the same interactions were found (TV/DVD, p = 0.03 and computer/games, p = 0.02). No interactions were found for girls. Based on these findings we proceeded to explore gender differences by WS for the behavioural variables, and the stratified analyses are presented in Table 4. No moderating effect was found for parental education and no stratified analyses were conducted.

Among the normal weight girls there were significant differences between the intervention and control group for the sedentary behaviours. The normal weight girls in the intervention group spent significantly less time on watching TV/DVD and computer/game-use compared to the normal weight girls in the control group (Table 4). For intake of SSB during weekend days the results were borderline significant (p = 0.06). We found the same trends among the overweight/obese girls, except for use of computer/games during week days, but the differences between the intervention and control groups were not significant.

For the boys, no significant differences were found neither among the boys with normal weight nor the overweight/obese boys (Table 4). Even though not significant, the overweight/obese boys in the intervention group spent more time on watching TV/DVD and computer/game-use compared to the control group after the intervention. Time used for computer/games during week days was borderline significant among the overweight/obese boys in the intervention group compared to the overweight/obese boys in the control group (p = 0.06). We made a magnitude-based inference about the true effect of the intervention on computer/game-use in week days among overweight/obese boys, which provided the uncertainty in the effect as 95% confidence limits and as likelihoods that the true value of the effect represented a harmful, trivial or beneficial change in the experimental group compared with that in the control group. After log-transformation of the dependent variable adjusted for pre-test (daily hours used for computer/games on weekdays), the mean effect was expressed in standardized units (fraction of the between-subject standard deviation at pre-test). The smallest standardized change was assumed to be 0.20 [31]. There was an 85% chance that the true effect was positive, 15% chance that it was trivial, and 0.3% chance that it was negative (standardized difference in the mean as Cohen units = 0.43, confidence interval -0.01 to 0.87, p = 0.06). Thus the intervention likely produced an increase in time used for computer/game-use in week days in overweight/obese boys.

No significant differences were found in age, height, BMI, pubertal development, parental education and sedentary behaviours at pre-test between overweight/obese boys in the intervention group and overweight/obese boys in the control group. The only exception was time used for TV/DVD during weekend days which was higher among overweight/obese boys in the intervention group (p = 0.03) (data not shown).

No differences were found in parental involvement when stratifying by the adolescents' WS and the parental educational level. However, parental awareness of the intervention was significantly higher among the parents of girls, while the parents of boys were more satisfied with the fact sheets (Table 5).

14.4 DISCUSSION

Data from the 8 month mid-way assessment indicated that girls in the intervention group spent significantly less time on watching TV/DVD and using computer/games compared to the girls in the control group, and the intake of SSB during weekend days was significantly lower among the girls in the intervention group. Girls' WS did not moderate these findings. No significant differences between the intervention and control group were found for outcome variables among the boys with normal weight or the overweight/obese boys, but moderation effects were found for WS (TV/DVD and computer/games during week days). There were no moderating effects of parental education for neither boys nor girls with respect to any of the three behaviours. The process evaluation showed that parental awareness was significantly higher among the parents of girls, while the parents of boys were more satisfied with the fact sheets. No other differences in the parental process evaluation were found.

The effects found were both in a desired direction (girls) and an undesired direction (overweight/obese boys). However, it may be questioned whether the effects were large enough to have any public health impact. One review suggests that in children an imbalance over time of about 2% (125 KJ or 15 minutes of play replaced by TV-viewing) may lead to obesity [32]. Based on these estimates two groups did benefit from the HEIA study. The decrease in intake of SSB among the overweight girls was 0.4 dl for week days and 0.5 dl for weekend days. This represents a decrease in calorie intake equal to 68-85 KJ per day (0.4 or 0.5 dl and 170 KJ/dl). By reducing the time used for TV/DVD during week days by 0.3 hours (about 18 minutes) and time used for computer/games during week days by 0.2 hours (about 12 minutes) among normal weight girls, the total sedentary screen time was reduced by 30 minutes, indicating a decrease in sedentary behaviour with a possible public health impact.

Further, we found that the overweight/obese boys in the intervention group had a non-significant tendency towards an undesired effect with regards to more time used for computer/games during week days compared to the overweight/obese boys in the control group (p = 0.06). By the use of magnitude-based inference as an alternative approach for this variable, we explored to what extent this change was of relevance. A confidence interval or p-value does not address the question of the clinical or practical importance of an outcome; a magnitude-based inference does [33]. It was possible to estimate the chances or probabilities that the true effect was harmful, trivial or beneficial, and the chances were estimated using the same assumptions about the outcome statistic as when estimating p-values or confidence intervals. The result indicated that the intervention likely produced an increase in time used for computer/game-use in week days in overweight/obese boys. This was an effect of clinical/practical importance, however, it was an unintended and undesired consequence of the intervention.

TABLE 3: Effects at 8 months mid-way assessment of the HEIA study, for all and by gender

	8 months mid-way assessment					8 months mid-way assessment									
	Total sample					Girls					Boys				
	Control		Intervention			Control		Intervention			Control		Intervention		
	Mean†	CI	Mean†	CI	p	Mean†	CI	Mean†	CI	p	Mean†	CI	Mean†	CI	p
	n‡ = 840		n‡ = 469			n‡ = 416		n‡ = 241			n‡ = 424		n‡ = 228		
SSB, dl/d															
- week	1.1	(1.0,1.2)	1.0	(0.9,1.1)	0.19	0.9	(0.8,1.0)	0.8	(0.6,0.9)	0.23	1.4	(1.2,1.5)	1.3	(1.1,1.5)	0.52
Group × WS					0.80					0.30					0.71
Group × PE					0.81					0.92					0.76
- weekend	2.4	(2.3,2.5)	2.3	(2.1,2.4)	0.20	2.1	(2.0,2.3)	1.9	(1.7,2.1)	0.04	2.6	(2.5,2.8)	2.6	(2.4,2.9)	1.00
Group × WS					0.77					0.83					0.97
Group × PE					0.35					0.47					0.77
TV/DVD, hours/d															
- week	1.6	(1.6,1.7)	1.5	(1.4,1.5)	0.002	1.6	(1.5,1.6)	1.3	(1.2,1.5)	0.001	1.7	(1.6,1.8)	1.6	(1.5,1.7)	0.20
Group × WS					0.05					0.36					0.03
Group × PE					0.26					0.83					0.26
- weekend	2.3	(2.3,2.4)	2.2	(2.1,2.3)	0.04	2.3	(2.2,2.3)	2.1	(1.9,2.2)	0.03	2.4	(2.3,2.5)	2.3	(2.2,2.5)	0.44
Group × WS					0.68					0.86					0.37
Group × PE					0.23					0.75					0.18
Computer/games, hours/d															
- week	1.2	(1.1,1.2)	1.1	(1.0,1.2)	0.06	1.0	(1.0,1.1)	0.9	(0.8,0.9)	0.004	1.3	(1.2,1.4)	1.3	(1.2,1.4)	0.76
Group × WS					0.01					0.08					0.02
Group × PE					0.31					0.34					0.73
- weekend	1.6	(1.6,1.7)	1.5	(1.4,1.6)	0.003	1.4	(1.3,1.5)	1.1	(1.0,1.3)	<.001	1.9	(1.8,1.9)	1.8	(1.7,1.9)	0.58
Group × WS					0.19					0.78					0.09
Group × PE					0.14					0.10					0.90

SSB = Sugar-sweetened beverages, Group = intervention and control, WS = weight status, PE = parental educational level Analyses: Overall for all and by gender, one-way ANCOVA. Group × WS/group × PE: separate interaction analyses for weight status and for parental education, two-way ANCOVA †Adjusted for pre-test behaviour ‡n vary slightly

TABLE 4: Effects at 8 months mid-way assessment of the HEIA study, by gender and weight status

	GIRLS Normal weight Mean†	CI	Overweight/obese Mean†	CI	BOYS Normal weight Mean†	CI	Overweight/Obese Mean†	CI
SSB, dl/d					**SSB, dl/d**			
- week	n = 545		n = 92		n = 550		n = 85	
Control	0.9	(0.8,1.0)	0.9	(0.6,1.3)	1.4	(1.3,1.6)	1.1	(0.8,1.5)
Intervention	0.8	(0.7,1.0)	0.5	(0.0,1.0)	1.3	(1.1,1.5)	1.2	(0.6,1.8)
- weekend	n = 572		n = 98		n = 600		n = 90	
Control	2.1	(2.0,2.3)	2.0	(1.5,2.4)	2.6	(2.5,2.8)	2.5	(2.0,3.0)
Intervention	1.9#	(1.7,2.1)	1.5	(0.9,2.2)	2.6	(2.4,2.9)	2.5	(1.6,3.4)
TV/DVD, hours/d					**TV/DVD, hours/d**			
- week	n = 579		n = 100		n = 630		n = 93	
Control	1.6	(1.5,1.6)	1.6	(1.4,1.8)	1.6	(1.5,1.7)	2.0	(1.7,2.2)
Intervention	1.3**	(1.2,1.4)	1.6	(1.3,1.9)	1.5	(1.4,1.6)	2.4	(1.9,2.8)
- weekend	n = 570		n = 99		n = 619		n = 93	
Control	2.2	(2.1,2.3)	2.3	(2.0,2.6)	2.4	(2.3,2.5)	2.6	(2.4,2.9)
Intervention	2.1*	(1.9,2.2)	2.1	(1.7,2.5)	2.3	(2.2,2.4)	2.9	(2.4,3.4)
Computer/games, hours/d					**Computer/games, hours/d**			
- week	n = 578		n = 101		n = 628		n = 94	
Control	1.0	(1.0,1.1)	1.0	(0.8,1.2)	1.3	(1.2,1.4)	1.5	(1.2,1.7)
Intervention	0.8***	(0.7,0.9)	1.1	(0.8,1.3)	1.2	(1.1,1.3)	2.0#	(1.5,2.4)
- weekend	n = 570		n = 100		n = 62		n = 93	
Control	1.4	(1.3,1.5)	1.7	(1.4,1.9)	1.8	(1.7,1.9)	2.0	(1.8,2.3)
Intervention	1.1***	(1.0,1.2)	1.4	(1.1,1.8)	1.8	(1.6,1.9)	2.4	(1.9,2.9)

SSB = Sugar-sweetened beverages, Overweight including obese. One-way ANCOVA. †Adjusted for pre-test behaviours *** p = <.001, ** p = 0.001, * p = 0.04, # p = 0.06

TABLE 5: Parental involvement at 8 months mid-way assessment of the HEIA study

Parents	%	Daughter %	Son %	p	Normal weight %	Over-weight/obese %	p	12 years or less %	Between 13 and 16 year%	More than 16 years %	p
Parental awareness	n	169	145	0.001	263	33	0.86	70	119	117	0.33
Low to moderate	104	23.7	26.9		33.3	33.3		22.9	35.0	35.0	
Moderate to high	97	34.3	44.1		31.6	27.3		35.7	27.7	32.5	
High	113	42.0	29.0		35.4	39.4		41.4	36.1	32.5	
Dose received	n	164	139	0.36	253	32	0.67	64	118	113	0.10
Low to moderate	88	25.6	33.1		28.9	31.2		37.5	25.4	27.4	
Moderate to high	109	37.8	33.8		36.0	28.1		26.6	44.1	32.7	
High	106	36.6	33.1		35.2	40.6		35.9	30.5	39.8	
Satisfaction - overall	n	158	150	0.55	286	37	0.98	78	130	123	0.57
Low to moderate	22	7.1	5.7		6.3	5.4		7.7	3.8	8.9	
Moderate to high	174	53.0	48.7		51.4	51.4		51.3	51.5	50.4	
High	145	39.9	45.6		42.3	43.2		41.0	44.6	40.7	
Satisfaction - fact sheets	n	179	150	0.01	274	36	0.70	74	125	121	0.20
Low to moderate	130	44.1	34.0		39.8	38.9		37.8	32.8	47.1	
Moderate to high	81	18.4	32.0		24.5	30.6		24.3	26.4	24.0	
High	118	37.4	34.0		35.8	30.6		37.8	40.8	28.9	

Only adolescents and parents at the intervention schools were included in the analyses. p = Pearson Chi-Square. Parental awareness: parental awareness of program activities for adolescents at school. Dose received: fact sheets received by parents. Satisfaction - overall: parental satisfaction of the project in general. Satisfaction - fact sheets: parental satisfaction of the fact sheets for parents (appreciation of receiving them/interesting content/useful tips)

We can only speculate in why the overweight/obese boys did not respond to the intervention in a desired direction and why the overweight/obese girls did so. The same goes for why we found an overall effect in girls and not in boys. With respect to the former, it could well be that boys being overweight/obese show evidence of reactance by responding with less functional strategies (becoming more sedentary) when confronted with messages concerning healthy eating and enhanced physical activity [34]. As to the latter, one possible explanation is that both the development and implementation of the intervention were dominated by a female approach. The intervention was to a large degree developed by women (mainly female researchers and pedagogues involved), it was mainly women who implemented the intervention at school (mostly female teachers) and process evaluation findings indicated that mothers were more involved than fathers at home (more than 80% of the parent answering the process evaluation questionnaire were women). Furthermore, Haug et al. [35] found that boys across Europe and USA were more likely to be overweight than girls, indicating that preventive initiatives may be inadequate and/or less effective for boys. A third explanation may be difference in parental involvement. The process evaluation indicated that parents of girls were more aware of the project compared to parents of boys, which could result in more parental support for the girls. Finally, analyses of the pre-test data from the HEIA study indicate that the girls may have better role models in their mothers compared to boys with regard to weight [29]. Parents, and in particular fathers, should be made aware of their potential to improve as role models [36,37].

When comparing the results from our study with other intervention studies aimed at reducing the consumption of SSB among children/adolescents, only two of the four identified studies reported effects by gender [38-41]. Haerens et al. [40] found no effect, while Singh et al. [41] reported a significant lower intake in the intervention group both for girls and boys. In total, eight [41-48] out of nine [49] identified studies that aimed at reducing the time used for screen activities among both boys and girls aged 9-15 assessed the moderating effect of gender or reported effect in boys and girls separately. Five of the studies [42-44,47,48] reported effects both for boys and girls, while one reported effect for boys only [41]. Harrison et al. [45] found no effect, while Salmon et al. [46] found an effect in the undesired direction in one of the intervention groups. Three of the studies checked the moderating effect of WS for sedentary behaviour [43,45,48]. Harrison et al. [45] found no interaction for screen time. In Planet Health [43], a reduction in TV-viewing predicted obesity change and mediated the intervention effect among the girls. Finally, obese children reported higher screen time at the post-test than overweight and normal weight adolescents in the study by Gentile et al. [48]. These findings are inconsistent and no clear pattern in the behavioural measures emerges, as reported in recent reviews as well [3,9]. The results from our study support that interventions work better for girls than for boys [3,15,16].

Because of the weak evidence of effective school-based obesity prevention interventions, Lytle [4] suggests that it may be time to re-evaluate where the research needs to move. Lytle points out that an investigation of how study participants receive the intervention rarely is examined [4]. The process evaluation in the HEIA study indicates that girls to a larger extent "bring the project home" compared to boys. This result is supported by previous process evaluations [50,51], and studies on gender differences in parent-child communication reporting that girls' self-disclosure at home about every day life is higher than for boys [52]. Parents of boys are more dependent on getting information from others than their sons [53]. This might explain why parents of boys appreciated the fact sheets more than parents of girls. Qualitative studies have found that parents are in need of effective communication strategies about ways to improve positive health behaviours, and that fact sheets may be a useful tool [54,55].

14.5.1 STRENGTHS AND LIMITATIONS

Our research has some limitations. The SSB consumption variables have not been validated, but our results are in line with data from a national representative study [56]. The measures of sedentary behaviour consisted of single items, resulting in crude estimates only [57]. Still, the mean behavioural outcomes are in line with the trends described by Marshall et al. [58]. The gender differences in time spent on watching TV were small, but boys spent more time on computer/games compared to girls. Furthermore, the test-retest correlation coefficients for the outcome measures were moderate to high (r = 0.46-0.78) [27]. The potential for generalization of our findings is limited because a local sample was recruited from a limited geographic area, mainly in small towns and their close surroundings. The recruitment of schools and participants may have caused a sampling bias, restricting the number of overweight/obese participants and resulting in reduced precision (larger confidence intervals). Finally, some degree of social desirability may be present in the data [59,60]. Still, the effects found should be taken into consideration because of the design of the HEIA study. One of the strengths of the present study is the large sample with objective measures of weight and height. Another strength is that parental education was reported by the parents themselves, and that we were able to collect these data from nearly all the parents giving their adolescent consent to participate in the study, and not only from those parents answering a questionnaire.

14.6 CONCLUSIONS

The evaluation of the HEIA study after 8 month revealed that young adolescent boys and girls responded differently to the intervention, and that preventive initiatives thus seem to work better for girls than for boys. Further, it seems important to conduct subgroup analyses to explore potential beneficial or negative effects of interventions. In future research the parental involvement should be evaluated, investigating possible differences in maternal and paternal support and role modelling. More focus on gender and initial WS in the formative evaluation phase of obesity prevention studies also seem warranted in order to enhance the effectiveness of preventive initiatives.

REFERENCES

1.   Kremers SP, de Bruijn GJ, Visscher TL, van Mechelen W, De Vries NK, Brug J: Environmental influences on energy balance-related behaviors: a dual-process view. Int J Behav Nutr Phys Act 2006, 3:9.

2. Kremers SP, Van der Horst K, Brug J: Adolescent screen-viewing behaviour is associated with consumption of sugar-sweetened beverages: the role of habit strength and perceived parental norms. Appetite 2007, 48:345-350.

3. Brown T, Summerbell C: Systematic review of school-based interventions that focus on changing dietary intake and physical activity levels to prevent childhood obesity: an update to the obesity guidance produced by the National Institute for Health and Clinical Excellence. Obes Rev 2009, 10:110-141.

4. Lytle LA: School-based interventions: where do we go next? Arch Pediatr Adolesc Med 2009, 163:388-389.

5. Doak C, Heitmann BL, Summerbell C, Lissner L: Prevention of childhood obesity - what type of evidence should we consider relevant? Obes Rev 2009, 10:350-356.

6. Chin A Paw MJM, Singh AS, Brug J, van Mechelen W: Why did soft drink consumption decrease but screen time not? Mediating mechanisms in a school-based obesity prevention program. Int J Behav Nutr Phys Act 2008, 5:41.

7. Naylor PJ, McKay HA: Prevention in the first place: schools a setting for action on physical inactivity. Br J Sports Med 2009, 43:10-13.

8. Thomas H: Obesity prevention programs for children and youth: why are their results so modest? Health Educ Res 2006, 21:783-795.

9. De Bourdeaudhuij I, Van Cauwenberghe E, Spittaels H, Oppert JM, Rostami C, Brug J, van Lenthe F, Lobstein T, Maes L: School-based interventions promoting both physical activity and healthy eating in Europe: a systematic review within the HOPE project. Obes Rev 2011, 12:205-216.

10. Birch LL, Ventura AK: Preventing childhood obesity: what works? Int J Obes (Lond) 2009, 33(Suppl 1):74-81.

11. Gruber KJ, Haldeman LA: Using the family to combat childhood and adult obesity. Prev Chronic Dis 2009, 6:1-10.

12. Rosenkranz RR, Dzewaltowski DA: Model of the home food environment pertaining to childhood obesity. Nutr Rev 2008, 66:123-140.

13. Granich J, Rosenberg M, Knuiman M, Timperio A: Understanding children's sedentary behaviour: a qualitative study of the family home environment. Health Educ Res 2010, 25:199-210.

14. Maziak W, Ward KD, Stockton MB: Childhood obesity: are we missing the big picture? Obes Rev 2008, 9:35-42.

15. Kremers SP, de Bruijn GJ, Droomers M, van Lenthe F, Brug J: Moderators of environmental intervention effects on diet and activity in youth. Am J Prev Med 2007, 32:163-172.

16. Stice E, Shaw H, Marti CN: A meta-analytic review of obesity prevention programs for children and adolescents: the skinny on interventions that work. Psychol Bull 2006, 132:667-691.

17. Rey-Lopez JP, Vicente-Rodriguez G, Biosca M, Moreno LA: Sedentary behaviour and obesity development in children and adolescents. Nutr Metab Cardiovasc Dis 2008, 18:242-251.

18. Robinson TN: Does television cause childhood obesity? JAMA 1998, 279:959-960.

19. Van der Horst K, Oenema A, Ferreira I, Wendel-Vos W, Giskes K, van Lenthe F, Brug J: A systematic review of environmental correlates of obesity-related dietary behaviors in youth. Health Educ Res 2007, 22:203-226.

20. Van der Horst K, Chin A Paw MJM, Twisk JW, van Mechelen W: A brief review on correlates of physical activity and sedentariness in youth. Med Sci Sports Exerc 2007, 39:1241-1250.

21. Stattin H, Kerr M: Parental monitoring: a reinterpretation. Child Dev 2000, 71:1072-1085.

22. Kerr M, Stattin H: What parents know, how they know it, and several forms of adolescent adjustment: further support for a reinterpretation of monitoring. Dev Psychol 2000, 36:366-380.

23. Riesch SK, Anderson LS, Krueger HA: Parent-child communication processes: preventing children's health-risk behavior. J Spec Pediatr Nurs 2006, 11:41-56.

24. Steckler A, Ethelbah B, Martin CJ, Stewart D, Pardilla M, Gittelsohn J, Stone E, Fenn D, Smyth M, Vu M: Pathways process evaluation results: a school-based prevention trial to promote healthful diet and physical activity in American Indian third, fourth, and fifth grade students. Prev Med 2003, 37(Suppl 1):80-90.

25. Haerens L, Deforche B, Maes L, Cardon G, Stevens V, De Bourdeaudhuij I: Evaluation of a 2-year physical activity and healthy eating intervention in middle school children. Health Educ Res 2006, 21:911-921.

26. Saunders RP, Evans MH, Joshi P: Developing a process-evaluation plan for assessing health promotion program implementation: a how-to guide. Health Promot Pract 2005, 6:134-147.

27. Lien N, Bjelland M, Bergh IH, Grydeland M, Anderssen SA, Ommundsen Y, Andersen LF, Henriksen HB, Randby JS, Klepp KI: Design of a two year comprehensive, multi-coponent school-based intervention to promote healthy weight development amog 11-13 year olds: the HEIA study. Scand J Public Health 2010, 38(Suppl 5):38-51.

28. Cole TJ, Bellizzi MC, Flegal KM, Dietz WH: Establishing a standard definition for child overweight and obesity worldwide: international survey. BMJ 2000, 320:1240-1243.

29. Bjelland M, Lien N, Bergh IH, Grydeland M, Anderssen SA, Klepp KI, Ommundsen Y, Andersen LF: Overweight and waist circumference among Norwegian 11-year-olds and associations with reported parental overweight and waist circumference: The HEIA study. Scand J Public Health 2010, 38(Suppl 5):19-27.

30. Hopkins WG: Spreadsheets for Analysis of Controlled Trials, with Adjustment for a Subject Characteristic. Sportscience 2006, 10:46-50.

31. Cohen J: Statistical Power Analysis for the Behavioral Sciences. 2nd edition. Hillsdale (NJ): Lawrence Erlbaum; 1988:19-74.

32. Goran MI: Metabolic precursors and effects of obesity in children: a decade of progress, 1990-1999. Am J Clin Nutr 2001, 73:158-171.

33. Batterham AM, Hopkins WG: Making meaningful inferences about magnitudes. Int J Sports Physiol Perform 2006, 1:50-57.

34. Brehm JW: A Theory of Psychological Reactance. New York: Academic Press; 1966.

35. Haug E, Rasmussen M, Samdal O, Iannotti R, Kelly C, Borraccino A, Vereecken C, Melkevik O, Lazzeri G, Giacchi M, Ercan O, Due P, Ravens-Sieberer U, Currie

C, Morgan A, Ahluwalia N: Overweight in school-aged children and its relationship with demographic and lifestyle factors: results from the WHO-Collaborative Health Behaviour in School-aged Children (HBSC) study. Int J Public Health 2009, 54(Suppl 2):167-179.

36. He M, Piche L, Beynon C, Harris S: Screen-related sedentary behaviors: children's and parents' attitudes, motivations, and practices. J Nutr Educ Behav 2010, 42:17-25.

37. Elfhag K, Tynelius P, Rasmussen F: Family links of eating behaviour in normal weight and overweight children. Int J Pediatr Obes 2010, 5:491-500.

38. James J, Thomas P, Cavan D, Kerr D: Preventing childhood obesity by reducing consumption of carbonated drinks: cluster randomised controlled trial. BMJ 2004, 328:1237.

39. Ebbeling CB, Feldman HA, Osganian SK, Chomitz VR, Ellenbogen SJ, Ludwig DS: Effects of decreasing sugar-sweetened beverage consumption on body weight in adolescents: a randomized, controlled pilot study. Pediatrics 2006, 117:673-680.

40. Haerens L, De Bourdeaudhuij I, Maes L, Vereecken C, Brug J, Deforche B: The effects of a middle-school healthy eating intervention on adolescents' fat and fruit intake and soft drinks consumption. Public Health Nutr 2007, 10:443-449.

41. Singh AS, Chin A Paw MJM, Brug J, van Mechelen W: Dutch obesity intervention in teenagers: effectiveness of a school-based program on body composition and behavior. Arch Pediatr Adolesc Med 2009, 163:309-317.

42. Robinson TN: Reducing children's television viewing to prevent obesity: a randomized controlled trial. JAMA 1999, 282:1561-1567.

43. Gortmaker SL, Peterson K, Wiecha J, Sobol AM, Dixit S, Fox MK, Laird N: Reducing obesity via a school-based interdisciplinary intervention among youth: Planet Health. Arch Pediatr Adolesc Med 1999, 153:409-418.

44. Patrick K, Calfas KJ, Norman GJ, Zabinski MF, Sallis JF, Rupp J, Covin J, Cella J: Randomized controlled trial of a primary care and home-based intervention for physical activity and nutrition behaviors: PACE+ for adolescents. Arch Pediatr Adolesc Med 2006, 160:128-136.

45. Harrison M, Burns CF, McGuinness M, Heslin J, Murphy NM: Influence of a health education intervention on physical activity and screen time in primary school children: 'Switch Off - Get Active'. J Sci Med Sport 2006, 9:388-394.

46. Salmon J, Ball K, Hume C, Booth M, Crawford D: Outcomes of a group-randomized trial to prevent excess weight gain, reduce screen behaviours and promote physical activity in 10-year-old children: switch-play. Int J Obes (Lond) 2008, 32:601-612.

47. Simon C, Schweitzer B, Oujaa M, Wagner A, Arveiler D, Triby E, Copin N, Blanc S, Platat C: Successful overweight prevention in adolescents by increasing physical activity: a 4-year randomized controlled intervention. Int J Obes (Lond) 2008, 32:1489-1498.

48. Gentile DA, Welk G, Eisenmann JC, Reimer RA, Walsh DA, Russell DW, Callahan R, Walsh M, Strickland S, Fritz K: Evaluation of a multiple ecological level child obesity prevention program: Switch what you Do, View, and Chew. BMC Med 2009, 7:49.

49. Gortmaker SL, Cheung LW, Peterson KE, Chomitz G, Cradle JH, Dart H, Fox MK, Bullock RB, Sobol AM, Colditz G, Field AE, Laird N: Impact of a school-based in-

terdisciplinary intervention on diet and physical activity among urban primary school children: eat well and keep moving. Arch Pediatr Adolesc Med 1999, 153:975-983.

50. Wind M, Bjelland M, Perez-Rodrigo C, Te Velde SJ, Hildonen C, Bere E, Klepp K-I, Brug J: Appreciation and implementation of a school-based intervention are associated with changes in fruit and vegetable intake in 10- to 13-year old schoolchildren - the Pro Children study. Health Educ Res 2008, 23:997-1007.

51. Nader PR, Sellers DE, Johnson CC, Perry CL, Stone EJ, Cook KC, Bebchuk J, Luepker RV: The effect of adult participation in a school-based family intervention to improve Children's diet and physical activity: the Child and Adolescent Trial for Cardiovascular Health. Prev Med 1996, 25:455-464.

52. Waizenhofer RN, Buchanan CM, Jackson-Newsom J: Mothers' and fathers' knowledge of adolescents' daily activities: its sources and its links with adolescent adjustment. J Fam Psychol 2004, 18:348-360.

53. Crouter AC, Bumpus MF, Davis KD, McHale SM: How do parents learn about adolescents' experiences? Implications for parental knowledge and adolescent risky behavior. Child Dev 2005, 76:869-882.

54. Borra ST, Kelly L, Shirreffs MB, Neville K, Geiger CJ: Developing health messages: qualitative studies with children, parents, and teachers help identify communications opportunities for healthful lifestyles and the prevention of obesity. J Am Diet Assoc 2003, 103:721-728.

55. Kaplan M, Kiernan NE, James L: Intergenerational family conversations and decision making about eating healthfully. J Nutr Educ Behav 2006, 38:298-306.

56. Øverby NC, Andersen LF: Ungkost 2000: A national representative dietary survey among Norwegian children and adolescents (In Norwegian). 2000. Oslo: Directorate for Health and Social Affairs

57. Bryant MJ, Lucove JC, Evenson KR, Marshall S: Measurement of television viewing in children and adolescents: a systematic review. Obes Rev 2007, 8:197-209.

58. Marshall SJ, Gorely T, Biddle SJ: A descriptive epidemiology of screen-based media use in youth: a review and critique. J Adolesc 2006, 29:333-349.

59. Klesges LM, Baranowski T, Beech B, Cullen K, Murray DM, Rochon J, Pratt C: Social desirability bias in self-reported dietary, physical activity and weight concerns measures in 8- to 10-year-old African-American girls: results from the Girls Health Enrichment Multisite Studies (GEMS). Prev Med 2004, 38(Suppl 1):78-87.

60. Jago R, Baranowski T, Baranowski JC, Cullen KW, Thompson DI: Social desirability is associated with some physical activity, psychosocial variables and sedentary behavior but not self-reported physical activity among adolescent males. Health Educ Res 2007, 22:438-449.

CHAPTER 15

AVERTING OBESITY AND TYPE 2 DIABETES IN INDIA THROUGH SUGAR-SWEETENED BEVERAGE TAXATION: AN ECONOMIC-EPIDEMIOLOGIC MODELING STUDY

SANJAY BASU, SUKUMAR VELLAKKAL, SUTAPA AGRAWAL, DAVID STUCKLER, BARRY POPKIN, AND SHAH EBRAHIM

15.1 INTRODUCTION

Sugar-sweetened beverage (SSB) consumption is established as a major risk factor for overweight and obesity, as well as an array of cardio-metabolic conditions, especially type 2 diabetes [1],[2]. The individual risk of type 2 diabetes attributable to SSB consumption remains statistically significant after adjustment for total energy consumption and body mass index (BMI) [3],[4]. While taxes on SSBs have been proposed in high-income countries to lower obesity and type 2 diabetes risks given limited success from other population measures and individual-level interventions

Averting Obesity and Type 2 Diabetes in India through Sugar-Sweetened Beverage Taxation: An Economic-Epidemiologic Modeling Study. © *Basu S, Vellakkal S, Agrawal S, Stuckler D, Popkin B, and Ebrahim S.* PLoS Medicine *11,1 (2014), doi:10.1371/journal.pmed.1001582. Licensed under Creative Commons Attribution 4.0 International License, http://creativecommons.org/licenses/by/4.0/.*

[5], recent assessments reveal a majority of SSB sales now occur outside the US and Europe, where marketing efforts appear most focused [6]–[8]. SSB sales in India, for example, have increased by 13% year-on-year since 1998, exceeding 11 liters per capita per year (Figure 1) [9]. At the population level, the acceleration of SSB consumption among middle-income country populations has been statistically associated with increased obesity, overweight, and type 2 diabetes prevalence rates, independent of concurrent changes in other caloric consumption, physical inactivity, and aging [6],[10],[11].

While econometric and modeling studies suggest the potential effectiveness of large (e.g., penny-per-ounce, or 20%–25%) but not smaller excise taxes on SSBs in the United States [12]–[15], and UK [16], a key unknown is whether such fiscal strategies will be wise to implement in middle-income nations like India and China, where several aspects of SSB consumption and disease risk are uniquely different from Western populations [17]. Asian countries' populations appear to be internally heterogeneous in their "nutrition transition" towards Western dietary patterns high in salt, sugar, and fat content [17],[18]. This implies that nationwide taxation may be perverse if benefits accrue among only select populations while monetary penalties apply universally, especially if the tax burden but not the tax benefit falls disproportionately on the poor. In India, processed foods make up a substantial portion of dietary consumption overall, but with marked variations between men and women and among age groups, income classes, and urban versus rural populations [19],[20]. Type 2 diabetes is similarly more prevalent among urban, higher-income men, but lower-income groups and women increasingly face a heightened burden of obesity and low diagnosis rates associated with poor health care access [21]–[23]. Furthermore, the beverages that people consume apart from SSBs also contain high caloric and glycemic loads in India and much of Asia [6], indicating that if a tax were to induce substitutions from SSBs to other beverages, the net health impacts on obesity and type 2 diabetes may be limited and, possibly, perverse [24].

We sought to characterize the influence of an SSB tax on overweight, obesity, and type 2 diabetes trajectories among multiple demographic groups in India. To perform the analysis, we first used a standard microeconomic approach to calculate how changes in SSB price relate to changes in SSB consumption ("own-price elasticity") and substitution of SSBs for other beverages ("cross-price elasticity"), using per capita consumption and price variations data from a nationally representative household survey [25]. We then estimated how changes in overall calories and glycemic load induced by a 20% excise tax on SSBs would be expected to alter overweight, obesity, and type 2 diabetes incidence over the period 2014–2024. We chose the 20% rate for comparability against tax simulations in Western populations, where a penny-per-ounce tax amounts to an ~20%–25% price increase [15]; the 20% change is also within the 35% SSB price variation range in the survey data employed for our assessment. We nevertheless varied the tax rate from 10% to 30% in sensitivity analyses to explore alternative forecasts. We constructed and validated a microsimulation model to estimate changes in weight and diabetes risk from the tax, examining how changes in modeled outcomes resulted from a variety of alternative assumptions. Our a priori hypothesis was that urban populations would be the primary beneficiaries of SSB taxation, given their high SSB exposure as well as elevated obesity and type 2 diabetes prevalence rates [9],[26].

15.2 METHODS

Our analysis proceeded in three steps. First, we calculated changes to overall beverage expenditure as well as own-price and cross-price elasticities between SSBs and the other major beverage types consumed in India (milk, fresh fruit juices, coffee, and tea) using survey data relating price to consumption. We next used these elasticity estimates to calculate per capita kilocalorie and glycemic load changes expected from a 20% excise tax on SSBs. Finally, constructing a discrete-time microsimulation model, we simulated changes in overweight, obesity, and type 2 diabetes incidence and prevalence over the period 2014–2023 given changes in caloric intake and glycemic load. Each component of our analysis was stratified by age-band, sex, income, and urban/rural residence, in order to analyze disparities between demographic subpopulations in India.

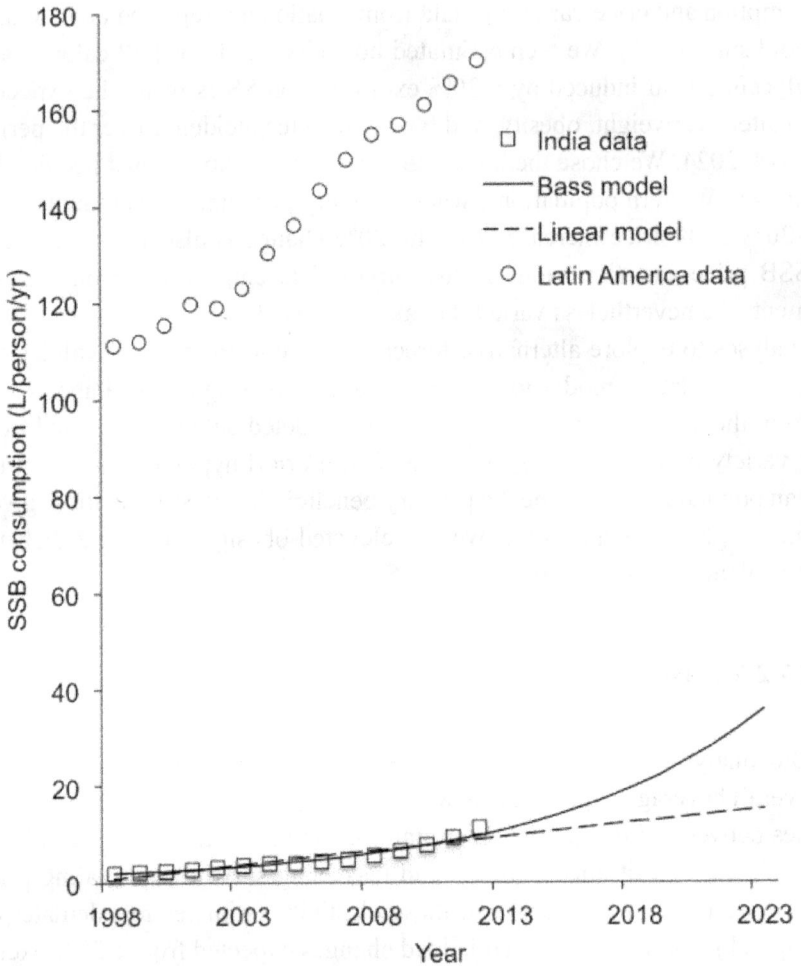

FIGURE 1: SSB consumption in liters per capita per year in India, 1998–2012 [9]. The Latin American average consumption is plotted for comparison, reflecting the population-weighted average per capita consumption from 13 countries (Argentina, Bolivia, Brazil, Chile, Colombia, Costa Rica, Dominican Republic, Ecuador, Guatemala, Mexico, Peru, Uruguay, and Venezuela).

15.2.1 DATA SOURCES

15.2.1.1 ELASTICITY CALCULATIONS.

The Indian National Sample Survey (NSS), wave 2009/2010 (the most recent data available), was used to calculate own- and cross-price elasticities corresponding to changes in SSB price in each demographic subgroup, controlling for changes in SSB availability [25]. The NSS Consumer Expenditure module is a widely used repeated quinquennial cross-sectional survey of household food consumption data from a nationally representative sample in terms of age and income distribution [25]. NSS data include beverage amount consumed and prices paid for each of the beverage categories, based on surveys of 100,855 households interviewed through a validated interviewer-assisted questionnaire with district-level validation of reported prices and oversampling of low-income, rural, and female-headed households. Our power calculations estimated that we could detect the odds ratio equivalent of a 10 kcal/person/day change with >80% power in each subgroup given a survey design effect of two [27]. We converted grams of consumption per capita into kilocalories per capita (mean and 95% confidence intervals) using a standard nutrient tables [28],[29]. Kilocalorie and glycemic load conversions included both mean and 95% confidence intervals reflecting the distribution of milk among whole, skim, and toned varieties [20]; the available fresh fruit juices on the Indian market [9]; and typical added sugar content to consumer-brewed coffee and tea [28]. Price was expressed in 2010 Indian rupees, adjusted through GDP price deflators [30].

15.2.1.2 BMI DISTRIBUTION AND TYPE 2 DIABETES STATUS.

While the NSS provides data on consumption and price, it does not provide data on health parameters such as BMI and type 2 diabetes status. To analyze the covariance of SSB consumption with BMI and type 2 diabetes status, we used data from the Public Health Foundation of India's Indian Migration Study (IMS) 2007–2010, a national sample of

7,049 men and women from all three income tertiles and both urban and rural residency status (Figure 2). These individuals were evaluated through interviewer-administered food frequency questionnaires and anthropometric and medical assessments published previously [20],[31]. The dietary assessment was validated against independent surveys and a subsample analysis of 418 participants subjected to three 24-hour dietary recalls [20].

15.2.2 ELASTICITY CALCULATION DETAILS

Given the absence of a suitable instrumental variable to link with SSB prices, we calculated elasticities among the beverages using the classical Quadratic Almost Ideal Demand System [32], a standardized microeconomic system of equations that estimate how price variations affect expenditure, substitution between goods, and overall consumption (the inflationary effects of taxation). The equations are detailed in Text S1, and complete elasticity results are presented for each demographic subgroup in Table 1. A standard two-step procedure was also used to first estimate the probability of consumption, to account for censoring and zero consumption, and then estimate the share of expenditures spent on each beverage, controlling for availability and a series of socioeconomic variables detailed in Text S1 [33]–[35]. The system allows us to estimate shifting out of the purchased beverage market in the context of prices (e.g., to tap water), versus the degree of substitution between beverage classes following a price change in each beverage. The demand system was estimated in Stata version MP12.1 (StataCorp). The face validity of own-price SSB elasticity was compared against an international systematic review of elasticities [36]; our demand system revealed an own-price elasticity of SSBs of −0.94 (95% CI −0.90 to −0.98), within the review-based 95% confidence interval of −0.33 to −1.24. Cross-elasticities, as tabulated in Text S1, were also similar to published estimates, although the published estimates available have not included India [37].

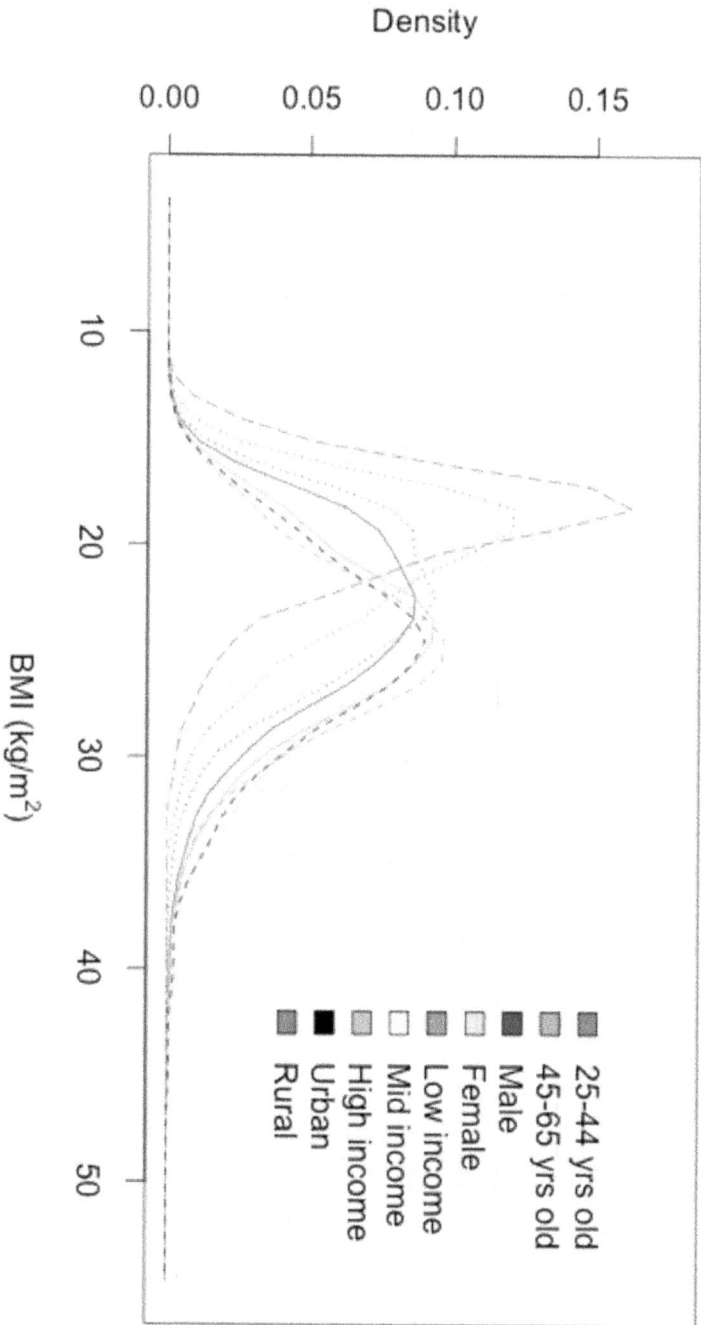

FIGURE 2: Body mass index (BMI) distributions among cohorts (kg/m²), 2010 [31].

TABLE 1: Elasticity given 1% change in SSB price, calculated from [25].

Beverage	Income Level			Residential Sector		Overall Population (95% CI)
	Low (95% CI)	Mid (95% CI)	High (95% CI)	Urban (95% CI)	Rural (95% CI)	
n	28,207	50,989	21,659	59,119	41,736	100,855
Milk	0.055 (0.013–0.096)*	0.046 (0.010–0.083)*	0.046 (0.010–0.083)*	0.049 (0.010–0.087)*	0.049 (0.012–0.087)*	0.049 (0.011–0.087)*
SSBs	−0.90 (−0.86 to −0.93)*	−0.96 (−0.92 to −1.00)*	−0.96 (−0.92 to −1.00)*	−0.94 (−0.90 to −0.98)*	−0.94 (−0.90 to −0.98)*	−0.94 (−0.90 to −0.98)*
Fresh fruit juice	0.32 (0.31–0.36)*	0.30 (0.25–0.35)*	0.30 (0.25–0.35)*	0.31 (0.27–0.35)*	0.31 (0.27–0.35)*	0.31 (0.27–0.35)*
Coffee	0.0016 (−0.077 to 0.051)	0.0054 (−0.058 to 0.084)	0.0054 (−0.058 to 0.084)	0.0041 (−0.064 to 0.073)	0.0041 (−0.064 to 0.073)	0.0041 (−0.064 to 0.073)
Tea	0.10 (0.062–0.131)*	0.14 (0.12–0.18)*	0.14 (0.12–0.18)*	0.13 (0.098–0.16)*	0.13 (0.098–0.16)*	0.13 (0.098–0.16)*

*$p<0.05$

15.2.3 TAX EFFECT ESTIMATES

To examine the kilocalorie changes attributable to a 20% SSB tax, the price elasticity for each beverage (percent change in consumption for each 1% change in SSB price) was multiplied by the change in SSB price (20% in the baseline case) and multiplied by baseline daily kilocalorie intake among multiple Indian subpopulations to estimate the change in individual daily intake for each beverage (Table 2).

TABLE 2: Kilocalorie consumption per day from beverages, overweight and obesity prevalence (% BMI$\geq$25 kg/m^2), and baseline diabetes incidence (per 100,000 persons) among cohorts, used for model initialization [20],[25],[31],[41],[42].

Cohorts		Milk (SD)	SSBs (SD)	Fresh Fruit Juice (SD)	Coffee (SD)	Tea (SD)	% BMI $\geq$25 kg/ m^2 (SD)	Diabetes Incidence (per 100,000)
Age	25–44	200 (5)	51 (1)	36 (0.3)	19 (2)	83 (5)	156 (35)	34 (8)
	45–65	226 (5)	37 (1)	30 (0.7)	24 (2)	81 (6)	379 (50)	48 (11)
Sex	M	220 (4)	50 (1)	34 (0.3)	21 (2)	85 (5)	507 (46)	32 (8)
	F	193 (5)	42 (1)	34 (0.5)	21 (2)	79 (6)	103 (44)	46 (10)
Income	Low	139 (6)	44 (1)	29 (0.8)	17 (2)	82 (6)	105 (67)	11 (2)
	Mid	173 (6)	48 (1)	40 (0.5)	26 (2)	81 (6)	157 (50)	16 (4)
	High	220 (6)	47 (1)	32 (0.7)	19 (2)	85 (6)	350 (45)	43 (10)
Residence	Urban	223 (6)	48 (1)	38 (2)	25 (2)	83 (6)	372 (50)	48 (11)
	Rural	187 (6)	45 (2)	28 (2)	16 (2)	82 (7)	242 (42)	21 (5)
Overall		207 (5)	46 (1)	34 (0.4)	21 (2)	82 (5)	38 (8)	307 (45)

Note that "income" here is measured using the Standard of Living Index (SLI), a household level assed-based scale devised for Indian surveys [38]. SD = standard deviation.

To estimate the potential effects of the tax on overweight and obesity prevalence (BMI$\geq$25 kg/m^2) and type 2 diabetes incidence, we constructed a microsimulation model, which simulates 10,000 adults for each cohort defined by every combination of: age (25–44, 45–65 years old), sex, income (low, middle, and high Standard of Living Index [SLI], a household-level asset-based scale devised for Indian surveys [38]), and urban/rural status (using the World Bank definition of urban residence [39]). Model details are itemized here according to ISPOR reporting guidelines [40], and the model flow diagram is depicted in Figure 2.

Sampling from the joint distribution of weight, height, consumption of each beverage type, and type 2 diabetes status from the IMS study, the model assigns simulated individuals a baseline profile of these factors, updating the estimates for secular trends (Table 2) [31],[41],[42]. Unlike a typical Markov model, the microsimulation approach can capture the impact of interventions on individual risk factor profiles, not just the average population effect of an intervention—allowing for complex relationships among multiple co-morbid risk factors to be incorporated into the experiment. This is important because reducing SSB consumption in an individual who has a high baseline intake of SSBs but also a high consumption of other beverages may have different outcomes than reducing SSB consumption for someone with less consumption of other beverages. The model was validated by comparing historical projections of 2000–2010 obesity and type 2 diabetes prevalence in India given year 2000 input values against independent World Health Organization survey-based estimates (Figure S1) [26].

We first simulated a baseline (no tax) case in which secular trends in kilocalorie consumption, glycemic load intake, and associated BMI and type 2 diabetes incidence changes were estimated. Two baseline scenarios were modeled: (1) a linear rise in SSB consumption of 13% per annum, fitting the secular trend from 1998–2012 (the longest time series available), and (2) a nonlinear rise predicted by a Bass marketing model used commonly by industry for projecting sales growth [43] (both shown in Figure 1; Bass model equation in Text S1). The model also incorporated secular trends in non-beverage calorie intake given by UN Food and Agricultural Organization estimates, to account for other caloric changes; linear trends in non-SSB beverage consumption were not statistically significant (Text S1) [9],[44]. Consumption changes were also converted into changes in glycemic load using standard glycemic index tables (Table 3) [45]. Note that these estimates include the typical distribution of sugars added by consumers to coffee and tea.

To convert the calorie change estimates into changes in weight over time (Figure 3), we used a validated set of equations developed by the National Institutes of Health to estimate individual body weight change after a change in calorie consumption (reproduced in Text S1 with parameter values in Table S1) [46]. While there are many potential alternative models relating caloric intake changes to body weight, we chose this model as these equations were validated against experimental controlled feeding studies among humans in the age groups included in this simulation, and more accurately predicted changes in body weight from measured changes in energy intake than did alternative published models in head-to-head comparisons [47]. The equations account for the time delay between consumption changes and weight changes, assuming that energy must be conserved, and that changes in body composition and body weight result from imbalances between the intake and utilization rates of calories along with shifts between intracellular and extracellular compartments.

TABLE 3: Effective glycemic load (g) per kcal when accounting for typical serving sizes (g) and energy content (kcals) of beverages [45].

Beverage	Glycemic Load (g) per kcal (95% CI)
Milk	0.0311 (0.0235–0.0387)
SSBs	0.1584 (0.1408–0.1759)
Fresh fruit juice	0.0870 (0.0758–0.0981)
Coffee	0.0919 (0.0850–0.0989)
Tea	0.0553 (0.0497–0.0608)

To estimate type 2 diabetes incidence (Figure 4), we employed a standard, validated hazard calculation method (Text S1) [48]. This calculation estimates how much an individual's risk of type 2 diabetes changes given changes in their beverage intake, employing an estimate of the relative risk of type 2 diabetes contributed by glycemic load, adjusted for an exponential rate of effect of $1/7.6$ years^{-1} (95% CI $1/2.8^{-1}/14.7$ years^{-1}) [49]. We used a type 2 diabetes relative risk estimate of 1.45 (95% CI 1.31–1.61) for each 100-g increment in glycemic load, based on a meta-analysis of 24 prospective cohort studies (p<0.001; 7.5 million person-years of follow-up) [50]. This relative risk estimate incorporates both the type 2 diabetes incidence risk associated with adiposity due to consumption, and the indirect pancreatic and hepatic effects of glycemic consumption that are obesity-independent (both obesity-mediated and non-obesity-mediated pathways) [51],[52]. We chose to use glycemic load relative risk estimates rather than relative risk estimates of diabetes specifically calculated only for SSBs [3], to account for the metabolic effects of beverages substituted for SSBs. This would be expected to produce conservative results from our simulation. Furthermore, the glycemic load calculation accounts for the fact that the impact on diabetes of different types of calories is different; that is, because the glycemic load per calorie is much higher for SSBs than other beverages (Table 3), a net change in calories alone does not predict type 2 diabetes risk, and the glycemic load estimate is used to account for the fact that some calories confer higher risk than others.

For prospective simulation of the period 2014–2023, 10,000 simulations were performed of the overall model (10,000 simulations each with 10,000 individuals per cohort) in MATLAB version R2013b (Math-Works), sampling repeatedly from the probability distributions of the input parameter values to estimate 95% confidence intervals around modeled outcomes (Figure 5). All model parameters—including kilocalorie consumption, elasticities, glycemic load, relative risks, and the metabolic parameters—were included in the uncertainty analysis.

To simulate the 20% excise SSB tax, we simulated full country-wide tax coverage starting at the beginning of the year 2014. In sensitivity analyses, we varied the SSB tax rate from 10% to 30%. In a further sensitivity analysis, SSB consumption trends were simulated using a standard Bass diffusion model employed by industry to project sales growth (Figure 1, $R^2 = 0.98$) [43], rather than the baseline linear trend also shown in Figure 1.

For outcomes analysis, we computed both overweight and obesity prevalence, because the threshold of 25 kg/m^2 has been the Indian government standard for BMI surveillance [53], given elevated risk of type 2 diabetes among South Asians at lower BMI levels (>24 kg/m^2) [54] than the international obesity threshold of 30 kg/m^2.

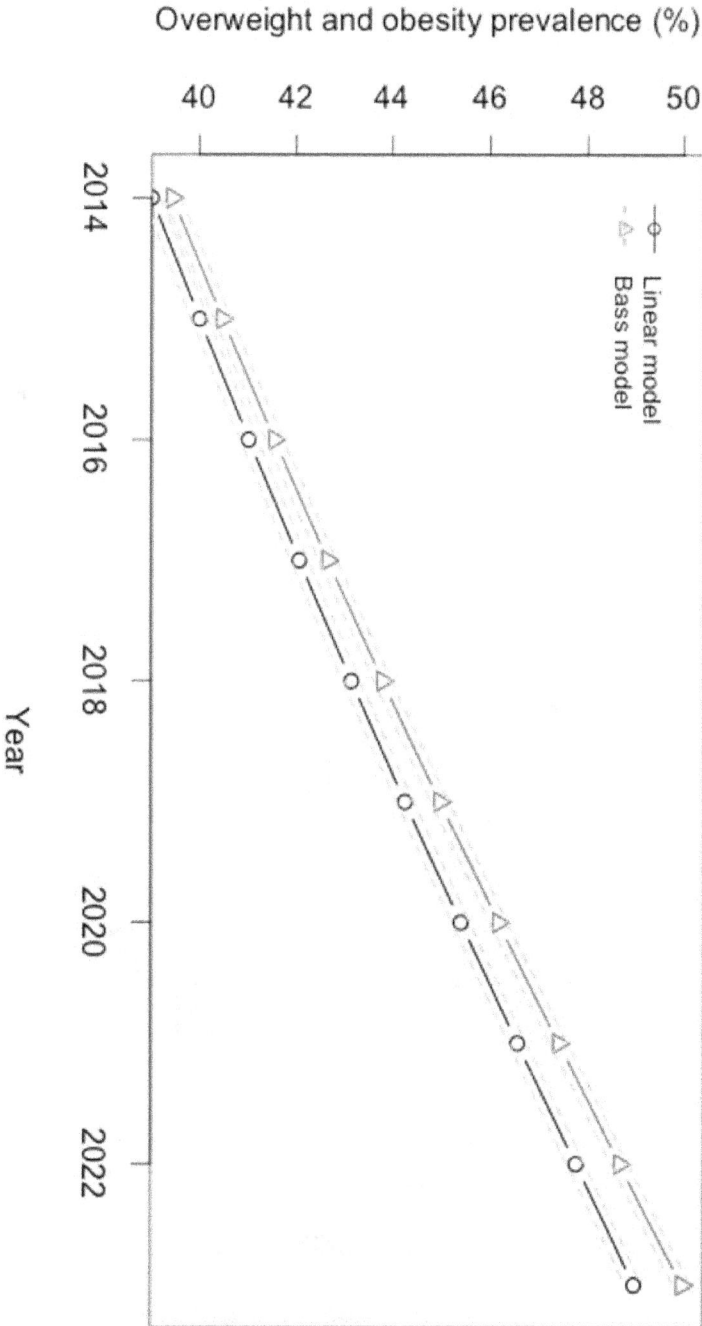

FIGURE 3. Projected trajectory of overweight, obesity in India, 2013–2024.

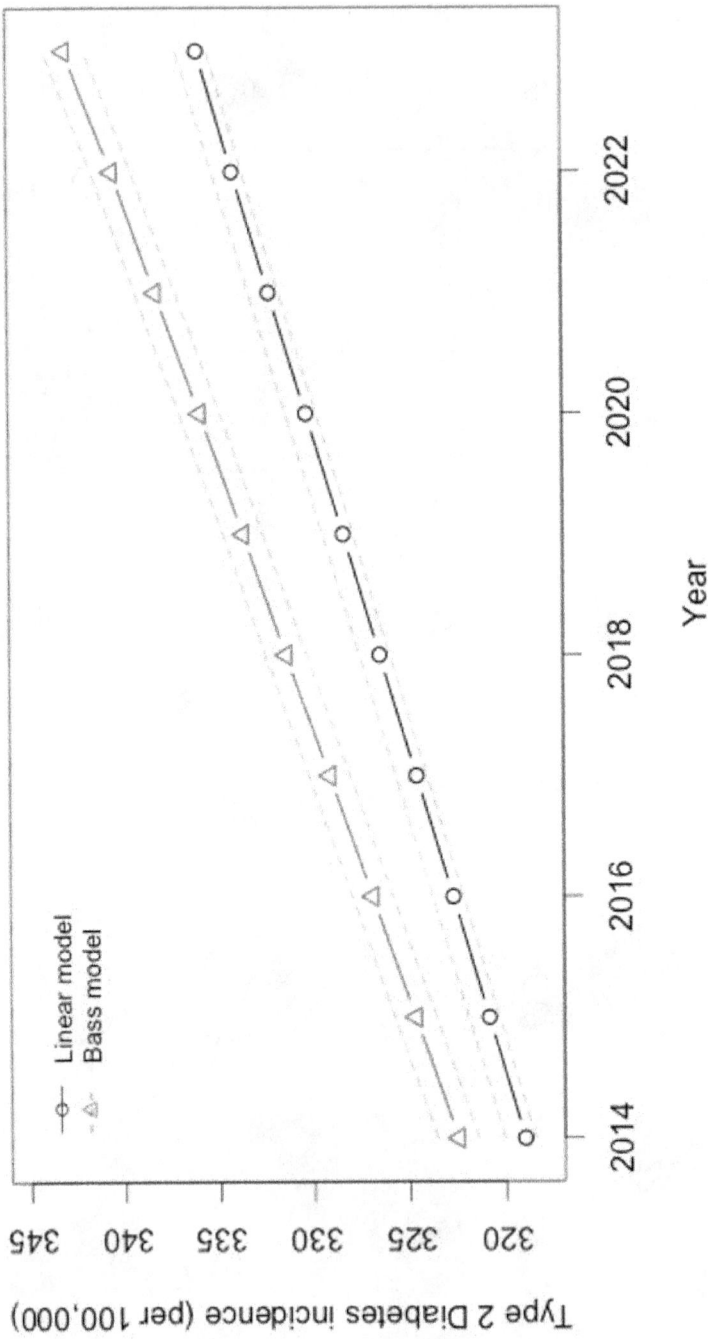

FIGURE 4: Projected trajectory of type 2 diabetes incidence in India, 2013–2024.

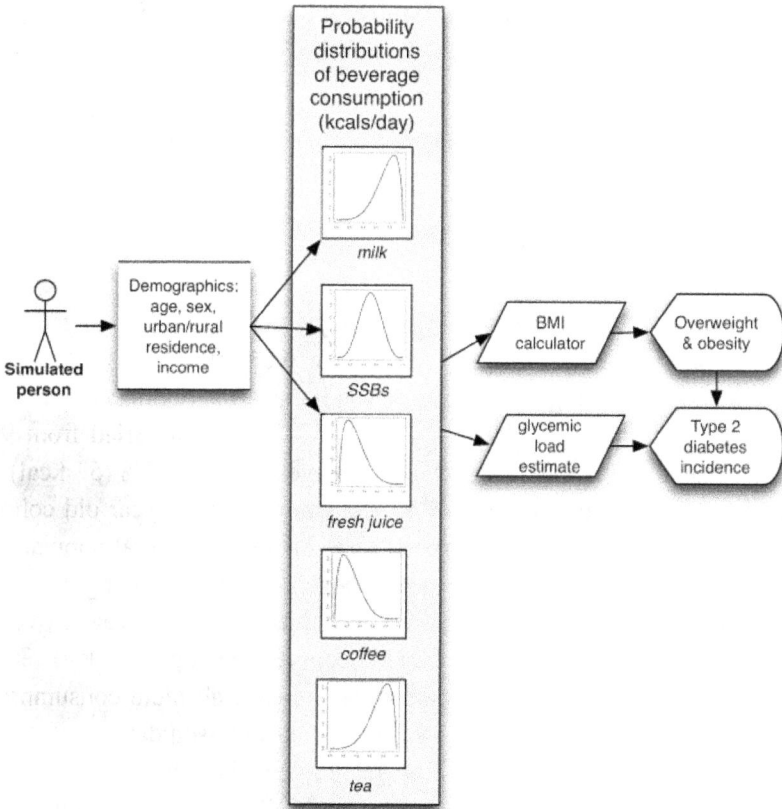

FIGURE 5: Model diagram.

15.2.4 ETHICS STATEMENT

Ethics committee approval for the IMS Study that was used to inform the model was obtained from the All India Institute of Medical Sciences Ethics Committee, reference number A-60/4/8/2004; for the overall modeling research, ethics committee approval was obtained from the Stanford University Institutional Review Board, reference number eP-28811.

15.3 RESULTS

15.3.1 SSB CONSUMPTION, OBESITY, AND TYPE 2 DIABETES RATES

We observed little variation in SSB consumption levels among demographic cohorts in India (Table 2). Among the 390 kcal/person/day typically consumed from beverages among surveyed Indians, approximately 12% (46 kcal/person/day) were conferred by SSBs. Consumption varied from 9% (37 kcal) among the older cohort of 45–65 year olds to 13% (52 kcal) of overall beverage consumption among the younger 25–44 year old cohort, and was roughly equal among urban (12%, 48 kcal) and rural populations (12%, 45 kcal). SSBs composed 14% of beverage calories among the poorest income tertile and 12% among the wealthiest tertile. However, overall beverage calories were lowest among the poor (310 kcal/person/day) versus the wealthiest tertile (404 kcal/person/day), hence absolute consumption varied insignificantly by wealth (44 versus 47 kcal/person/day).

Rates of obesity and type 2 diabetes universally increased across cohorts in our projections over the period 2014–2023. We observed that if linear secular trends in SSB consumption continued in the absence of a tax (Figure 1), Indian overweight and obesity prevalence (percent adults 24–65 with BMI$\geq$25 kg/m^2) would be expected to increase from 39% to 49% and type 2 diabetes incidence would be expected to rise in parallel from 319 to 336 per 100,000 per year over the period 2014–2023. Amplification of these trends to 50% overweight prevalence and 343 per 100,000 type 2 diabetes incidence by year 2023 were observed in the Bass diffusion scenario, in which SSB consumption followed the curvilinear rise of marketing model projections (Figure 1), which forecast consumption increasing from 12.8 l/person/year in 2014 to 36.3 l/person/year in 2023 (approximately one-fourth the 2012 rates in Latin American countries [9]; Figure 1).

15.3.2 ELASTICITIES

Much of the rise in SSB consumption would be expected to shift toward other beverage consumption in the context of an SSB tax. On the basis of microeconomic demand system estimates of expenditure data, SSB consumption was observed to decline by 0.94% for each 1% increase in SSB price (95% CI, a 0.90%–0.98% reduction). Substitution among beverages revealed a 0.049% (0.011%–0.087%) increase in milk consumption, 0.31% (0.27%–0.35%) increase in fresh fruit juice consumption, and a 0.13% (0.098%–0.16%) increase in tea consumption for each 1% rise in SSB price in the overall population, with small variations between groups (Table 1), but a non-significant degree of substitution with coffee (0.004%, −0.064% to 0.073%). Full elasticity estimate details are provided in Table 1.

15.3.3 TAX EFFECTS

Using the calculated elasticities to project the effects of a 20% excise tax on SSBs (Figures S2–S6), we estimated obesity and type 2 diabetes rate changes among demographic cohorts (Figures 6–8). Overweight and obesity prevalence declined by 1.6% to 5.9% and type 2 diabetes incidence by 1.2% to 1.9% from the baseline estimates among the Indian subpopulations under a 20% SSB tax (Figures 7 and 8; 3.0% overweight/obesity reduction and 1.6% type 2 diabetes reduction in the overall population). Different sensitivities to the tax among cohorts were driven primarily by differences in the distribution of BMI, such that groups with lower current median BMIs were more easily able to maintain members of the cohort below the threshold of 25 kg/m^2 (Table 2). In the setting of linear consumption increases in SSBs, younger (25–44 year olds), male, low-income, and rural populations were observed to experience the largest relative decline in kilocalorie consumption from beverages and associated declines in overweight and obesity prevalence (Figures 6–8). When differential glycemic load among beverages and different baseline incidence rates of type 2 diabetes were accounted for, urban rather than rural populations experienced the largest relative declines in type 2 diabetes incidence (Figure 8). As shown in Figures 6, 7, and 8, a large confidence interval was observed among females and low-income populations due to imprecision in current diabetes incidence estimates among these groups, resulting from less robust surveillance quality among these cohorts.

Converting the relative rate declines into absolute numbers of averted overweight, obesity, and type 2 diabetes cases—accounting for population size differences and demographic trends in population growth [55]—revealed large variations among population subgroups. The largest number of prevalent overweight and obesity cases averted from 2014–2023 would still be expected among the younger cohort (3.9 million people avoiding overweight in the 25–44 year group versus 1.1 million in the 45–65 year old group), as well as males (2.9 million versus 2.1 female), and rural populations (3.1 million versus 1.4 million urban), but also among the highest income tertile (1.7 million versus 1.4 million in the mid tertile and 1.1 million among the lowest tertile). In absolute numbers, the most type 2 diabetes cases averted from 2014–2023 were among the older cohort (573,000 among 45–65 year olds versus 477,000 in 25–44 year olds over 2014–2023), men (1.6 million versus 1.2 million women), the highest income tertile (603,000 versus 248,000 in lowest tertile), and rural populations (877,000 versus 741,000 urban). In total, 11.2 million overweight and obesity cases (−3.0%, 95% CI 7.5–15.0 million) and 400,000 type 2 diabetes cases (−1.6%, 95% CI 300,000–500,000) would be averted from 2014–2023 by a 20% SSB excise tax, according to our model.

15.3.4 SENSITIVITY ANALYSES

The preventive impact of the tax was amplified by 40% to 60% when we shifted our assumptions from a linear trend in SSB consumption to a Bass diffusion model of SSB consumption trends, but qualitative differences between population subgroups were unaltered (Figures 6–8). Should consumer trends in SSB consumption increase according to the Bass trajectory, the preventive efficacy of a 20% SSB tax would rise by 40% to 60% over the baseline forecast, reducing overweight and obesity prevalence by 2.5%–10.0% and averting 1.0%–2.8% of incident type 2 diabetes (a 4.2% reduction in overweight/obesity prevalence, or 15.8 million people, 95% CI 10.4–21.1 million, and 2.5% reduction in type 2 diabetes incidence in the overall population, or 600,000 people, 95% CI 400,000–800,000; Figures 7 and 8).

The sensitivity of overweight, obesity, and type 2 diabetes to tax rate variations was linear in the case of overweight and obesity rates, but nonlinear for type 2 diabetes incidence, such that reducing the tax from 20% to 10% reduced the projected impact of the tax on overweight and obesity by 50% and on type 2 diabetes incidence by 62%. Conversely, increasing the tax from 20% to 30% increased the projected impact of the tax on overweight and obesity by 50% and on type 2 diabetes incidence by 33%. The nonlinearity in diabetes rates arose from complex changes in glycemic load intake when accounting for substitutions between beverages; increasing the SSB tax, for example, produces diminishing returns as substituted goods contribute to total glycemic load consumption to varying degrees, conditional on their price and total per capita expenditures on beverages.

15.4 DISCUSSION

An excise tax on SSBs would be expected to mitigate increases in overweight, obesity, and type 2 diabetes cases in India under numerous alternative scenarios and assumptions, even after accounting for beverage substitution patterns. Under the conservative scenario of a linear rise in SSB consumption, a 20% SSB excise tax would be expected to prevent 11.2 million new cases of overweight and obesity (a 3.0% decline), and 400,000 cases of type 2 diabetes (a 1.6% decline) over the decade 2014–2023, according to a microsimulation model informed by nationally representative consumer expenditure, price, BMI, and type 2 diabetes incidence data. Under the case in which consumption follows business marketing models, which mirror recent SSB sales increases, a 20% SSB tax would be expected to avert 4.2% of prevalent overweight/obesity and 2.5% of incident type 2 diabetes from 2014–2023. As compared to other population-level obesity interventions (e.g., nutrition labels and consumer education) that have been studied to date, which typically result in <1% reductions in overweight and obesity and non-significant changes in diabetes rates [56]–[60], this implies a comparatively large population-level impact from SSB taxation. While a number of low- and middle-income countries are creating an array of large-scale interventions to address increased obesity and diabetes, to date none have sustained reductions in BMI [18].

The SSB tax appeared likely to significantly lower both BMI and type 2 diabetes incidence among all demographic cohorts, without perverse increases in BMI or type 2 diabetes due to substitution effects. However, the effect sizes of the tax varied notably among different demographic groups. Contrary to our a priori hypothesis, the largest relative declines in overweight and obesity prevalence were observed among young rural men, as this group with lower current BMI more easily maintained itself below the BMI threshold of 25 kg/m^2 in scenarios with SSB taxation than without such taxation. The BMI threshold of 25 kg/m^2 corresponds to a critical inflexion point of increasing type 2 diabetes risk among Indians [54].

These findings offer substantial contributions to the existing literature on non-communicable disease prevention in low- and middle-income countries. Our assessment is the first to our knowledge to study the impact of SSB taxation in India, which is expected to experience more deaths from non-communicable diseases than any other country in the world over the next decade, and is considered a policy leader among developing nations devising chronic disease interventions [61]. Unlike most assessments of large-scale interventions in developing countries, our study is based on disaggregated population-representative data specific to different income groups, urban/rural residence, both sexes, and both middle-aged and older adults, accounting for within-country heterogeneity in consumption behavior and disease risk. Prior policy models have been criticized for either projecting results from Western populations onto other countries, or aggregating large, heterogeneous developing country populations into a single population average, which can produce perverse outcomes when policies benefit one segment of the population while potentially risking poor outcomes among others [17],[62].

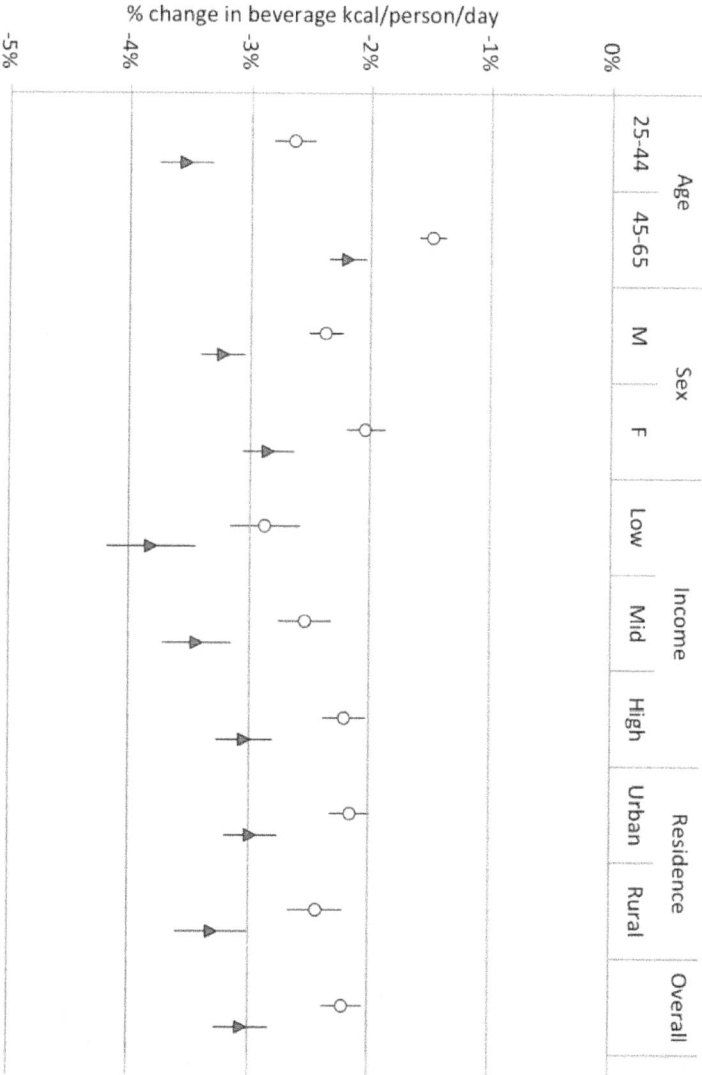

FIGURE 6: Projected changes in kilocalories per person per day consumed from all beverages. Open circles, linear model; triangles, Bass model of changes in SSB consumption over time.

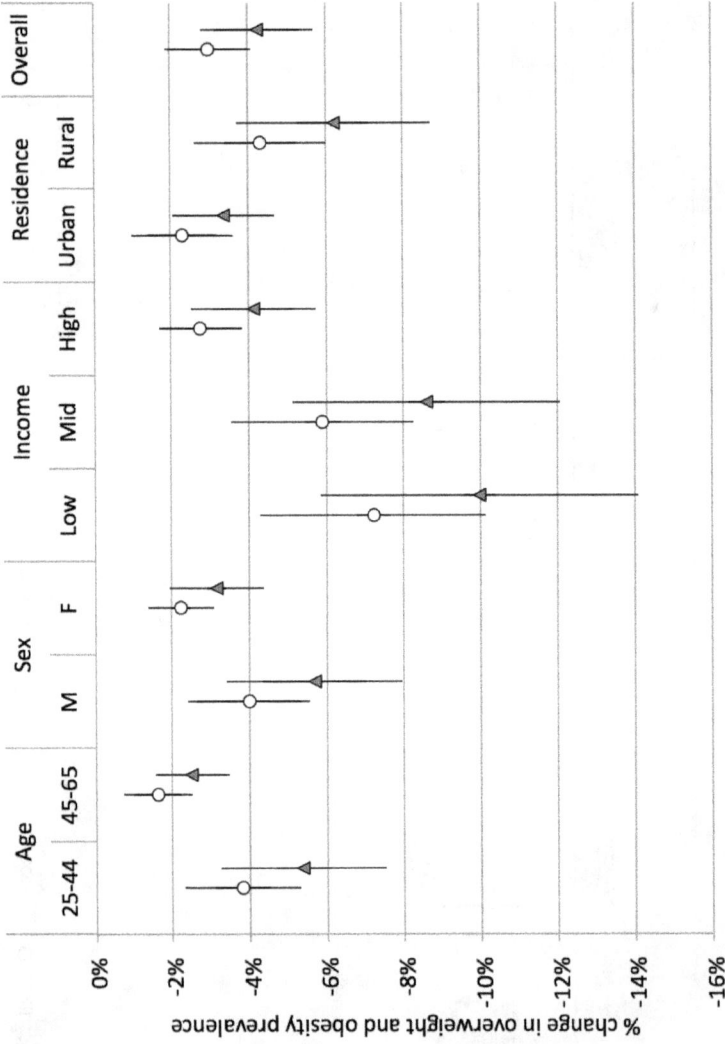

FIGURE 7: Change in overweight and obesity prevalence (relative change in percent of adults with body mass index >25 kg/m²). Open circles, linear model; triangles, Bass model of changes in SSB consumption over time.

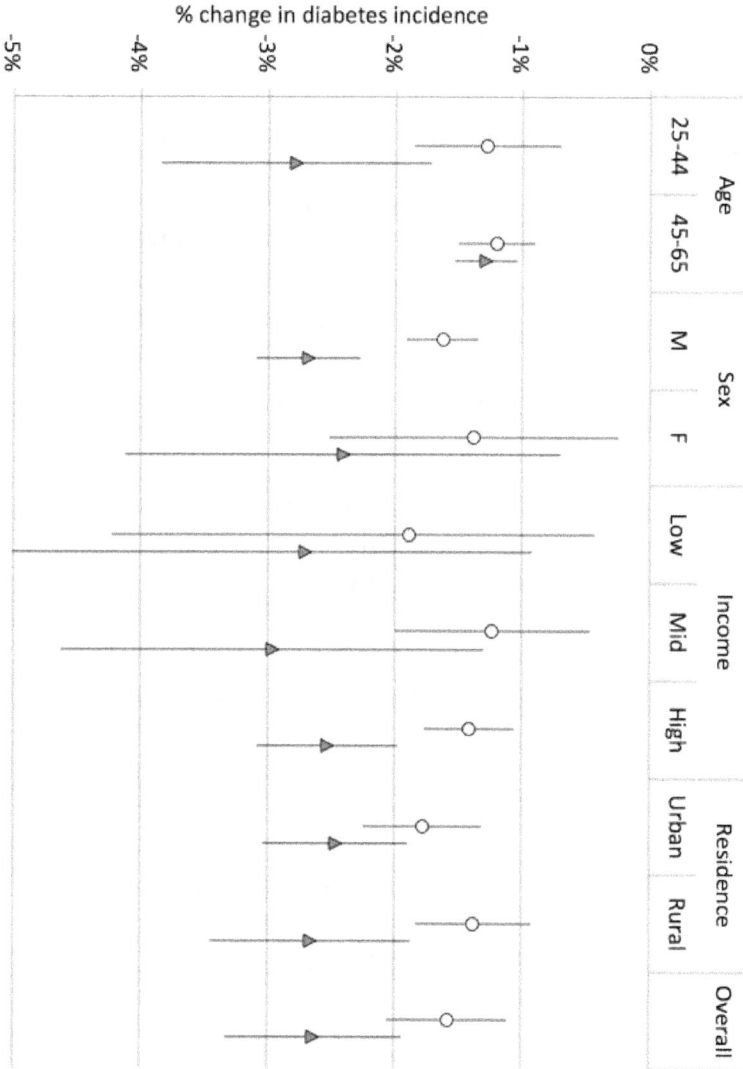

FIGURE 8: Change in type 2 diabetes incidence (per 100,000) under a 20% excise tax on SSBs. Open circles, linear model; triangles, Bass model of changes in SSB consumption over time.

Our results also incorporate the effects of substitution among beverage classes through a direct estimation method rather than assumptions alone, an advance over most models of fiscal policy that have been criticized for ignoring this issue or assuming arbitrary levels of substitution [63]. The research also lends insights into the fact that obesity and diabetes impacts of SSB taxes may not be entirely parallel, in light of the glycemic load effects of food intake on type 2 diabetes risk. This glycemic load factor incorporates the differential impact of each calorie of SSBs versus other beverages on diabetes risk, given that glycemic load per calorie of SSBs is about 5.3 times that of milk, for example (Table 3).

The impact of BMI on chronic disease among Indians is notably different than among other populations. A large literature suggests that Indians at BMIs ranging from 20–22 kg/m^2 have percent body fats equivalent to non-Hispanic white Americans or British adults with BMIs of 27–30 kg/m^2, and Indians have an increased risk type 2 diabetes at much lower BMI levels than these other populations [64]–[68]. Our estimates therefore relied directly on both adiposity-related and direct metabolic impact estimates of type 2 diabetes risk associated with glycemic load consumption changes. The estimates incorporate the glycemic load impact of fruit juices as substitutes for SSBs, given the literature suggesting that fruit juice consumption may have adverse metabolic effects consistent with glycemic load contributions, even if having lower calories than SSBs [69].

As with other projections of fiscal policy interventions, our assessment relies on mathematical modeling, which inherently requires several assumptions and limitations. First, we employ the assumption that consumer expenditure behavior from prior years, captured in price elasticities, will reflect future behavior among consumers. This abstraction makes it impossible to account for the potential increased willingness-to-pay for SSBs in the context of social trends in popularity and income increases. Second, our metabolic equations calculating weight change in the context of caloric change does not account for diet beverages (which are currently <0.1 l/person/year in India [9]) that have unclear relationships to metabolic syndrome [70]–[72], and assumes that physical activity will not change directly as a result of soda taxation, even though compensatory activity after substitution may also occur (e.g., individuals who change their diet may decide to exercise more or less based on perceptions of the healthfulness of their dietary change). Third, we abstract from dietary food frequency questionnaires that are validated against 24-hour dietary recalls and independent databases [20], but are still subject to recall bias and underreporting. Fourth, our model produced wide confidence intervals among the lowest-income tertile and women due to undersampling of rural low-income populations. Nevertheless, our purpose in employing this model was not to predict exact future rates of disease, which is impossible from any model, but to understand potential demographic differences in taxation impact and estimate the sensitivity of forecasts to varying assumptions about future SSB consumption. A consistent finding among all cohorts was that a rise in SSB consumption in accordance with recent trends would portend increasing overweight, obesity, and type 2 diabetes rates, but also render an excise tax on SSBs differentially more effective as a preventive population strategy. Finally, we did not account for safety concerns if SSB taxation shifts to increasing tap water usage in the context of some populations have unsafe water supplies in India; however, this is unlikely to produce a true epidemiological shift in disease burden as populations already exposed to non-potable water-based pathogens would likely to continue to be exposed, and unexposed populations are unlikely to be newly exposed because of an SSB tax given that nearly all populations drink some tap water in their locality. Similarly, we did not track the vitamin and mineral-related implications of SSB taxation as it implies differential consumption of fruit juices that may have other nutritional benefits but that also contribute to type 2 diabetes risks [69].

Another limitation of our analysis is that our treatment of the SSB taxation strategy is unable to quantify the attendant ethical, political, and social dilemmas presented by taxation strategies. Sufficient data are not available on changes in beverage intake behaviors among Indian children, or the long-term metabolic and cardiovascular consequences of SSB consumption changes among children aside from weight gain [73]. Hence, we focused on validated models of adult metabolism, since the cardiovascular and metabolic disease burden and health care cost would be expected to accrue most among adults over the near-term policy window that we simulated here. Excise taxation on foods can also be viewed as discriminatory, paternal, or regressive (in an economic sense). An alternate perspective is that preventing obesity and diabetes among lowest-income populations, who are among the most affected over time, will produce the greatest social benefit as low-income populations are also least likely to obtain diagnosis and treatment for chronic disease [5]. Another unresolved political issue is the administrative challenge of enforcing taxes on purchases in informal settings, given that SSBs are often sold by small vendors, with potential implications for household income, economic growth, and poverty given the employment impact of SSB sales. Excise taxes at the manufacturing level would allow bypassing of some enforcement obstacles, but remain politically opposed by beverage companies. Studies of existing SSB taxes in Western populations have highlighted that the taxes imposed have been generally too small to have meaningful effect size, while imposing larger taxes at equivalent levels to those simulated here may confer greater benefits [14],[15]. Future research should replicate the findings observed here in other rapidly developing middle-income countries where SSB consumption is increasing at a rapid rate [6].

For policy, our research indicates that SSB price increases are likely to generate substantial reductions in overweight, obesity, and type 2 diabetes through pathways affecting caloric intake and glycemic load. Fiscal strategies could mitigate obesity and type 2 diabetes in India over the next decade, even for more remote and low-income populations that are less likely to have transitioned to other components of Western diets in the near term.

REFERENCES

1. Malik VS, Schulze MB, Hu FB (2006) Intake of sugar-sweetened beverages and weight gain: a systematic review. Am J Clin Nutr 84: 274–288.
2. Malik VS, Popkin BM, Bray GA, Després J-P, Willett WC, et al. (2010) Sugar-sweetened beverages and risk of metabolic syndrome and type 2 diabetes: a meta-analysis. Diabetes Care 33: 2477–2483. doi: 10.2337/dc10-1079
3. Schulze MB, Manson JAE, Ludwig DS, Colditz GA, Stampfer MJ, et al. (2004) Sugar-sweetened beverages, weight gain, and incidence of type 2 diabetes in young and middle-aged women. JAMA 292: 927–934. doi: 10.1001/jama.292.8.927
4. The InterAct consortium (2013) Consumption of sweet beverages and type 2 diabetes incidence in European adults: results from EPIC-InterAct. Diabetologia 56: 1520–1530. doi: 10.1007/s00125-013-2899-8

5. Brownell KD, Farley T, Willett WC, Popkin BM, Chaloupka FJ, et al. (2009) The public health and economic benefits of taxing sugar-sweetened beverages. N Engl J Med 361: 1599–1605. doi: 10.1056/nejmhpr0905723

6. Basu S, McKee M, Galea G, Stuckler D (2013) Relationship of soft drink consumption to global overweight, obesity, and diabetes: a cross-national analysis of 75 countries. Am J Public Health: e1–e7.

7. Kleiman S, Ng SW, Popkin B (2012) Drinking to our health: can beverage companies cut calories while maintaining profits? Obes Rev Off J Int Assoc Study Obes 13: 258–274. doi: 10.1111/j.1467-789x.2011.00949.x

8. Barquera S, Hernandez-Barrera L, Tolentino ML, Espinosa J, Ng SW, et al. (2008) Energy intake from beverages is increasing among Mexican adolescents and adults. J Nutr 138: 2454–2461. doi: 10.3945/jn.108.092163

9. Euromonitor International (2013) Passport Global Market Information Database. New York: Euromonitor.

10. Basu S, Stuckler D, McKee M, Galea G (2012) Nutritional determinants of worldwide diabetes: an econometric study of food markets and diabetes prevalence in 173 countries. Public Health Nutr 1: 1–8. doi: 10.1017/s1368980012002881

11. Basu S, Yoffe P, Hills N, Lustig RH (2013) The relationship of sugar to population-level diabetes prevalence: an econometric analysis of repeated cross-sectional data. PLoS ONE 8: e57873 doi:10.1371/journal.pone.0057873.

12. Finkelstein EA, Zhen C, Nonnemaker J, Todd JE (2010) Impact of targeted beverage taxes on higher- and lower-income households. Arch Intern Med 170: 2028–2034. doi: 10.1001/archinternmed.2010.449

13. Powell LM, Chaloupka FJ (2009) Food prices and obesity: evidence and policy implications for taxes and subsidies. Milbank Q 87: 229–257. doi: 10.1111/j.1468-0009.2009.00554.x

14. Sturm R, Powell LM, Chriqui JF, Chaloupka FJ (2010) Soda taxes, soft drink consumption, and children's body mass index. Health Aff (Millwood) 29: 1052–1058. doi: 10.1377/hlthaff.2009.0061

15. Wang YC, Coxson P, Shen YM, Goldman L, Bibbins-Domingo K (2012) A Penny-per-ounce tax on sugar-sweetened beverages would cut health and cost burdens of diabetes. Health Aff (Millwood) 31: 199–207. doi: 10.1377/hlthaff.2011.0410

16. Briggs ADM, Mytton OT, Kehlbacher A, Tiffin R, Rayner M, et al. (2013) Overall and income specific effect on prevalence of overweight and obesity of 20% sugar sweetened drink tax in UK: econometric and comparative risk assessment modelling study. BMJ 347: f6189. doi: 10.1136/bmj.f6189

17. Ebrahim S, Pearce N, Smeeth L, Casas JP, Jaffar S, et al. (2013) Tackling non-communicable diseases in low- and middle-income countries: is the evidence from high-income countries all we need? PLoS Med 10: e1001377 doi:10.1371/journal. pmed.1001377.

18. Popkin BM, Adair LS, Ng SW (2012) Global nutrition transition and the pandemic of obesity in developing countries. Nutr Rev 70: 3–21. doi: 10.1111/j.1753-4887.2011.00456.x

19. Reardon T, Timmer CP, Minten B (2012) Supermarket revolution in Asia and emerging development strategies to include small farmers. Proc Natl Acad Sci U S A 109: 12332–12337. doi: 10.1073/pnas.1003160108

20. Bansal D, Satija A, Khandpur N, Bowen L, Kinra S, et al. (2010) Effects of migration on food consumption patterns in a sample of Indian factory workers and their families. Public Health Nutr 13: 1982–1989. doi: 10.1017/s1368980010001254

21. Subramanian S, Corsi DJ, Subramanyam MA, Davey Smith G (2013) Jumping the gun: the problematic discourse on socioeconomic status and cardiovascular health in India. Int J Epidemiol 42: 1410–1426. doi: 10.1093/ije/dyt017

22. Vellakkal S, Subramania SV, Millett C, Basu S, Stuckler D, et al. (n.d.) Socioeconomic inequalities in non-communicable diseases prevalence in India: disparities between self-reported diagnoses and standardized measures. PLoS ONE 8: e68219 doi:10.1371/journal.pone.0068219.

23. Deepa M, Anjana RM, Manjula D, Narayan KMV, Mohan V (2011) Convergence of prevalence rates of diabetes and cardiometabolic risk factors in middle and low income groups in urban India: 10-year follow-up of the Chennai Urban Population Study. J Diabetes Sci Technol 5: 918–927. doi: 10.1177/193229681100500415

24. Fletcher JM, Frisvold DE, Tefft N (2010) The effects of soft drink taxes on child and adolescent consumption and weight outcomes. J Public Econ 94: 967–974. doi: 10.1016/j.jpubeco.2010.09.005

25. Ministry of Statistics and Programme Implementation (2012) National Sample Survey. Delhi: Government of India.

26. World Health Organization (2012) WHO Global InfoBase.Geneva: WHO.

27. Cohen J (1988) Statistical power analysis for the behavioral sciences. New York: Routledge Academic.

28. US Department of Agriculture (2013) National Nutrient Database for Standard Reference. Release 25. Washington (D.C.): National Agricultural Library.

29. Gopalan C, Sastri BVR, Balasubramanian SC (1971) Nutritive value of Indian foods. Hyderabad: Hyderabad Natl Inst Nutr.

30. OECD (2013) Main Economic Indicators - complete database. Paris: Organisation for Economic Co-operation and Development. Available: http://www.oecd-ilibrary.org/content/data/data-00052-en. Accessed 9 June 2013.

31. Ebrahim S, Kinra S, Bowen L, Andersen E, Ben-Shlomo Y, et al. (2010) The effect of rural-to-urban migration on obesity and diabetes in India: a cross-sectional study. PLoS Med 7: e1000268 doi:10.1371/journal.pmed.1000268.

32. Banks J, Blundell R, Lewbel A (1997) Quadratic Engel curves and consumer demand. Rev Econ Stat 79: 527–539. doi: 10.1162/003465397557015

33. Shonkwiler JS, Yen ST (1999) Two-step estimation of a censored system of equations. Am J Agric Econ 81: 972–982. doi: 10.2307/1244339

34. Haines PS, Guilkey DK, Popkin BM (1988) Modeling Food Consumption Decisions as a Two-Step Process. Am J Agric Econ 70: 543–552. doi: 10.2307/1241492

35. Pollak RA, Wales TJ (1978) Estimation of complete demand systems from household budget data: the linear and quadratic expenditure systems. Am Econ Rev 68: 348–359.

36. Andreyeva T, Long MW, Brownell KD (2010) The impact of food prices on consumption: a systematic review of research on the price elasticity of demand for food. Am J Public Health 100: 216–222. doi: 10.2105/ajph.2008.151415

37. Dharmasena S, Capps O (2012) Intended and unintended consequences of a proposed national tax on sugar-sweetened beverages to combat the US obesity problem. Health Econ 21: 669–694. doi: 10.1002/hec.1738

38. International Institute for Population Sciences (IIPS) (2007) National Family Health Survey (NFHS-3). Mumbai: IIPS.

39. World Bank (2012) World Development Indicators. Washington (D.C.): IBRD.

40. Caro JJ, Briggs AH, Siebert U, Kuntz KM (2012) Modeling Good Research Practices—Overview A Report of the ISPOR-SMDM Modeling Good Research Practices Task Force–1. Med Decis Making 32: 667–677. doi: 10.1177/0272989x12454577

41. Sadikot SM, Nigam A, Das S, Bajaj S, Zargar AH, et al. (2004) The burden of diabetes and impaired glucose tolerance in India using the WHO 1999 criteria: prevalence of diabetes in India study (PODIS). Diabetes Res Clin Pract 66: 301–307. doi: 10.1016/j.diabres.2004.04.008

42. Danaei G, Finucane MM, Lu Y, Singh GM, Cowan MJ, et al. (2011) National, regional, and global trends in fasting plasma glucose and diabetes prevalence since 1980: systematic analysis of health examination surveys and epidemiological studies with 370 country-years and 2.7 million participants. Lancet 378: 31–40. doi: 10.1016/s0140-6736(11)60679-x

43. Bass FM (2004) Comments on "A New Product Growth for Model Consumer Durables The Bass Model.". Manag Sci 50: 1833–1840. doi: 10.1287/mnsc.1040.0300

44. Food and Agricultural Organization (2013) FAOSTAT database. Rome: United Nations.

45. Atkinson FS, Foster-Powell K, Brand-Miller JC (2008) International Tables of Glycemic Index and Glycemic Load Values: 2008. Diabetes Care 31: 2281–2283. doi: 10.2337/dc08-1239

46. Hall KD, Sacks G, Chandramohan D, Chow CC, Wang YC, et al. (2011) Quantification of the effect of energy imbalance on bodyweight. Lancet 378: 826–837. doi: 10.1016/s0140-6736(11)60812-x

47. Hall KD, Jordan PN (2008) Modeling weight-loss maintenance to help prevent body weight regain. Am J Clin Nutr 88: 1495–1503. doi: 10.3945/ajcn.2008.26333

48. Lim SS, Gaziano TA, Gakidou E, Reddy KS, Farzadfar F, et al. (2007) Prevention of cardiovascular disease in high-risk individuals in low-income and middle-income countries: health effects and costs. Lancet 370: 2054–2062. doi: 10.1016/s0140-6736(07)61699-7

49. CDC (n.d.) CDC's Diabetes Program - Data & Trends - Duration of Diabetes - Distribution of Diabetes Duration Among Adults Aged 18–79 Years, United States, 1997–2009. Available: http://www.cdc.gov/diabetes/statistics/duration/fig2.htm. Accessed 19 December 2012.

50. Livesey G, Taylor R, Livesey H, Liu S (2013) Is there a dose-response relation of dietary glycemic load to risk of type 2 diabetes? Meta-analysis of prospective cohort studies. Am J Clin Nutr 97: 584–596. doi: 10.3945/ajcn.112.041467

51. Bremer AA, Mietus-Snyder M, Lustig RH (2012) Toward a unifying hypothesis of metabolic syndrome. Pediatrics 129: 557–570. doi: 10.1542/peds.2011-2912

52. Teff KL, Grudziak J, Townsend RR, Dunn TN, Grant RW, et al. (2009) Endocrine and metabolic effects of consuming fructose- and glucose-sweetened beverages with

meals in obese men and women: influence of insulin resistance on plasma triglyceride responses. J Clin Endocrinol Metab 94: 1562–1569. doi: 10.1210/jc.2008-2192

53. Indian Consensus Group (1996) Indian consensus for prevention of hypertension and coronary heart disease. A joint scientific statement of Indian Society of Hypertension and International College of Nutrition. J Nutr Env Med 6: 309–318. doi: 10.3109/13590849609007257

54. Chiu M, Austin PC, Manuel DG, Shah BR, Tu JV (2011) Deriving ethnic-specific BMI cutoff points for assessing diabetes risk. Diabetes Care 34: 1741–1748. doi: 10.2337/dc10-2300

55. Registrar General & Census Commissioner (2011) Census of India. Delhi: Ministry of Home Affairs.

56. Tuah NA, Amiel C, Qureshi S, Car J, Kaur B, et al. (2011) Transtheoretical model for dietary and physical exercise modification in weight loss management for overweight and obese adults. Cochrane Database Syst Rev 10: CD008066. doi: 10.1002/14651858.cd008066.pub2

57. Shaw K, O'Rourke P, Del Mar C, Kenardy J (2005) Psychological interventions for overweight or obesity. Cochrane Database Syst Rev 2: CD003818. doi: 10.1002/14651858.cd003818.pub2

58. Waters E, de Silva Sanigorski A, Hall BJ, Brown T, Campbell KJ, et al. (2012) Interventions for preventing obesity in children (review). Cochrane Collab 1–212. doi: 10.1002/14651858.cd001871.pub3

59. Thomas DE, Elliott EJ, Baur L (2007) Low glycaemic index or low glycaemic load diets for overweight and obesity. Cochrane Database Syst Rev Online CD005105. doi: 10.1002/14651858.cd005105.pub2

60. Prevention I of M (US) C on AP in O, Glickman D (2012) Accelerating Progress in Obesity Prevention: Solving the Weight of the Nation. Washington (D.C.): National Academies Press.

61. World Health Organization (2011) United Nations high-level meeting on noncommunicable disease prevention and control. Geneva: WHO.

62. Basu S, Babiarz KS, Ebrahim S, Vellakkal S, Stuckler D, et al. (2013) Palm oil taxes and cardiovascular disease mortality in India: economic-epidemiologic model. BMJ 347: f6048. doi: 10.1136/bmj.f6048

63. Eyles H, Mhurchu CN, Nghiem N, Blakely T (2012) Food pricing strategies, population diets, and non-communicable disease: a systematic review of simulation studies. PLoS Med 9: e1001353 doi:10.1371/journal.pmed.1001353.

64. Misra A, Khurana L (2009) The metabolic syndrome in South Asians: epidemiology, determinants, and prevention. Metab Syndr Relat Disord 7: 497–514. doi: 10.1089/met.2009.0024

65. Misra A, Vikram NK (2004) Insulin resistance syndrome (metabolic syndrome) and obesity in Asian Indians: evidence and implications. Nutr Burbank Los Angeles Cty Calif 20: 482–491. doi: 10.1016/j.nut.2004.01.020

66. Bhat DS, Yajnik CS, Sayyad MG, Raut KN, Lubree HG, et al. (2005) Body fat measurement in Indian men: comparison of three methods based on a two-compartment model. Int J Obes 2005 29: 842–848. doi: 10.1038/sj.ijo.0802953

67. Deurenberg-Yap M, Schmidt G, van Staveren WA, Deurenberg P (2000) The paradox of low body mass index and high body fat percentage among Chinese, Malays

and Indians in Singapore. Int J Obes Relat Metab Disord J Int Assoc Study Obes 24: 1011–1017. doi: 10.1038/sj.ijo.0801353

68. Kesavachandran CN, Bihari V, Mathur N (2012) The normal range of body mass index with high body fat percentage among male residents of Lucknow city in north India. Indian J Med Res 135: 72–77. doi: 10.4103/0971-5916.93427

69. Bazzano LA, Li TY, Joshipura KJ, Hu FB (2008) Intake of fruit, vegetables, and fruit juices and risk of diabetes in women. Diabetes Care 31: 1311–1317. doi: 10.2337/dc08-0080

70. De Koning L, Malik VS, Kellogg MD, Rimm EB, Willett WC, et al.. (2012) Sweetened beverage consumption, incident coronary heart disease, and biomarkers of risk in men. Circulation 125: 1735–1741, S1.

71. De Koning L, Malik VS, Rimm EB, Willett WC, Hu FB (2011) Sugar-sweetened and artificially sweetened beverage consumption and risk of type 2 diabetes in men. Am J Clin Nutr 93: 1321–1327. doi: 10.3945/ajcn.110.007922

72. Duffey KJ, Steffen LM, Van Horn L, Jacobs DR Jr, Popkin BM (2012) Dietary patterns matter: diet beverages and cardiometabolic risks in the longitudinal Coronary Artery Risk Development in Young Adults (CARDIA) Study. Am J Clin Nutr 95: 909–915. doi: 10.3945/ajcn.111.026682

73. De Ruyter JC, Olthof MR, Seidell JC, Katan MB (2012) A trial of sugar-free or sugar-sweetened beverages and body weight in children. N Engl J Med 367: 1397–1406. doi: 10.1056/nejmoa1203034

There are several supplemental files that are not available in this version of the article. To view this additional information, please use the citation on the first page of this chapter.

CHAPTER 16

BIG FOOD, FOOD SYSTEMS, AND GLOBAL HEALTH

DAVID STUCKLER AND MARION NESTLE

This article was commissioned for the PLoS Medicine series on Big Food that examines the activities and influence of the food and beverage industry in the health arena.

Let's begin this essay with a blunt conclusion: Global food systems are not meeting the world's dietary needs [1]. About one billion people are hungry, while two billion people are overweight [2]. India, for example, is experiencing rises in both: since 1995 an additional 65 million people are malnourished, and one in five adults is now overweight [3],[4]. This coexistence of food insecurity and obesity may seem like a paradox [5], but over- and undernutrition reflect two facets of malnutrition [6]. Underlying both is a common factor: food systems are not driven to deliver optimal human diets but to maximize profits. For people living in poverty, this means either exclusion from development (and consequent food insecurity) or eating low-cost, highly processed foods lacking in nutrition and rich in sugar, salt, and saturated fats (and consequent overweight and obesity).

Big Food, Food Systems, and Global Health. © *Stuckler D and Nestle M.* PLoS Medicine *9,6 (2012), doi:10.1371/journal.pmed.1001242. Licensed under Creative Commons Attribution License.*

To understand who is responsible for these nutritional failures, it is first necessary to ask: Who rules global food systems? By and large it's "Big Food," by which we refer to multinational food and beverage companies with huge and concentrated market power [7],[8]. In the United States, the ten largest food companies control over half of all food sales [9] and worldwide this proportion is about 15% and rising. More than half of global soft drinks are produced by large multinational companies, mainly Coca-Cola and PepsiCo [10]. Three-fourths of world food sales involve processed foods, for which the largest manufacturers hold over a third of the global market [11]. The world's food system is not a competitive marketplace of small producers but an oligopoly. What people eat is increasingly driven by a few multinational food companies [12].

Virtually all growth in Big Food's sales occurs in developing countries [13] (see Figure 1). The saturation of markets in developed countries [14], along with the lure of the 20% of income people spend on average on food globally, has stimulated Big Food to seek global expansion. Its rapid entry into markets in low- and middle-income countries (LMICs) is a result of mass-marketing campaigns and foreign investment, principally through takeovers of domestic food companies [15]. Trade plays a minimal role and accounts for only about 6% of global processed food sales [15]. Global producers are the main reason why the "nutrition transition" from traditional, simple diets to highly processed foods is accelerating [16],[17].

Big Food is a driving force behind the global rise in consumption of sugar-sweetened beverages (SSBs) and processed foods enriched in salt, sugar, and fat [13]. Increasing consumption of Big Food's products tracks closely with rising levels of obesity and diabetes [18]. Evidence shows that SSBs are major contributors to childhood obesity [19],[20], as well as to long-term weight-gain, type 2 diabetes, and cardiovascular disease [21],[22]. Studies also link frequent consumption of highly processed foods with weight gain and associated diseases [23].

Of course, Big Food may also bring benefits—improved economic performance through increased technology and know-how and reduced risks of undernutrition—to local partners [24]. The extent of these benefits is debatable, however, in view of negative effects on farmers and on domestic producers and food prices [25].

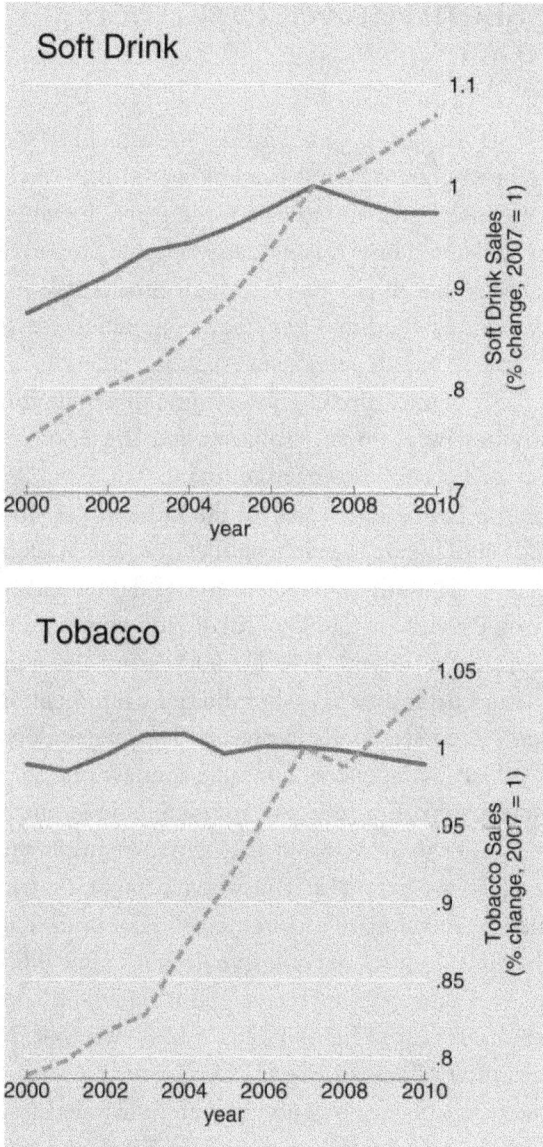

FIGURE 1: Growth of Big Food and Big Tobacco sales in developing countries: An example. Solid line is developed countries, dashed grey line is developing countries. Source: Passport Global Market Information Database: EuroMonitor International, 2011 [12].

16.1 PUBLIC HEALTH RESPONSE TO BIG FOOD: A FAILURE TO ACT

Public health professionals have been slow to respond to such nutritional threats in developed countries and even slower still in developing countries. Thanks to insights from tobacco company documents, we have learned a great deal about how this industry sought to avoid or flout public health interventions that might threaten their profits. We now have considerable evidence that food and beverage companies use similar tactics to undermine public health responses such as taxation and regulation [26],[27],[28],[29], an unsurprising observation given the flows of people, funds, and activities between Big Tobacco and Big Food. Yet the public health response to Big Food has been minimal.

We can think of multiple reasons for the failure to act [30]. One is the belated recognition of the importance of obesity to the burden of disease in LMICs [13]. The 2011 Political Declaration of the United Nations High-Level Meeting on Prevention and Control of Non-communicable Diseases (NCDs) recognized the urgent case for addressing the major avoidable causes of death and disability [31], but did not even mention the roles of agribusiness and processed foods in obesity. Despite evidence to the contrary, some development agencies continue to view obesity as a "disease of affluence" and a sign of progress in combating undernutrition [32].

A more uncomfortable reason is that action requires tackling vested interests, especially the powerful Big Food companies with strong ties to and influence over national governments. This is difficult terrain for many public health scientists. It took five decades after the initial studies linking tobacco and cancer for effective public health policies to be put in place, with enormous cost to human health. Must we wait five decades to respond to the similar effects of Big Food?

If we are going to get serious about such nutritional issues, we must make choices about how to engage with Big Food. Whether, and under what circumstances, we should view food companies as "partners" or as part of the solution to rising rates of obesity and associated chronic diseases is a matter of much current debate, as indicated by the diverse views of officials of PepsiCo and nutrition scientists [24],[27],[28],[33],[34].

16.2 ENGAGING WITH BIG FOOD—THREE VIEWS

We see three possible ways to view this debate. The first favors voluntary self-regulation, and requires no further engagement by the public health community. Those who share this view argue that market forces will self-correct the negative externalities resulting from higher intake of risky commodities. Informed individuals, they say, will choose whether to eat unhealthy foods and need not be subjected to public health paternalism. On this basis, UN secretary-general Ban Ki Moon urged industry to be more responsible: "I especially call on corporations that profit from selling processed foods to children to act with the utmost integrity. I refer not only to food manufacturers, but also the media, marketing and advertising companies that play central roles in these enterprises" [35]. Similarly, the UK Health Minister recently said: "the food and drinks industry should be seen, not just as part of the problem, but part of the solution...An emphasis on prevention, physical activity and personal and corporate responsibility could, alongside unified Government action, make a big difference" [36].

The second view favors partnerships with industry. Public health advocates who hold this view may take jobs with industry in order to make positive changes from within, or actively seek partnerships and alliances with food companies. Food, they say, is not tobacco. Whereas tobacco is demonstrably harmful in all forms and levels of consumption, food is not. We can live without tobacco, but we all must eat. Therefore, this view holds that we must work with Big Food to make healthier products and market them more responsibly.

The third approach is critical of both. It recognizes the inherent conflicts of interest between corporations that profit from unhealthy food and public health collaborations. Because growth in profit is the primary goal of corporations, self-regulation and working from within are doomed to fail. Most proponents of this viewpoint support public regulation as the only meaningful approach, although some propose having public health expert committees set standards and monitor industry performance in improving the nutritional quality of food products and in marketing the products to children.

We support the critical view, for several reasons. First, we find no evidence for an alignment of public health interest in curbing obesity with that of the food and beverage industry. Any partnership must create profit for the industry, which has a legal mandate to maximize wealth for shareholders. We also see no obvious, established, or legitimate mechanism through which public health professionals might increase Big Food's profits.

Big Food attains profit by expanding markets to reach more people, increasing people's sense of hunger so that they buy more food, and increasing profit margins through encouraging consumption of products with higher price/cost surpluses [28]–[31],[37]. Industry achieves these goals through food processing and marketing, and we are aware of no evidence for health gains through partnerships in either domain. Although in theory minimal processing of foods can improve nutritional content, in practice most processing is done so to increase palatability, shelf-life, and transportability, processes that reduce nutritional quality. Processed foods are not necessary for survival, and few individuals are sufficiently well-informed or even capable of overcoming marketing and cost hurdles [38]. Big Food companies have the resources to recruit leading nutritional scientists and experts to guide product development and reformulation, leaving the role of public health advisors uncertain.

To promote health, industry would need to make and market healthier foods so as to shift consumption away from highly processed, unhealthy foods. Yet, such healthier foods are inherently less profitable. The only ways the industry could preserve profit is either to undermine public health attempts to tax and regulate or to get people to eat more healthy food while continuing to eat profitable unhealthy foods [33],[39]. Neither is desirable from a nutritional standpoint. Whereas industry support for research might be seen as one place to align interests, studies funded by industry are 4- to 8-fold more likely to support conclusions favorable to the industry [40].

Our second reason to support the critical view has to do with the "precautionary principle" [41]. Because it is unclear whether inherent conflicts of interest can be reconciled, we favor proceeding on the basis of evidence. As George Orwell put it, "saints should always be judged guilty until they are proved innocent." We believe the onus of proof is on the food industry. If food companies can rigorously and independently establish self-regulation or private–public partnerships as improving both health and profit, these methods should be extended and replicated. But to date self-regulation has largely failed to meet stated objectives [42],[43],[44],[45],[46],[47], and instead has resulted in significant pressure for public regulation. Kraft's decision to ban trans fats, for example, occurred under pressure of lawsuits [48]. If industry believed that self-regulation would increase profit, it would already be regulating itself.

We believe the critical view has much to offer. It is a model of dynamic and dialectic engagement. It will increase pressures on industry to improve health performance, and it will encourage those who are sympathetic to the first or second views to effect change from within large food and beverage companies.

Public health professionals must recognize that Big Food's influence on global food systems is a problem, and do what is needed to reach a consensus about how to engage critically. The Conflicts of Interest Coalition, which emerged from concerns about Big Food's influence on the U.N. High-Level Meeting on NCDs, is a good place to start [29],[49]. Public health professionals must place as high a priority on nutrition as they do on HIV, infectious diseases, and other disease threats. They should support initiatives such as restrictions on marketing to children, better nutrition standards for school meals, and taxes on SSBs. The central aim of public health must be to bring into alignment Big Food's profit motives with public health goals. Without taking direct and concerted action to expose and regulate the vested interests of Big Food, epidemics of poverty, hunger, and obesity are likely to become more acute.

REFERENCES

1. De Schutter O (2011) Report submitted by the Special Rapporteur on the right to food. Geneva: United Nations. Available: http://www2.ohchr.org/english/issues/foo d/docs/A-HRC-16-49.pdf.

2. Patel R (2008) Stuffed and starved: The hidden battle for the world food system: Melville House. 448 p.

3. Doak C, Adair LS, Bentley M (2005) The dual burden household and nutrition transition paradox. Int J Obesity 29: 129–136.

4. Stein AD, Thompson AM, Waters A (2005) Childhood growth and chronic disease: evidence from countries undergoing the nutrition transition. Matern Child Nutr 1: 177–184. Available: http://www.ncbi.nlm.nih.gov/entrez/query.fcgi?cmd=Retrieve &db=PubMed&dopt=Citation&list_uids=16881898.

5. Caballero B (2005) A nutrition paradox – underweight and obesity in developing countries. N Engl J Med 352: 1514–1516.

6. Eckholm E, Record F (1976) The two faces of malnutrition. Worldwatch. Available: http://www.worldwatch.org/bookstore/publication/worldwatch-paper-9-two-faces-malnutrition.

7. Pollan M (2003) The (agri)cultural contradictions of obesity. New York Times. Available: http://www.nytimes.com/2003/10/12/magazine/12WWLN.html.

8. Brownell K, Warner KE (2009) The perils of ignoring history: Big Tobacco played dirty and millions died. How similar is Big Food? Milbank Quarterly 87: 259–294.

9. Lyson T, Raymer AL (2000) Stalking the wily multinational: power and control in the US food system. Agric Human Values 17: 199–208.

10. Alexander E, Yach D, Mensah GA (2011) Major multinational food and beverage companies and informal sector contributions to global food consumption: Implications for nutrition policy. Global Health 7: 26.

11. Alfranca O, Rama R, Tunzelmann N (2003) Technological fields and concentration of innovation among food and beverage multinationals. International Food and Agribusiness Management Review 5.

12. EuroMonitor International (2011) Passport Global Market Information Database: EuroMonitor International.

13. Stuckler D, McKee M, Ebrahim S, Basu S (2012) Manufacturing Epidemics: The Role of Global Producers in Increased Consumption of Unhealthy Commodities Including Processed Foods, Alcohol, and Tobacco. PLoS Med. 6. doi:10.1371/journal.pmed.1001235.

14. Hawkes C (2002) Marketing activities of global soft drink and fast food companies in emerging markets: A review. Geneva: World Health Organization. Available: http://www.who.int/hpr/NPH/docs/globalization.diet.and.ncds.pdf.

15. Regmi A, Gehlhar M (2005) Processed food trade pressured by evolving global supply chains. Amberwaves: US Department of Agriculture. Available: http://www.ers.usda.gov/amberwaves/february05/features/processedfood.htm.

16. Popkin B (2002) Part II: What is unique about the experience in lower- and middle-income less-industrialised countries compared with the very-high income countries? The shift in the stages of the nutrition transition differ from past experiences! Public Health Nutr. 5. : 205–214. doi:10.1079/PHN2001295.

17. Hawkes C (2005) The role of foreign direct investment in the nutrition transition. Public Health Nutri 8: 357–365.

18. Basu S, Stuckler, D McKee M, Galea G (2012) Nutritional drivers of worldwide diabetes: An econometric study of food markets and diabetes prevalence in 173 countries. Public Health Nutrition. In press.

19. Maliv V, Schulze MB, Hu FB (2006) Intake of sugar-sweetened beverages and weight gain: A systematic review. Am J Clin Nutr 84: 274–288.

20. Moreno L, Rodriguez G (2007) Dietary risk factors for development of childhood obesity. Curr Opin Clin Nutr Metab Care 10: 336–341.

21. Hu F, Malik VS (2010) Sugar-sweetened beverages and risk of obesity and type 2 diabetes. Physiol Behav 100: 47–54.

22. Malik V, Popkin BM, Bray GA, Despres JP, Hu F (2010) Sugar-sweetened beverages, obesity, type 2 diabetes mellitus, and cardiovascular disease risk. Circulation 121: 1356–1364.

23. Pereira M, Kartashov AI, Ebbeling CB, Van Horn L, Slattery ML, et al. (2005) Fast food habits, weight gain and insulin resistance in a 15-year prospective analysis of the CARDIA study. Lancet 365: 36–42.

24. Yach D, Feldman ZA, Bradley DG, Khan M (2010) Can the food industry help tackle the growing burden of undernutrition? Am J Public Health 100: 974–980.

25. Evenett S, Jenny F (2011) Trade, competition, and the pricing of commodities. Washington D.C.: Center for Economic Policy Research. Available: http://www.voxeu.org/reports/CEPR-CUTS_report.pdf.

26. Chopra M, Darnton-Hill I (2004) Tobacco and obesity epidemics: Not so different after all? BMJ 328: 1558–1560.

27. Ludwig D, Nestle M (2008) Can the food industry play a constructive role in the obesity epidemic? JAMA 300: 1808–1811.

28. Wiist W (2011) The corporate playbook, health, and democracy: The snack food and beverage industry's tactics in context. In: Stuckler D, Siegel , K , editors. Oxford: Oxford University Press.

29. Stuckler D, Basu S, McKee M (2011) UN high level meeting on non-communicable diseases: An opportunity for whom? BMJ. 343. d5336 p. doi:10.1136/bmj.d5336.

30. Stuckler D (2008) Population causes and consequences of leading chronic diseases: A comparative analysis of prevailing explanations. Milbank Quarterly 86: 273–326.

31. UN General Assembly (2011) Political declaration of the High-level Meeting of the General Assembly on the Prevention and Control of Non-communicable Diseases (NCDs). New York: UN. Available: http://www.un.org/en/ga/ncdmeeting2011/.

32. Mitchell A (2011) Letter to National Heart Forum about 'Priority actions for the NCD crisis'. In: Lincoln P, editor. London: UK DFID.

33. Monteiro C, Gomes FS, Cannon G (2009) The snack attack. Am J Public Health 100: 975–981.

34. Acharya T, Fuller AC, Mensah GA, Yahc D (2011) The current and future role of the food industry in the prevention and control of chronic diseases: The case of PepsiCo. In: Stuckler D, Siegel , K , editors. Oxford: Oxford University Press.

35. Ki-Moon B (2011) Remarks to the General Assembly meeting on the prevention and control of non-communicable disease. Geneva: UN. Available: http://www.un.org/apps/news/infocus/sgspeeches/statments_full.asp?statID=1299.

36. Lansley A (2011) 4th plenary meeting. Geneva: UN. Available: http://www.ncdalliance.org/sites/default/files/rfiles/Monday%20Sep%2019%203pm.pdf.

37. Koplan J, Brownell KD (2010) Response of the food and beverage industry to the obesity threat. JAMA 304: 1487–1488.

38. Wansink B (2007) Mindless eating: Why we eat more than we think. Bantam Books.

39. Wilde P (2009) Self-regulation and the response to concerns about food and beverage marketing to children in the United States. Nutr Rev 67: 155–166.

40. Lesser L, Ebbeling CB, Goozner M, Wypij D, Ludwig DS (2008) Relationship between funding source and conclusion among nutrition-related scientific articles. PLoS Med. 4. e5 p. doi:10.1371/journal.pmed.0040005.

41. Raffensperger C, Tickner J (1999) Protecting public health and the environment: implementing the precautionary principle. Washington D.C.: Island Press.

42. Lewin A, Lindstrom L, Nestle M (2006) Food industry promises to address childhood obesity: Preliminary evaluation. J Public Health Policy 27: 327–348.

43. Lang T (2006) The food industry, diet, physical activity and health: A review of reported commitments and prctice of 25 of the world's largest food companies. London: Oxford Health Alliance.

44. Sharma L, Teret SP, Brownell KD (2010) The food industry and self-regulation: Standards to promote success and to avoid public health failures. Am J Public Health 100: 240–246.

45. Bonell C, McKee M, Fletcher A, Haines A, Wilkinson P (2011) The nudge smudge: misrepresentation of the "nudge" concept in England's public health White Paper. Lancet 377: 2158–2159.

46. Campbell D (2012) High street outlets ignoring guidelines on providing calorie information. The Guardian. London. Available: http://www.guardian.co.uk/business/2012/mar/15/high-street-guidelines-calorie-information.

47. Hawkes C, Harris JL (2011) An analysis of the content of food industry pledges and marketing to children. Public Health Nutr 14: 1403–1414.

48. Zernike K (2004) Lawyers shift focus from Big Tobacco to Big Food. New York Times. New York. Available: http://www.nytimes.com/2004/04/09/us/lawyers-shift-focus-from-big-tobacco-to-big-food.html.

49. Conflicts of Interest Coalition (2011) Statement of Concern.

AUTHOR NOTES

CHAPTER 1

Conflict of Interests
The authors state that there is no conflict of interests.

Author Contributions
Maria del Mar Bibiloni and Josep A. Tur contributed to the design of the strategy for the literature search and double screened and selected the retrieved documents. Antoni Pons provided previous literature searches and analysis. Maria del Mar Bibiloni and Josep A. Tur prepared the main outline of the paper and all authors contributed to the preparation of the paper.

Acknowledgments
The authors would like to thank the Spanish Ministry of Health and Consumption Affairs (Programme of Promotion of Biomedical Research and Health Sciences, Projects 05/1276 and 08/1259, and Red Predimed-RETIC RD06/0045/1004 and CIBERobn CB12/03/30038), Grant of support to research groups no. 35/2011 (Balearic Islands Government and EU FEDER funds), Spanish Ministry of Education and Science (FPU Programme, PhD fellowship to M.M.B.). The Research Group on Community Nutrition and Oxidative Stress, University of Balearic Islands belongs to the Centre Català de la Nutrició (IEC).

CHAPTER 2

Acknowledgments
Completion of this secondary data analysis was partially supported by Robert Wood Johnson Foundation initiative, AACORN (African American Collaborative Obesity Research Network). Many thanks to Justin Moore, PhD, and Andrew Kaczynski, PhD, for their thoughtful reviews of the manuscript.

CHAPTER 3

Acknowledgments

This study was funded by a Canadian Diabetes Association Innovation Grant (#IG-1-07-2307-KA) and equipment was supplied through a CFI/ORF Leaders Opportunity. The funding source had no role in the study design, collection, analysis or interpretation of the data, writing the manuscript, or the decision to submit the paper for publication. Kristi Adamo holds a CIHR New Investigator Award and an MRI Early Researcher Award. Jean-Philippe Chaput holds a Junior Research Chair in Healthy Active Living and Obesity Research. The authors declare no conflict of interest.

CHAPTER 4

Funding

The present research work was funded by the Universiti Sains Malaysia (USM) Research University Grant (1001/PPSK/812015). The funders had no role in study design, data collection and analysis, decision to publish, or preparation of the manuscript.

Competing Interests

The authors have declared that no competing interests exist.

Acknowledgments

Nurul Fadhilah A is supported by the SLAB Program of Malaysia of Higher Education (MOHE) through its Academic Staff Training of the Universiti Pendidikan Sultan Idris (UPSI). The authors are grateful to all participants and their parents/guardians for their full commitments and co-operation in the study.

Author Contributions

Conceived and designed the experiments: AN LHF. Performed the experiments: AN PST. Analyzed the data: AN LHF. Wrote the paper: AN IH LHF.

CHAPTER 5

Conflict of Interest Statement
The authors declare no conflict of interest.

Acknowledgments
This study was supported by FCT-MCTES Grants nos: BPD/65180/2009, BD/44422/2008, BD/36796/2007, SFRH/BPD/76947/2011 and PTDC/DES/098309/2008, and by the Azorean Government

CHAPTER 6

Competing Interests
The authors declare that they have no competing interests.

Author Contributions
RW and PC conceived the study, participated in its design and coordination, and drafted the manuscript. WX, NW and BG carried out the pilot study and helped in the design of the current study. DL and XW participated in the design of the study and helped to draft the manuscript. All authors read and approved the final manuscript.

Acknowledgments
The study is supported by Research Fund for the Doctoral Program of Higher Education of China. Contract number: 20103156110003.

CHAPTER 7

Conflict of Interest
The authors declare no conflict of interest related to this manuscript.

Acknowledgments and Funding
We are extremely grateful to all the families who took part in this study, the midwives for their help in recruiting them, and the whole ALSPAC team, which includes interviewers, computer and laboratory technicians,

clerical workers, research scientists, volunteers, managers, receptionists and nurses. The United Kingdom Medical Research Council (Grant ref: 74882) the Wellcome Trust (Grant ref: 076467) and the University of Bristol provide core support for ALSPAC. SPG is funded by a Cancer Institute NSW Early Career Development Fellowship Grant (10/ECF/2-11).

The concept of the study was developed by SPG and CTC. NS managed laboratory assays. Data analysis and drafting the manuscript were primarily done by LG and SPG. CTC, LAB, AN, NS and DAL participated in data interpretation and preparation of the manuscript. We would like to thank Professor Jennifer Peat for statistical support and review of the manuscript.

CHAPTER 8

Acknowledgments

A Dunbar Research Scholarship, a University of Otago Research Grant and a bequest and strategic development funds from the Dunedin School of Medicine funded the current study. The authors thank Carmen Lobb and Phoebe Cleland for research assistance, as well as Anna Dawson and Dr Henry Pharo for the psychological assessments. The authors also thank the children, adolescents and families who participated in the study.

CHAPTER 9

Acknowledgments

The authors gratefully acknowledge the contributions of Judith Peters, MBA, HHSA, from the School District of Philadelphia for her work in leading the YRBS in Philadelphia. We also thank all the school principals, staff, and students who participated in this study. Our thanks go also to Adam Davey, PhD, Associate Professor, Department of Public Health, for his input on the data analysis.

CHAPTER 10

Competing Interests

The authors declare that they have no competing interests.

Author Contributions

Conception of the idea for the study: LBS. Development of the protocol, organization and funding: LBS, CM, AP, and SM. Responsible for the data analysis: AM. Supervision of the data analysis: SM and AP. Writing of the manuscript: AM and LBS. All authors have read the draft critically, to make contributions, and have approved the final text.

Acknowledgments

We thank the adolescents for their participation in the study, and the physical education teachers for their assistance in helping collecting data. We further thank to General Directorate of Education - Ministry of Education and Science for supporting the implementation of the school-based research project. This study was supported by the FCT – Science and Technology Foundation (Portugal), PTDC/DES/108372/2008.

CHAPTER 11

Conflict of Interest

No conflict of interest was declared.

Acknowledgments

The authors gratefully acknowledge the adolescents and their parents who participated in this study. The AVENA Study was supported by the Spanish Ministry of Health, FIS (00/0015) and grants from Panrico S.A., Madaus S.A. and Procter & Gamble S.A. The AFINOS Study was supported by grant DEP2006-56184-C03-01-02-03/PREV from the Spanish Ministry of Education and Science and co-funded by FEDER funds from European Union. DMG was supported by a scholarship from the Spanish Ministry of Education and Science AP2006-02464. FBO was supported by grants from the Spanish Ministry of Education (EX-2008-0641) and the Swedish Heart-Lung Foundation (20090635).

Contributors' Statement

Ana M Veses and David Martinez-Gomez wrote the paper and analysed the data. Sonia Gomez-Martinez wrote the paper and conducted the research. Germán Vicente-Rodriguez, Ruth Castillo and Francisco B Ortega provided essential reagents and other materials. María E Calle designed the research. Marcela Gonzalez-Gross and Oscar L Veiga designed and conducted the research, and Ascensión Marcos designed the research and had primary responsibility for final content. All authors read and approved the final manuscript.

CHAPTER 12

Competing Interest

The authors have no conflicts of interest to disclose.

Author Contributions

SBT was involved in study conception and design, data collection, data analysis and drafting and editing. SK was involved in data collection, data analysis, drafting and editing. BW was involved in data collection, data analysis and editing. DS was involved in study conception and design and editing. BZ was involved in study conception, design and implementation of the clinical trial, and editing. NS was involved in study conception, design and implementation of the clinical trial and the current study. He participated in the data interpretation and editing. All authors were involved in writing the paper and had final approval of the submitted and published versions.

Funding Source

Dr. Bout-Tabaku was funded by a T32 grant 5-T32-AR07442-23 and The Arthritis Foundation Clinical to Research Transition Award.
Primary grant for the clinical trial
NIH R01HD049701.

CHAPTER 13

Funding

P.P. was supported by NIH Grant GM076990 and salary awards from the Michael Smith Foundation for Health Research and the Canadian Institutes for Health Research. J.G. was supported by postdoctoral fellowships from the Canadian Institutes for Health Research, Michael Smith Foundation for Health Research and the MIND Foundation of British Columbia. IMAGEN received research funding from the European Community's Sixth Framework Programme (LSHM-CT-2007-037286).

Acknowledgments

We thank the following individuals for their contributions in acquiring data in the SYS: Jacynthe Tremblay and her team of research nurses (Saguenay Hospital), Helene Simard and her team of research assistants (Cégep de Jonquière), Rosanne Aleong (program manager, Rotman Research Institute) and Nick Qiu (MR image processing, Rotman Research Institute). The Canadian Institutes of Health Research (Z.P., T.P.), Heart and Stroke Foundation of Quebec (Z.P.) and the Canadian Foundation for Innovation (Z.P.) supported the SYS.

Conflict of Interest

M.A. is a James McGill Professor of Biostatistics at McGill University. T.P. is the Tanenbaum Chair in Population Neuroscience at the Rotman Research Institute, University of Toronto. This paper reflects only the authors' views and the Community is not liable for any use that may be made of the information contained therein.

CHAPTER 14

Competing Onterests

The authors declare that they have no competing interests.

Author Contributions

All authors are responsible for the reported research. M.B. worked on the statistical analyses, wrote the first draft of the manuscript and made the greatest contribution to the paper. All authors participated in designing the study and project planning. N.L. was the project coordinator and participated in all parts of the work. All authors provided critical revision of the paper, and read and approved the final manuscript.

Acknowledgments and Funding

The study HEalth In Adolescents (HEIA) was funded by the Norwegian Research Council [grant number 155323/V50] with supplementary funds from the Throne Holst Nutrition Research Foundation, University of Oslo and also from the Norwegian School of Sport Sciences. Many thanks go to the participants, the project staff, and to Linda Selje Sunde for her work on the process evaluation data.

CHAPTER 15

Funding

Funded by the National Institute on Aging (P30 AG017253, SB), the International Development Research Center (SB, SV, DS, SE), Wellcome Trust (SE), and the Stanford University Department of Medicine (SB). DS is funded by an ERC investigator award 313590-HRES. The funders had no role in study design, data collection and analysis, decision to publish, or preparation of the manuscript.

Competing Interests

BP spoke on hydration at a symposium sponsored by Danome Water at The Nutrition Society (British), assisted colleagues at the National Institute of Public Health in Mexico with a grant on SSBs vs. water funded by Danome Water, and was a coinvestigator on another RCT of water vs. diet beverages vs. SSB funded by Nestlé. DS is a member of the Editorial Board of *PLOS Medicine*.

Author Contributions

Conceived and designed the experiments: SB DS SE. Performed the experiments: SB SV SA. Analyzed the data: SB SV SA BP. Contributed reagents/materials/analysis tools: SB SV SA BP. Wrote the first draft of the manuscript: SB. Contributed to the writing of the manuscript: SB SV SA DS BP SE. ICMJE criteria for authorship read and met: SB SV SA DS BP SE. Agree with manuscript results and conclusions: SB SV SA DS BP SE.

CHAPTER 16

Funding
No specific funding was received for writing this article.

Competing Interests
MN and DS are the guest editors of the *PLoS Medicine* series on Big Food.

Author Contributions
Analyzed the data: DS. Wrote the first draft of the manuscript: DS. Contributed to the writing of the manuscript: DS MN. ICMJE criteria for authorship read and met: DS MN. Agree with manuscript results and conclusions: DS MN.

INDEX

For Product Safety Concerns and Information please contact our EU
representative GPSR@taylorandfrancis.com
Taylor & Francis Verlag GmbH, Kaufingerstraße 24, 80331 München, Germany